W9-CHP-989

# Artemis Speaks:
## VBAC*Stories and Natural Childbirth Information

*Dear Abby!*
*You are a great midwife -*
*I love the vision of*
*stopping the war -*
*let's see if I can*
*↑ maintain it! ♡ Nan*
*temp tations abound!!*

# Artemis Speaks:
## VBAC*Stories and Natural Childbirth Information

written and compiled by Nan Koehler, M.S., T.B.A.**

*Vaginal Birth After Cesarean Section
**Traditional Birth Attendant

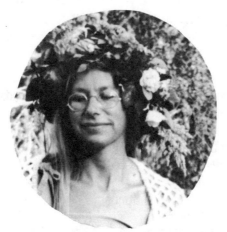

Nan Koehler
13140 Frati Lane
Sebastopol, CA 95472
(707) 874-2315 home
(707) 829-1131 work

Published by
Jerald R. Brown, Inc.
Occidental, California, U.S.A.

Publisher: NAN ULLRIKE KOEHLER
13140 FRATI LANE
SEBASTOPOL, CA 95472

Copy Editor: Sahedran Sattizahn
Galley Proofreaders: Boz Williams and Leonore Hollander
Typesetting: Taber Type, Sebastopol, California
Production and Design Manager: Jerald R. Brown
Designed and produced by Nan Koehler at home.
Cover Painting: Stanley Mouse. Used by permission.
Cover Lettering: Ayala
Principal Photographer: David Burns
Printer: Haddon Craftsman
First printing: 1985, 3000 copies.
Second printing: 1989, 3000 copies
Nan would like to credit and thank Radha Malasquez, Juanita Ingle, and Marilyn Murphy for help and support in creating this book.

Library of Congress Catalog Card Number: 85-70586

ISBN 0-9623851-0-7

## Dedicated to Carolyn Schroth

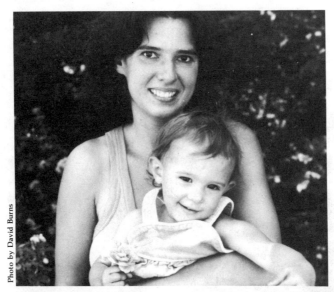

Photo by David Burns

and Sandra Sato.

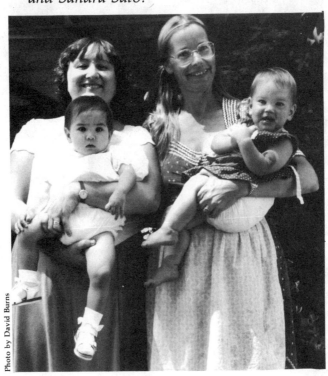

Photo by David Burns

iii

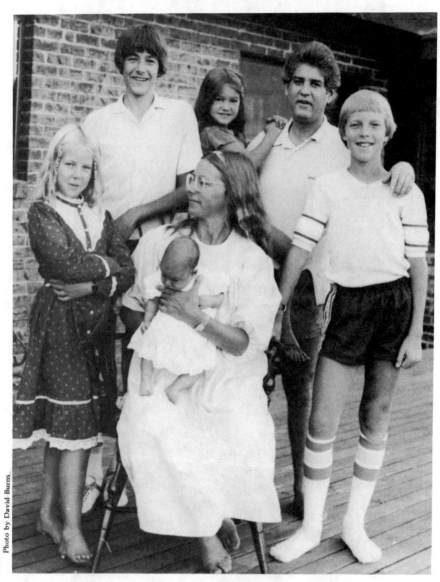

*Jubilee, Ethan, Nan and Sarah, Shayna and Don, and Joshua.*

# TABLE OF CONTENTS

## Part I:

# VBAC Information

# PART II:

# *VBAC Stories and Pictures*

# PART III:

# *Preparing the Body*

# PART IV:

# *Preparing the Mind*

# PART V:

# *Preparing the Spirit*

# PART VI:

# *Taking Care of the Baby, Husband and Yourself*

# PART VII:

# Conclusion — What You Really Need to Know!

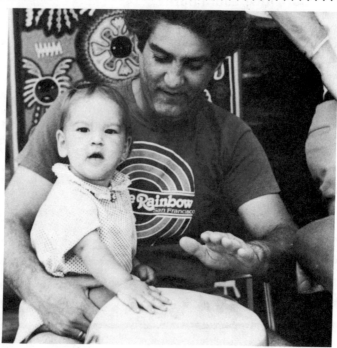

Nan's husband, Dr. Donald A. Solomon, and their youngest daughter, Sarah

xii

# *About the Author*

Nan Koehler was born in Darmstadt, Germany, on April 22, 1941, and moved to the States with her mother and brother after WW II in 1946. She grew up in the Philadelphia area, and attended Earlham College, a Quaker school in Indiana. After spending her junior year at the Art Academy in Vienna, she returned to earn a degree in biology, marry her first husband and earn an M.S. in Ecology at the University of Chicago.

Nan did scientific research in pathology, botany, and embryology before teaching high school biology. After moving to the San Francisco Bay Area in 1967, she taught in private alternative schools. Her first pregnancy was the springboard for Nan to launch a scholarly investigation of natural childbirth. After the birth of Ethan, Nan's first child, her husband died in a motorcycle accident.

Her next two children, Joshua and Jubilee, by her second husband were born at home, and Nan found the experiences so rewarding that she began promoting home birth as a serious alternative to doctor-manipulated hospital births. She was also gaining a reputation as an expert in the use of herbal teas and other natural remedies and health-enhancing practices, shared during her increasingly popular group "herb walks" and informal classes.

Nan's inclinations as a teacher have favored the development of her approach to the birthing process as one where the couple should have a thorough understanding of the physiology and psychology of birthing. After training as a labor coach, Nan was approached by more and more women for information and support in their choice of a home birth. In 1976 she met Dr. Donald A. Solomon, an Obstetrician/Gynecologist who was seeking a midwife with whom to work, and who eventually became Nan's third husband. Nan says, "I've learned a lot of obstetrics from him, and he has learned a lot about diet and herbs from me." They now have two girls, Shayna and Sarah, who were born at home, of course.

As a Traditional Birth Attendant, Nan has helped two-thirds of the nearly 800 women seen in the last twelve years in the Solomon/Koehler practice, with Don providing medical backup as required. Nan has helped thirty women who previously had cesarean births through successful home births (two of whom had had three previous c-sections), as well as twenty-five breech births. Nan only helps high risk women if they are fully cognizant of the risks, and says, "My limits come when something medical has to happen to protect mother or baby; then Don takes over." They will not do medical procedures, such as administration of drugs, at home births; in such cases, they transport the woman to a hospital, where Nan often continues her supporting role.

During her years of work with pregnant women, Nan has written and gathered from wide-ranging sources the educational materials appearing in this book. As xeroxed "handouts," the materials were used to complement the Sunday afternoon repeating cycle of ten classes that Nan continues to conduct for pregnant women and their partners. Originally conceived as two books, one on natural childbirth information and the other on V.B.A.C.s (Vaginal Birth After C-section), they have been combined in one comprehensive volume designed by the author with large, easy-to-read type.

Artemis Speaks:

## Carry Me Earthside

Carry me earthside passion
let heaven roll over me.
Love throws me Here
now caught, then free
to give birth gracefully.

Carry me earthside labor
let my midwife guide us well
through the ring of fire
the bonds of illusion
to see the one who births me.

Carry me earthside childbirth
let my love-fruit fall so gently.
Turn me inside out re-born
and at service
for my babe, my mate and Thee.

—Jeannine Parvati Baker
© *Psyche's Midwife*, 1985.

Jeannine Parvati Baker, MA, founder of Hygieia
College of Womancraft & Lay Midwifery (available as a
correspondence course); author of *Hygieia: A Woman's
Herbal*, and *Prenatal Yoga* (Freestone Publishing Co.)
P.O. Box 398, Monroe, UT 84754.

# Preface

## Artemis and Apollo: V/BAC

### by Jeannine Parvati Baker

The present V/BAC movement has within its body politic an earlier mythological base — the story of Artemis and Apollo. Long, long ago we find the beautiful immortal Leto in process of giving birth to divinely sired twins, Artemis and Apollo. As legend has it, two midwives attended that birth, flying to it in the forms of white doves.

They assist Leto in the deliverance of her first-born twin, Artemis, who immediately receives Her Brother, Apollo, acting as newborn midwife. From here the divine twins grow into the patrons of healing, each in their unique ways. Artemis is known as the wild herbalist and universal midwife, healing and soothing all mothers in giving birth, be they human or animal. Apollo goes on to become the father of the archetypal medical doctor of our times, Asclepius.

Where Apollo approaches healing as a medical science, dissecting through analysis, Artemis heals through ecstatic dance with language and the plant familiars as Her allies. Science and Art have at their source the same mother.

The trend feminism suffered through "blaming" the medical establishment (i.e. patriarchy and all its priesthoods) for the world's problems and specifically the alarming cesarean epidemic, is coming to an end. My second title, *Hygieia: A Woman's Herbal* (Freestone Publishing, 1978) supported the realization that assuming the classical victim stance was not empowering to women. The best "preventative" medicine feminists can practice is forgiveness. Anger and bitterness are not the best healing mode — and an ineffective way to transform our dominant culture. V/BAC is the perfect metaphor for this cultural healing. That it is Artemis who leads the way back into wholeness is not surprising.

I met Nan Koehler Solomon a decade ago when she asked me to come lecture her labor coaching group on prenatal yoga and spiritual midwifery. This was the beginning of our guerilla theatre and growing relationship. She reminds me keenly of the archetypal Artemisian midwife in so many ways that I began to dub Nan this Goddess' name. Nan's subsequent partnership with Dr. Donald A. Solomon, Ob/Gyn, made the connection all the more apparent. Here was the marriage of the two perspectives on healing birth. Through Artemis we find the focus on natural plant allies and through Apollo the "objective" and empirical perspective. The perfect meeting ground for the twins' reunion is in healing cesarean families. Together they aid in mothers' empowerment to give natural birth after the medical drama of surgery.

This healing of birth can best be done when there is a sense of completion and peace about past cesareans. This forgiveness can be extended not only to the medical men, the primal father, and the patriarchy at large, but fully to oneself. As Hygieia says, "Healing one mother is healing our Earth". Through recognition of the natural relationship between Artemis and Apollo, this full forgiveness can be granted. They come from the same source.

So, dear reader, if you are healing a cesarean scar, take heart. Herein is an amazing array of tools to empower you in realizing your vision of V/BAC. Both Nan and I are "pushy visionaries," for we forsee a time when all women can know the bliss of giving unattended, natural birth. This book contains many secrets to heal body/soul/spirit after a cesarean operation and prepare you, if you are ever called to give birth or be in attendance at one again, to deliver in the way that is best-for-life.

Let me close this introduction with a prayer to the powers that be: To the BIRTHFORCE ItSelf, we thank you for bringing us to our primal knees and humbling the prideful; we thank you for turning us inside out in our passion; for granting us an opportunity to meet the God(Us) at the place where space and time come apart—and for the equal opportunity to heal ourSelves forever by giving conscious birth. We thank you for all our babies and for those yet to come—whose faces we have yet to see rising in the ground. We thank you for making us co-creators and letting our bodies and souls be temples for the greatest work there is. What we ask of you is to let us see you all the more clearly at birth and beyond; to hear your voice in the spaces between the breaths; to worship You in the ways which heal our families and bring peace to us all. In Your Name, our Divine Parents, we dedicate our good work. Blessed Be.

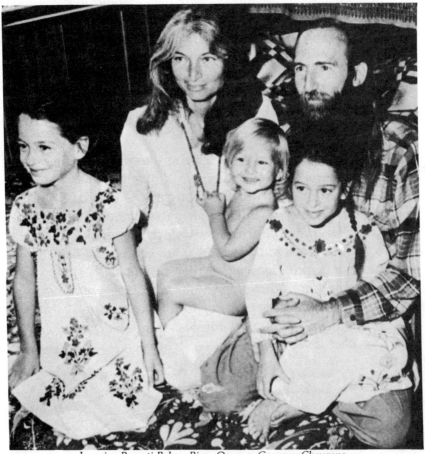

*Jeannine Parvati Baker, Rico, Oceana, Gannon, Cheyenne*

Artemis Speaks:

*At this time, an old woman approached the crowd, but was pushed back. Then Issa said, "Reverence Woman, mother of the universe; in her lies the truth of creation. She is the foundation of all that is good and beautiful. She is the source of life and death. Upon her depends the existence of man, because she is the sustenance of his labors. She gives birth to you in travail, she watches over your growth. Bless her. Honor her. Defend her. Love your wives and honor them, because to-morrow they shall be mothers, and later — progenitors of a whole race. Their love ennobles man, soothes the embittered heart and tames the beast. Wife and mother — they are the adornments of the universe."*

*"As light divides itself from darkness, so does woman possess the gift to divide in man good intent from the thought of evil. Your best thoughts must belong to woman. Gather from them your moral strength, which you must possess to sustain your near ones. Do not humiliate her, for therein you will humiliate yourselves. And all which you will do to mother, to wife, to widow or to another woman in sorrow — that shall you also do for the Spirit."*

From: *The Lost Years of Jesus*

Article published in *Heart*, Spring, 1983, Vol. 3, No. 1, p. 110.

# Foreward

*by Nancy Wainer Cohen*

For many years a number of enlightened and determined individuals have been working to reduce the outrageous number of unnecessary cesareans that are performed in this country, and to help increase the number of VBACs (vaginal birth after cesareans) among the women who have already been sectioned. The way for these travelers is often difficult. It is paved with attitudes and policies that dehumanize birth, and blocked by those who worship obstetrical technology and seek to discount and diminish the time-tested and miraculous process of birth.

Nan Koehler is one of the courageous, conscious and determined individuals who has ground the stones along the way into gravel, and who has converted the incorrigible by her knowledge, love, expertise and example. A midwife among midwives, she has rejected a system that labels healthy women high risk and has refused to be influenced by a political/obstetrical structure that serves neither mothers nor their infants. She is unafraid — of birth, of death, of life. She is also unafraid of VBAC, and as a spokesperson for thousands of cesarean and VBAC women, I wish to thank her for her commitment to birthing women and for the example she sets for others who attend births.

Sadly, it is not easy for women in our country to birth their babies these days. There is pressure to birth in institutions that are primarily constructed for the ill; pressure to utilize unproven, expensive, invasive equipment; pressure to allow pathology-oriented, medically trained robots to oversee the sacred and awesome act of birth. It is an act of courage for any pregnant woman to face the policies and procedures that await her in most American obstetrical units, even more so for VBAC women who must overcome the feelings of inadequacy, sadness, anger, confusion and disappointment that are often present as a result of an operative birth. VBAC women must also overcome the prejudice, impatience, chauvinism and ignorance of a medical establishment that sees them as "obstetrical cripples."

The National Institute of Health has designed VBAC a low risk, and even the American College of Obstetricians and Gynecologists has acknowledged that elective repeat cesarean is unwarranted in most situations. Every study that has ever been done on the subject of VBAC has supported the claims that it is safe. Still, the cutting persists. Only through accurate information that continue to defend the natural process of birth, support from birth attendants who are confident of this process, and the inspiration of women who have birthed their babies joyously and naturally, will the cesarean rate be reduced and the rate of VBACs increased. As women look inside and find the place that is fully capable of birthing, as they take responsibility for themselves, their babies, and their births, the rate of pure, natural, home births will increase.

*Artemis Speaks* helps women look inside and take responsibility. It is a compilation of materials that speak to the physiological, emotional, nutritional, sexual and spiritual aspects of birth. It is an encyclopedia for birthing! How wonderful to have, under one cover, so many excellent articles and stories that educate, inspire, and instill confidence. After reading the many varied excerpts, I felt as if I had just completed a bowl of hearty vegetable soup with dozens of different delicious tastes that were all mixed together to form a nourishing and complete meal.

I am grateful that my path crossed Nan's in the fall of 1982. I never think of my wonderful trip to California without seeing her beautiful face and feeling her dedication and love for birthing women. I am grateful for the time and care that went into bringing so many important resources together to form this book. Knowledge *is* power, and I invite you to set a ladle and take spoonsfuls of the "broth" offered here into your bowls and into your beings.

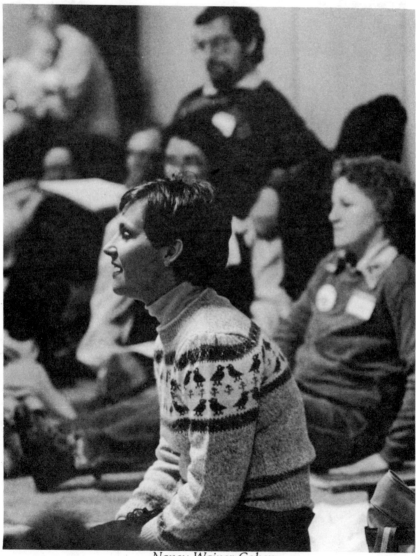

*Nancy Wainer Cohen*

*The Eastern woman's mind is such that many are completely satisfied with being Mothers. It's as if in the West we forget to valorize "love." What did we do today? "We 'loved', nourished and directed our children." From inside you can see what an accomplishment that really is. To love is to be near what is "real" in our life experience. Western minds want to see a materialization of what has been done but if we watch from our heart we can see that loving has been done but gone unattached and returned to the source: the infinite. Om.*

— Letter to Nan, April 4, 1983 from
Radha Malasquez, Varanasi, India

# Introduction

This collection of material grew from a few pages of diet and exercise advice into a packet especially designed for women planning a natural home birth. Now I want to extend this information to women attempting a VBAC (pronounced vee-back), a vaginal birth after Cesarean section. Any woman hoping for this experience will need to be as informed as a woman preparing for a home birth because she will have to overcome all the anxiety connected with this birth option. Hopefully, with all the interest, stories, workshops and support available today, having a VBAC will be as easy as having a home birth has become. Having a Cesarean section is, for the most part, a breakdown in the normal process of birth. In a few instances, cesareans are necessary, but not at the current rate of twenty-thirty percent of all deliveries. My horror and shock at watching this trend are what have motivated me to make this material available to a wider audience.

I have tried to keep my voice to a minimum and have included many other voices because, from my perspective, recipes and "dos and don'ts" often do not fit specific situations exactly. Each of us is unique and the more we consciously create what happens around us, even if our birth experiences are terrible (death or C-section or whatever), we don't feel "done-to" or victimized.

Remember: Knowledge is Power. You are beautiful, healthy women, the product of the survival of other men and women over millions of years. You wouldn't be here if you weren't perfect in every way. You certainly wouldn't be pregnant. Sometimes things do go wrong, but believe me, not very often! Interference with the natural process and our ignorance are usually the only culprits. I have been guilty of interference myself when I was not trusting nature or my skills.

The greatest achievement for all of us in the birthing community is to step aside and say, "Hey, wait a minute. I'm OK. My baby is OK. Back off. Leave me alone. We'll be fine, thanks." Just breathe and trust the process. Trust that the forces of the universe, the elements, God, whatever you call it, know what is right and proper for our survival. We certainly don't! And remember that death is part of life. It's our friend, our saviour. We will be all right. Then we can say, "Please surround me with lovers and friends who support me so I can relax and feel that my life and my baby's life are part of the flow of all life, wanted and needed by everyone."

And so, in that light, I want to offer: first, information to support your decision to attempt a VBAC; second, VBAC stories to inspire you and bolster your courage; third, information/handouts on Natural Childbirth and Parenting; and fourth, I've included a polemic about the more esoteric aspects of childbirth. My love and support to all of you.

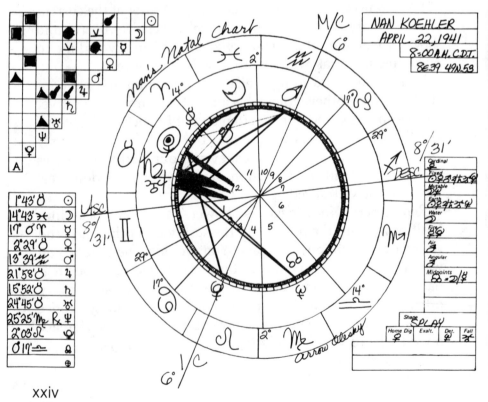

xxiv

The following is a summary of general instructions for *a VBAC at home or in the hospital.*

The following is a summary of general instructions for *a VBAC at home or in the hospital.*

1. Study, take classes and talk to people. Don't be shy about your situation!

2. Secure good physical support (a good doctor and birth environment) and emotional/social support (a good midwife and circle of friends).

3. Eat an exemplary diet, rest each day, and exercise. Walk two miles each day. Eat no dairy products, no sugar or honey, no desserts, and little wheat. (Eat whole wheat only.) Try to eat an alkaline diet and take the maximum vitamin dose recommended. Drink three to four quarts (this is for dry California, less elsewhere) of water a day plus a daily cup of red raspberry tea.

4. Massage vigorously: your abdomen, labia and perineum. Massage two times a day with olive oil. Keep the oil by your bedside and massage yourself when you awake in the morning and before you go to sleep at night. By the end of your pregnancy you should feel no scar tissue. This procedure improves the circulation of blood to these areas and helps give you confidence.

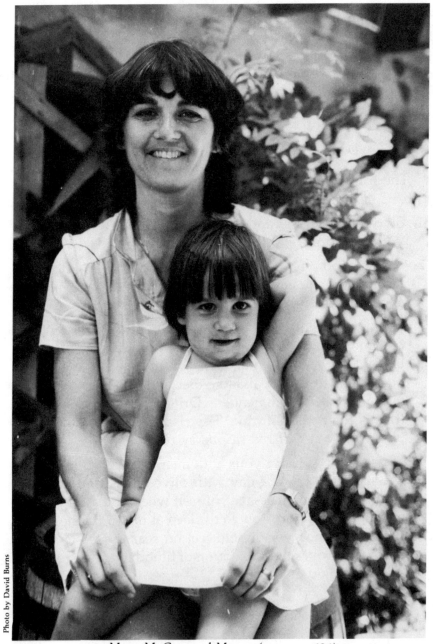

Photo by David Burns

*Mary McCoy and Megan (see page 121)*

xxvi

# PART I

# VBAC Information

Artemis Speaks, Part I: VBAC Information

# *The Decision To Birth VBAC*

*by Justine Clegg*

When a woman decides to have a VBAC (vaginal birth after cesarean), she's taking a big risk. It takes a lot of courage. The risks aren't medical. Those medical people who've been involved with VBAC births for a number of years readily admit VBAC isn't medically high risk. Politically and legally VBAC *is* high risk for the doctor. For the mother, it's high risk emotionally, mentally and spiritually. It's a whole lot easier to just go along with the system, to schedule a repeat cesarean and not have to deal with all the uncertainty. The mother going for a VBAC is told all those horror stories about her uterus rupturing, and when she finally finds a doctor who will support her, it's only if she satisfies certain requirements, and submits to all kinds of invasive tactics during labor such as internal fetal monitoring, frequent internals to make sure she's "progressing well enough," and after a lovely awake and aware vaginal birth and immediate bonding, some women will even be given a general anesthetic so the doctor can reach in and feel her scar!

OK, so she has found a doctor who will go along with what she wants, and she's come to terms with the trade-offs she's had to accept. Our mother settles down to relax, feeling confident that her doctor will give her a fair "trial of labor" (accepting that he is putting her "on trial"). She devotes her time to making sure her diet is top notch; she's exercising and preparing her body for labor and birth, attending refresher courses in some childbirth technique or another, and generally nesting and getting ready for The Big Day.

Many times the doctor she thinks is supportive, somehow during the last few weeks of her pregnancy turns out to be less than he's portrayed himself all those months. The attitude for

2

the first six months is, "Sure, sure honey, don't worry; we'll do things the way you want," and then towards the end, "Well, there's this problem and that problem and so we'd better do it my way after all. You don't want to hurt your baby, do you, honey?" Women are very emotional during pregnancy, very vulnerable and suggestible, especially during those last weeks and labor and delivery. If she feels a hostile, untrusting, non-supportive environment, it's practically impossible to let go and birth. It's just a sign of how much we love our babies that when we perceive a threatening situation we don't want to let our babies out into the possibility of danger. This is largely unconscious, but it is a survival mechanism, which made women unable to birth if they somehow sensed a lion lurking around their cave, or that the midwife would obey Pharoah's order to destroy all boy babies born to Hebrew women in Egypt — we are not the first generation to have to birth in an atmosphere of danger and fear.

What makes us unique is that today no one acknowledges this fear. "Relax, honey, we'll take care of you; everything's going to be fine," they tell you. But they don't believe it. They are afraid. They look at childbirth as a risky situation; (you are either "low risk" or "high risk"). They are just waiting for something to go wrong. They are afraid of lawsuits. They are afraid of doing something contrary to medical protocol in their community. They are afraid of something happening to mother or baby; and most of all, they are afraid of death. They have no idea this climate of fear exists and how it is communicated to the birthing woman in a thousand little ways. They are so used to practicing defensive obstetrics, that it seems "natural" to them.

Why does this climate of fear have such an effect on birthing women? Well, first of all, the heightened emotional awareness and sensitivity during labor is a result of hormone changes and is built into us for a purpose — to help us respond first to our bodies so we can labor and birth more effectively, and later on to respond to our babies, to "bond."

3

This heightened sensitivity makes a laboring woman more perceptive to emotional undertones that are being communicated. Midwives have always intuitively known that women need emotional and spiritual security to birth successfully. That is because midwives were traditionally women who'd had children themselves and knew what it was all about. They knew that birth was not only the culmination of nine months of pregnancy, but also the beginning of a lifetime relationship; that the woman was being called upon to grow from being woman/wife to being mother. This growth is often difficult and requires much support, and midwives traditionally offered this support to the woman and her man during pregnancy and later on after the baby arrived, maybe for years afterwards. The birthing woman was surrounded by midwives experienced not only in birthing but in mothering; surrounded by the other women in her family who had birthed (not who had their babies pulled from them while they were unconscious, either with forceps as our mothers did, or surgically as our sisters and friends today); women who knew what birth was all about, and women who loved the mother-to-be.

In the days when emotional and spiritual awareness were considered witchcraft, midwives were burned at the stake. Today, emotional and spiritual awareness are considered unscientific and unimportant. Technology is where it's at. The technology involved with childbirth today is counterproductive to a relaxing birthing atmosphere. Women who've had previous cesareans usually don't believe in their abilities to birth successfully. When they go into labor, (and very often just going into labor is a difficult thing for VBAC women to do, because when labor starts, then it's all on the line), VBAC women need *more* emotional and spiritual security than the average woman. And they are *less* likely to get it, because the medical profession, considering birth to be so dangerous anyway, certainly considers VBAC to be frought with danger. After all, someone has already decided

4

that this woman couldn't birth vaginally so the doctor/nursing staff can't help but be prejudiced against a successful VBAC. It is the rare hospital situation, the rare doctors and labor room nurses who practice obstetrics without this fear permeating their every move, decision, expression, sentence. It's no wonder the cesarean rate is climbing.

Through technology, American's answer to religion, everyone is guaranteed a successful outcome: healthy mother and baby. (In our culture, what's produced must be the best, while the experience of producing it is considered unimportant.) And, in the event of a less than successful outcome, those involved can rest assured that "We did everything we could." In the "old days" when everyone accepted that occasionally mothers and babies died during childbirth, the birth attendants didn't feel so threatened by the possibility of death. Mothers, fathers and birth attendants mourned their losses then as today. Their hearts were no less broken than ours would be; but, then, it was not considered unexpected to lose a child at birth or during the early years. It was looked upon as an act of God. Now, doctors must be God, and they are to blame if something goes wrong. Of course this attitude has fostered the climate nowadays that if something does go wrong, the patient feels betrayed and sues someone. And, true to form, the medical profession blames the victim, "We have to practice lawsuit medicine, because people are so quick to sue." Well, who taught us that the doctor is God? Who taught us to "leave everything to the doctor, and don't worry your pretty little head about anything"? Just look at the doctor-patient relationship (midwives call their patients "clients"): the doctor acts like a benevolent/tyrannical father (depending on his style and the situation), and she is expected to act like a child. He is "Dr. Jones" while she is called by her first name. She asks him questions like: "Am I pregnant? When am I due? Is my baby all right? How big is my baby? Am I healthy? When will I go into labor? How am I doing in labor? Am I being a good patient?" When he answers, she is

5

either lying on an examining table or sitting across from a large desk, both situations further emphasizing the child-like status of the patient. (She knows the answers to her questions herself, if only someone will give her permission to tune in to her own body and trust her intutition!) All this helps the pregnant patient to turn responsibility, and therefore control, over to her doctor. Even if she has a terrific doctor, he is very limited by the hopsital, the nurses, the anesthesiologists, the administration — the whole system. But she doesn't know that. Not yet. Not until she goes into the hospital in labor.

Many women feel fortunate that someone was there with all that technology to rescue them and their babies from the horrible dangers of vaginal birth. They look upon their doctors as their saviors, their heros — the "masked man" of the '80's. And some few are justified, knowing their babies wouldn't be here without today's high technology. But, let's be honest, they are in the minority. The rest, wondering if their cesarean was really necessary, are bewildered, confused, angry, depressed, and feel like failures. They blame themselves, and feel inadequate. "If only I'd been stronger, tried harder, pushed longer, if only I hadn't taken that demerol; if only my body had worked better. . . ." The woman joins in the chorus of blaming the victim. We know a woman whose husband walked out on her after their daughter was born by cesarean. He told her all the women in his family push their babies out and she wasn't a real woman because she couldn't. (Incidentally, her second baby was a VBAC at home.)

If she believes her failure to deliver vaginally was due to her own inadequacies, how much worse does she feel when the VBAC turns into another cesarean: "A two-time loser," "My body can't seem to get it right," and "I'm actually embarrassed to tell anyone I've had a cesarean," are some of the letters we've received. Now she is in the situation her sisters were in 5-10 years ago. She's had two cesareans and no chance of a vaginal now. It used to be that if she'd had one, that was *it*. Finished. Now she gets two chances at bat. But she's still play-

6

ing in the same game, with the same rules. Considering everything, it's amazing that 50% of women attempting VBACs manage to pull it off!

If she was using her VBAC to atone for her previous failure, to prove that her body can work right, that she really is a woman in every sense of the word—how much more unworthy and inadequate she'll feel if the VBAC doesn't work out. And her friends and family, who wondered why she was so upset the first time ("After all, you have a healthy baby," "Aren't you lucky; you won't ever have to go through labor," "Next time you can pick your baby's birth day,") and thought she was crazy to try and have a vaginal after a cesarean ("I mean, everyone knows how dangerous that is!," "Just go along with your doctor and everything will be fine," "Who are you to question your doctor? Have you been to medical school?") aren't going to have any sympathy for her feelings. Who was she to think she knew more than her doctor? It's what she deserves, being such a smarty pants. What's so bad about a cesarean, anyway? Everyone's having them these days. And on and on. Expressing and dealing with feelings is the beginning of recovery. The end is surviving, stronger and more together than before. It may not seem that will ever happen, but it will.

A woman who's willing to get pregnant again and go for a VBAC is a sensitive, honest and courageous woman. She is every bit as heroic as the pioneer women of the frontier days; indeed she *is* a pioneer. She's willing to travel into the unknown, uncharted wilderness of her dreams, hopes and fears; to lay it all on the line and risk profound hurt and disappointment that few not in that situation can begin to comprehend. Regardless of the outcome, such a woman has emerged victorious. She has *nothing* to be ashamed of. We need to affirm our admiration for her, and she for herself. Those that need to be ashamed are those that perpetrate the frauds on women and seek to make us victims.

Reprinted by permission from Florida Midwives Association Newsletter, *Heart Tones*, Vol. 4, No. 1. 1509 Mantua Ave., Coral Gables, FL 33146.

*Excerpt From the Article*

# To Repeat Or Not To Repeat?

*by Jeffrey E. King, M.D.*
*Department of Obstetrics & Gynecology*

The decision whether or not to perform a repeat cesarean section is not so burdensome after careful review of available literature. The incidence of uterine rupture, the major danger resulting from a trial of labor, has been reported to range from 0.3% to 5.5%. No doubt this places the fetus at increased risk. In a recent report by Merrill of over 600 patients, the uterine rupture frequency was 0.5% and could not be directly related to perinatal mortality or morbidity. In analysis of maternal mortality it was discovered that death resulting from uterine rupture usually occurs in patients without a uterine scar in whom rupture was unexpected, undiagnosed, and inadequately managed.

The economic savings of a trial of labor are substantial with regard to hospital days and patient expense.

REFERENCES:
Merrill, B., Gibbs, C.. *"Vaginal Delivery After Cesarean Section."* OB/GYN, 52:50-52, 1978.
Morewood G., O'Sullivan, M., McConney, J.. *"Post-Cesarean Vaginal Delivery."* OB/GYN, 42:589-595, 1973.

P.C.C. NEWSLETTER
(502) 588-5817
FUNDED BY THE COMMONWEALTH OF KENTUCKY
DEPARTMENT OF HUMAN RESOURCES
DIVISION FOR MATERNAL AND CHILD HEALTH SERVICES

EDITORS:
John T. Queenan, M.D.
Larry N. Cook, M.D.
J. Patrick Lavery, M.D.

EDITORIAL STAFF:
Patricia Chappell, Coordinator
Jean Dean, Senior Secretary

*Reprinted by permission of the Perinatal Coordinating Center, Dept. of Obstetrics and Gynecology, University of Louisville, Louisville, Kentucky, 40292 and Jeffrey King, M.D., Obstetrics and Gynecology, Georgetown University, Washington, D. C.*

# *Birth*
## *A Commentary*

*by Nancy Wainer Cohen*

The United States has one of the highest rates of cesarean section birth in the world, and the number is increasing daily. In spite of expensive, sophisticated, ultra-modern equipment and technology, we still rank only sixteenth or seventeenth in fetal and maternal morbidity and mortality. Repeat cesareans, which are predominantly elective and unnecessary (although many women are not aware of this), account for a significant number of our "surgical insults." We call them cesarean "births," and cesarean "deliveries," and we have become, sadly, far too complacent about their occurrence. Research *clearly* supports the safety of vaginal birth after cesarean (VBAC) and yet the practice of cutting women persists. The National Institute of Health Consensus Development Task Force on Cesarean Childbirth announced full support of VBAC, yet our physicians continue to threaten us with death, uterine rupture, and statements such as, "Well, in your case . . ." or "If it were *my* wife . . ." Many obstetricians refuse to consider the N.I.H. statement, even though it was researched and documented by their respected colleagues.

When a cesarean is necessary, it is an important, often lifesaving, procedure. But far too many cesareans are done unnecessarily or when it has *become* necessary because of medical intervention; unnecessary obstetrical interference, invasive procedures, and attitudes about women, pregnancy and birth which affect a positive outcome. These factors often contribute negatively to the course of labor and delivery and ultimately to the outrageous number of women who are told that they must be cut open in order to have their babies "safely." In our country cesareans are glorified: they are referred to in medical jargon as "delivering from above" (vaginal births are called "delivering from below") and most of us are ignorant about the risks and the high number of complications and dangers inherent in the procedure.

I believe that most cesareans could be prevented. I believe that there is an attitude in our country on the part of most health professionals, that birth is impossible without tools, tubes, chemicals, and machines. We think that doctors deliver babies, not that women *give birth*. This attitude has been adopted and integrated by most people in our culture, and from it stem so many of the problems and complications that arise. Women come to their births believing that somehow someone will "get their baby out" for them, rather than trusting in themselves and their body's ability to open and give forth of their infant. Fear, anxiety, and lack of confidence are expressed by far too many women when asked to describe their feelings about giving birth. In answer to the question, "In my birth fantasy, my labor takes _____ hours," 79 out of 100 women I surveyed answered "between 20 minutes and 2 hours." They want to run away from the pain and "get it over with."

Even with prepared childbirth, many women are not feeling confident and secure. Traditional childbirth classes perpetuate many of the misdirected beliefs and activities that contribute to surgical birthing. Classes are often taught by medically-oriented individuals, within the hospital setting, where course content must be sanctioned by the obstetrical staff. Clearly, this is not a consumer-oriented situation. Many childbirth educators spend several weeks teaching breathing exercises, but do we need to *learn* how to breathe? Wouldn't that time be better spent on discussions of sexuality, nudity, pain confrontation, the marital relationship, etc., and how these affect birthing? Why aren't we taught that we can conserve our energy for the pushing stage of labor by breathing as slowly as possible through each contraction for the entire labor? Why is it that so many couples argue about the fact that they haven't practiced their breathing? Are not those few precious minutes

10

each day best spend on talking with each other, holding each other, and sharing our feelings at that particular moment in time? And why do women think they must be "in control?" Why isn't it taught that control is *not* essential and that it often *produces* body tension? Is a quiet, subdued woman more in control than another who is crying, loud, and active? Why is the famous "focal point" not another human being's loving face, or even the thought of one's baby? Why can't we *accept* our bodies' sensations, appreciate them, and focus on them? Many classes still imply that we must be good little birthing people; we must always listen to The Doctor and permit him to make all the decisions, and we must obey all of the hospital rules, most of which were designed for sick people. Some classes even teach couples how to "enjoy" surgery. When a cesarean is necessary it should be a good experience, but it seems very unfortunate to subject women and babies needlessly to the risks inherent in a major abdominal operative procedure, even if it can be a "good experience." I was once a proponent of cesarean classes; I now believe they are, for the most part, an insult to women.

Many classes still insist that the father be "the coach." This is like asking a fisherman to be a carpenter, or an accountant to be a dentist; for being an effective labor support person requires an objective viewpoint, familiarity and love for birth, patience, and an attitude that birth is normal. "Coaching" connotes standing at the sidelines, making quick decisions, acting as a cheerleader, yelling directions to a (perhaps dazed or exhausted) team player. Fathers often feel pressured by the role and have no one that they trust to whom they can look for new techniques or suggestions for helping their mate. They themselves often feel helpless and vulnerable at births, and frightened by these foreign, uncomfortable feelings. They may be in need of some gentle "cheerleading" themselves. They are part of the "team" that needs loving guidance. This is but one of many issues for men that needs to be addressed in childbirth classes. But there just doesn't seem to be enough time to talk about these things when all that "breathing" has to be taught.

It is a true test of nature's plan that so many women still manage to give birth vaginally in spite of our inane obstetrical ways in the United States. During labor we are deprived of food (yes, Virginia, you *can* have a chicken sandwich) even though our bodies can't possibly work effectively and to peak efficiency if we have not eaten for hours and hours (or sometimes days). Birth is a time of great energy. No one would be expected to run a marathon or swim the English Channel if she had been deprived of sustenance and was unable to continue to nourish herself from time to time during the experience. While women all over the rest of the world are encouraged to eat during labor, we in this country are not permitted to maintain our strength, energy and well-being by replenishing our bodies adequately (or at all) during this time.

We are put into hospital "jonnies" that speak to us of sickness, embarrassment, weakness. Once planted, the seeds of doubt grow nothing but weeds! We need to be wearing black negligees, or comfortable dungarees, or a pretty jumper—clothes that speak to us of a relaxation, femininity, openness.

We are put on our backs and hooked up to I.V.'s (can you see a marathoner running up Heartbreak Hill with a portable I.V. to give her energy, or see having an I.V. put into a woman's arm every time she gets into her car, *in case* she has an accident?), monitors, and anything else available at that moment, all of which can negatively alter the course of normal labor and adversely affect our unborn.

If we make too much noise we are given drugs that will quiet us down, even though these agents can quiet the baby's heartbeat or our uterine contractions as well. Or, if we aren't making enough noise we can always get some "Pit." (Pitocin is a synthetic hormone used to induce or augment labor.) We are deprived of the people in our lives whose presence would do more than any drug ever marketed to calm us down and

12

help us feel relaxed, nurtured, supported, and able to cope. Instead, we are asked to trust any staff member that happens to be assigned to us, having no idea what personal views on birth she might hold, whether they are compatible with ours, and knowing that at 11:00 P.M., when the shift changes, she will leave to rest up for the next day. United States obstetrics also surrounds us with men, who have never and will never give birth, and who tell us, "Don't worry, *I* know. *I'll* take care of things."

We are assigned to beds that are too slim to be shared by our mates, so that being caressed (good heavens, my dear!) and cuddled is impossible. We are confined in rooms that do not have hot soothing showers or large relaxing tubs. We are in institutions which are otherwise devoted to illness (in one of the major birthing hospitals in my area the labor rooms are *underground!!!*) and very few people believe that we are healthy, normal women capable of doing what our bodies have been doing for eons—working as they were designed.

We are subjected and exposed to ultrasound, x-rays, internal and external fetal monitors, none of which are either beneficial, necessary or safe in most circumstances. We endure countless vaginal exams, which are invasive and usually unnecessary. We are the recipients of comments such as, "You aren't dilating fast enought." (I wonder if telling a man he is not getting an erection fast enough would help him to ejaculate) or that, "I'll tell you when you can start pushing." (Don't you dare ejaculate until you are "checked"!) We are told (and many women *believe*) that it doesn't make any difference if the baby is artificially fed or breastfed, or if the mother doesn't want rooming-in. We are given strong messages that our bodies are unable to birth without interference. Those who avoid "the knife" for a cesarean will find it being used elsewhere (never mind that the Scandinavian countries have a $5\frac{1}{8}$ episiotomy rate while ours is $96\frac{1}{8}$). We are part of a twentieth century farce and sadly, most of us don't even know it yet.

13

Until we educate ourselves, believe in our bodies, and trust our babies' ability to get born, we will continue to be doing ourselves and our unborn a grave injustice. If our babies knew how to get in, we must assume that they know how to get out!

We must begin by teaching ourselves, and our sons and daughters as well, that birth is a natural, beautiful, physiological, spiritual event. We must embrace the concept of *healthy pain* and see labor as our healthy body's work to deliver our babies. We must give birth in a supportive environment that believes in women and nurtures them during birth. We must respect the complexity of the whole process of pregnancy and birth and tamper with it only when our actions are appropriate and justified. We must continually question the use of procedures that might *potentially* cause complications or produce sequelae. All interference must be considered guilty until proven innocent.

We must identify negative presences and remarks that tighten our minds and our bodies, and insist that they have no place at our birthday parties! We must understand that our pelves will release, they *will* open, if we can only give them the proper opportunity to do so. Numbers that measure our pelvic diameters are basically useless. (We are told so often that a small penis works as well as a large one, aren't we?) We have all seen women with totally adequate pelves have difficulty with 7 pound babies. We have also seen women with contracted pelves who open up and deliver 9 pound infants. *Clearly*, it is far more than simply the pelvic structure that permits an infant to be born.

We must learn to rely on our instincts again — the instincts which tell us when to eat, when to walk, when to squat, when to make noise, and when to be quiet. We must also rely on the instincts of others who *believe in birth* and are knowledgeable about it. We must take responsibility for our decisions. We must understand that birth is Birth, not just birth. Birth is a time for us as men and women to learn, grow, become — to grow ourselves up! It is a time to watch how we "do ourselves." It is a time for changing some relationships,

14

cementing and creating others.

We have a responsibility to each other as women and as a people to insure that women come to their birthing experiences confident, enthusiastic, well-nourished and energetic. We have a responsibility to help each other begin to trust our bodies and see birth as a normal experience. No more judgments and accusations. ("Home, you had your baby at home? or "You left the hospital three hours after the birth?") We must not insult ourselves, or our infants, or The Plan, by being cut open unnecessarily. (No one would argue that the health and well-being of both mother and child are not the most important considerations and it is precisely for this reason that we must avoid unnecessary surgery and procedures that can lead to it.) Having a baby by cesarean is a little like getting pregnant by artificial insemination — an important option for some, but not usually the method of choice. For many women, it's like ordering a filet mignon at the Ritz Carlton and getting a peanut butter and jelly sandwich for the same price. It's still nice to be at the Ritz, and it is a deluxe peanut butter and imported jelly, but somehow, it's not quite the same.

There is great understanding and sympathy for a man who is able to get an erection but not ejaculate. Most people understand that the ability to ejaculate is part of his total identity as a male. There is support for his feelings of inadequacy, frustration, failure, sadness, and guilt. But there is very little understanding for cesarean women who have feelings of disappointment and sadness, and feelings of failure and frustration at not being able to complete the normal physiological process of birth. For many women, becoming pregnant and giving birth are integrally and intricately linked with feelings of self-worth and identity. Is it any wonder that so many woman in our culture are grieving? To want to give birth in a way that unites us to other women, to all Woman, to want to experience each of the cycles of our lives — this is not *insane;* it is *normal!*

Birth is a significant life experience. It's effects are immeasurable and boundless. It can be — and needs to be — a time of peace, exhilaration and joy, and a time of love that can be reflected upon and treasured for a lifetime. Some people will read these words and not comprehend or appreciate what has been said. They will criticize, pull apart, extol the virtues of fetal monitors, argue for x-rays, defend the starving of women during labor, and insist upon chaining women to beds during labor by means of tubes and machines. For others, understanding simply *exists*, and did so before any of these words were written. For them, no explanation is necessary, and it is to them that I dedicate my work, my commitment to safer birthing in this country, and my boundless energy invested in preventing unnecessary cesareans.

## *Preventing Cesareans and Avoiding Repeat Cesareans by:*

- reading consumer oriented materials
- being nutritionally aware and eating well
- exercising
- learning about medical interventions and their consequences
- understanding that a woman's belief about herself and her labor determine the course of that labor
- learning what beliefs and attitudes you bring with you to your birth
- finding a midwife or labor coach who believes in birth without intervention
- selecting a doctor who understands and supports your wishes (and with whom you can communicate freely)
- clearing out your past birth experience
- developing positive attitudes and beliefs
- designing a hospital request list
- getting really in tune with your spouse

16

- developing a network of support (to encourage and applaud you)
- getting in touch with your strength and ability to open up and give birth
- constantly thinking how lucky your baby is going to be—born *naturally!*
- practicing relaxation exercises
- practicing visualization techniques (and using these to learn about yourself)
- realizing that women for centuries have been able to give birth
- loving your pregnant body
- practicing touching and massage
- understanding that childbirth is a beautiful way to learn about yourself
- remembering that you can depend on people who love you and care about you during labor
- avoiding medical interventions
- avoiding psychological interventions
- remaining clear about what your needs and rights are
- stamping on your "mind parasites"!
- preparing yourself physically, emotionally, psychologically, and spiritually
- remembering that your mind and your body work *together*
- keeping in mind you can help to create the kind of birthing environment you wish
- resting every day so you don't go into labor exhausted
- expending the least amount of energy possible to get you through each contraction
- taking each contraction one-at-a-time
- remembering that you can eat lightly during labor
- changing positions (and scenery!)—or tuning into your psychological state—when labor slows down
- remembering that labor doesn't necessarily progress at an even tempo
- knowing when fear, tension, inhibitions, embarrassment, anger, etc. are affecting your labor

- remembering that some babies take their *time* to be born
- keeping in mind the couples in your class and the couples in classes before yours who care about you and are supporting you
- thinking "baby baby baby" during contractions
- using a *loving* focal point!
- maintaining eye contact and touch contact
- forgetting your hang-ups about "transition"
- *not* thinking of labor as a performance
- going with your labor (doing whatever you need to do)
- realizing there is a "learning to labor" period
- remembering how safe VBAC is (pretend you are in Europe!)
- keeping in mind the baby's head need not be engaged
- letting this labor be its own unique experience—not your previous experience or a friend's experience, etc.
- learning, trusting, believing—trusting and feeling that you can do it!

Reprinted by permission of Nancy W. Cohen.

Nancy Wainer Cohen was a co-founder of C/SEC, Inc. and coordinator of that organization from 1973 to 1978. Since 1972, she has counseled hundreds of women on the subjects of cesarean childbirth, vaginal birth after cesarean, and cesarean prevention, and has spoken all over the country to health professionals, childbirth educators, and consumers. Ms.Cohen has been instrumental in the formation of cesarean awareness groups nationwide and conducts VBAC teacher training seminars. Her articles have appeared in numerous publications. She is a La Loche League leader and was Area Professional Liaison for New Hampshire from 1974 to 1976. In 1978 Ms. Cohen left C/SEC to teach classes and do individual childbirth counseling. She is a labor attendant and is currently studying midwifery. Her personal birth experiences include a cesarean delivery for her first child, a vaginal birth in the hospital for her second, and a home birth for her third.

Copyright © 1981 by Nancy Wainer Cohen

Reprinted from *Childbirth Alternatives Quarterly*, Fall 1981, Vol. III, No. 1.

## FOR FURTHER READING

The Report of the Consensus Development Task Force on Cesarean Childbirth of the National Institutes of Health may be ordered at no cost from Pamela Driscoll or Joan Miller, Office of Research Reporting, NICHD, Bldg. 31, Rm. 2A-32, Bethesda, MD 20205, 301/496-5133.

Unnecessary Cesareans: Ways to Avoid Them by Diony Young and Charles Mahan is available from the ICEA Bookcenter, Box 20048, Minneapolis, MN 55420. Write for current catalog.

"The Cesarean Epidemic: Who's Having This Baby, Anyway—You or the Doctor?" by Gena Corea appeared in the July 1980 issue of *Mother Jones* magazine and is available from the Mother Jones Reprint Service, 625 Third Street, San Francisco, CA 94107. Minimum order is 2 copies for $1. plus 35¢ for postage with additional copies 25¢ each. California residents add 6 percent sales tax.

"Cesarean Births: Why They Are Up 100 Percent" by Deborah Lamed appeared in the October, 1978 issue of *Ms.* magazine. See your local library for a copy.

## FOR MORE INFORMATION

Nancy Wainer Cohen offers classes on VBAC and cesarean prevention. For more information contact her at 10 Great Plain Terrace, Needham, MA 02192 or call 617/449-2490.

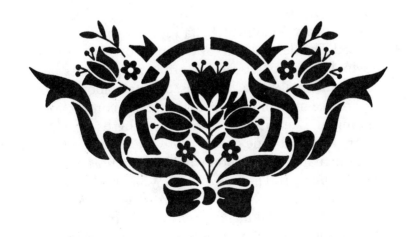

# Tips For Easing A Difficult Labor

*by Nan Koehler, Sandra Sato and Marilyn Murphy*

*(For the woman who has had a difficult time birthing in the past, or who is anticipating a difficult labor this time . . .)*

## Before Labor Begins:

1. Three weeks before birth, take Blue Cohosh daily to tone the uterus (in tea, tablet form, capsules, or as herbal tincture).

   Instructions for making a proper medicinal tea: Do not let the herbs or herb water touch metal! Place desired amount (usually 1 teaspoon is plenty) of fresh or dried herb in 1 or 2 quart glass jar, then pour boiling water into the jar over the herbs. Let steep and cool. Sip throughout the day to keep the essence of the herb present in the body all the time.

2. Drink Red Raspberry tea once a day throughout pregnancy, then in the last month drink it 3-4 times a day. A classic tea formula, used by our grandmothers in the last month of pregnancy, which can be added to the Red Raspberry and drunk 3-4 times a day is: Black Cohosh Root, Squaw Vine (Mitchella repens or partridge berry), Blessed Thistle, Lobelia, and Pennyroyal.

   Mix herbs in a 1:1 ratio, store in a tight glass jar in the dark, and make tea daily as directed above. You will experience more intense Braxton-Hicks contractions after sipping the tea. Don't panic. The herbs won't trigger labor, they just tone or stimulate the uterus so that when labor actually begins, you will be ready for it. (Like priming the pump!) The more work your body does before labor, the more effaced you are, the easier the actual labor will be. Making the teas and drinking them on a daily basis is also like a positive mantra or meditation. It's

20

affirming your positive intentions and affirming the power of the natural process by making and using Mother Nature's simple remedies. It takes an extra effort to use the teas, and as you drink them, you whisper to yourself the positive affirmations which will bring you the results you desire.

3. Take Evening Primrose oil (available in health food stores in capsule or oil form) 3 times a day beginning 3 weeks before the baby is due. Evening Primrose oil has in it the precursors of prostaglandins, the hormone which causes the cervical connective tissue fibers to soften and give.

4. Take pituitary extract tablets 3 times a day, with meals, or 2 teaspoons powdered Shiitake-Reishi mushrooms once a day, 3 weeks or so before baby is due, along with 100 mg. of the B vitamin complex. This will stimulate the pituitary gland to produce enough oxytocin during labor, and the B vitamins will strengthen the liver, which needs to break down this hormone to promote rhythmic surges of oxytocin release.

5. Emotional preparation is important, especially so that you don't repeat a previous bad experience. Some suggestions are visualization, yoga, meditation, written affirmations, exercise, diet.

6. It is very important for women who have had previous C-sections to take the vitamins to keep their tissue strong and healthy and eliminate any possibility of tears or rupture. Vitamin E–800 IU/day and Vitamin C–up to 10,000 mg./day before the birth, then return to taking about 2,000-4,000 mg./day during nursing. 2,000 mg. of calcium and 1,000 mg. of magnesium are also important to prevent muscle cramping and to reduce the amount of pain you experience.

7. A wonderful preparation for a VBAC attempt is to massage your abdomen twice daily at the scar site to improve circulation to the area and prevent rupture. Keep some vegetable oil by your bedside and vigorously mas-

21

sage your stomach, focusing on where you feel the ridge of tissue down by your pubic hair. Then rub some oil onto your vagina to help keep you from tearing. When you massage your abdomen, don't rub hard enough to hurt yourself or set off contractions, just hard enough to stimulate the blood flow to the area.

8. Keep your baby small by avoiding dairy products (no cow's milk), drinking teas and eating seeds, nuts and dried fruit for snacks. Read *Nature's Children* by Juliette De Bairacli Levy. Don't restrict food intake, just eat very well!

# *In Labor:*

1. *Eat!* If in early labor, eat a good meal and try to maintain your normal dietary rhythm. If in advanced labor, drink a pep drink or protein drink of juice or milk with 1 ripe banana, a raw egg, 3 tablespoons of protein powder and 1-2 teaspoons of magnesium oxide powder.

2. *Walk!* If labor begins during the day, take a long walk (2-3 miles) to stimulate the contractions. If labor starts at night, go back to sleep and if you can't sleep, then walk (outdoors, 2-3 miles, for at least an hour) to make the contractions come even harder and more frequently. It's also very effective while walking to squat with the contractions because the pressure of the baby's head on the cervix in this position intensifies the contractions. The more discomfort, pain, etc. you experience, the better! It means that the baby is coming. (However, pain between contractions may be a sign of uterine rupture.)

3. *Hot bath or shower.* The hot water relaxes the muscles better than anything and submergence in water does something to the women's energy. I've heard it said that water cleanses the aura. Whatever it does, in labor, it's like magic.

4. *Emotional support,* especially from an experienced woman and/or a brave husband is critical throughout labor. This includes visualization, encouragement, help with relaxation, massage and reminders that pain is normal and temporary.

5. *Sleep—Oil of celery seed.* If tired from a long prodromal labor, lay down on the left side and take 5-10 drops of oil of celery seed for sleep. (Oil of celery seed is a natural barbituate!)

6. *Pelvic presses.* If the baby's head doesn't descend (not engaged) have the midwife or husband try pushing on the pelvis at the top of the illium or hip bone during a contraction while the woman squats and pushes. (If this is going to work it will work after 3-4 tries.) You'll be able to feel the head moving down. (Use the pressure points shown in *Herbs, Helps and Pressure Points,* p. 31, to push on the pelvis).

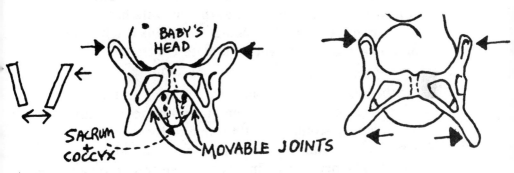

BABY'S HEAD

SACRUM + COCCYX — MOVABLE JOINTS

7. *Black Cohosh.* Use this tincture to stimulate contractions. (Preferred over blue cohosh, which is traditionally used to expel the placenta). Give the tincture when pitocin would normally be given. Give orally a dropper full every half hour or 10 drops in half a glass of water every half hour. (A note of caution: My experience with store bought tinctures was unsuccessful, but my homemade tincture works very well indeed. Make your own or get one from a very reliable source.)

23

# *More Things to Try in Labor:*

8. *Calcium or magnesium orotate,* Use this instead of calcium lactate as mentioned in *Herbs, Helps and Pressure Points.* Magnesium orotate is the most effective during labor, and is absorbed faster than lactate. Available in lozengers, May-O-Tabs, etc. Magnesium orotate will help the woman relax.

9. *Evening Primrose Oil—a natural source of prostaglandins,* applied directly on the cervix during labor will soften the cervix in women who have trouble dilating. Especially helpful for women who have had surgery on their cervix or who are DES daughters. You also might need to have the birth attendant "ream" the cervix to break any adhesion fibers from previous surgery, abortions, etc. I do this as a matter of course on almost all women when I first check them. It will also stimulate the contractions. Pressure on the front of the cervix makes a contraction come. Sometimes the midwife has to "manually" open the cervix or massage the cervix often to stretch or break scar tissue and stimulate contractions. Believe me—it's better than another C-section.

10. *Castor oil.* If the membranes are ruptured and the woman hasn't slept or can't be normal, take 4 ounces of castor oil on an empty stomach. Within one to five hours you will experience strong diarrhea which will stimulate the uterus. The nerves that innervate the lower colon also innervate the uterus. Castor oil also has the hormone prostaglandin that Evening Primrose oil has, which ripens the cervix. If you are at all ready to go into labor this is definitely the ultimate kicker. If you aren't ready for labor nothing, I repeat NOTHING, can get it started, and if you persist you will end up with a C-section. Castor oil can be taken more gradually, a teaspoon at a time, with the dose progressively increased over several days. If you are desperate, use the full dose.

24

11. *Change the energy*—easier said than done. This can be accomplished with threats, exchanging participants or simply clearing the room, playing music, going outside, getting into the bathtub or being brave enough to discuss possible underlying fears. An unconventional, but very effective, method I've discovered is to use marijuana at this time. I read somewhere that marijuana seeds make a good uterine stimulant. I prepared a tincture of it and used it with women who were stuck. To my surprise it did help tremendously, but in a way I hadn't expected. Usually it helped them bear the pain, stop complaining and begin to cry and open up. Of course I would only give this sort of remedy to a woman who was in agreement with it.

12. *Hydration* is another factor to be aware of—simple, but often neglected to the disadvantage of the laboring woman. Make sure that you drink often, a good sip between each contraction. If labor is protracted, be sure your fluid intake equals about a quart every 4-6 hours. Remember also to urinate every hour! To help with liquid intake, my favorite birthing tea is a 1:1 ratio of Basil, Nutmeg, Lavender, and Red Raspberry.

13. *Rupture of membranes.* Some women can't deliver without artificial rupture of the membranes. It's something you must be prepared to do. If the woman has been in good labor for many hours and is at least 5-6 centimeters dilated, then rupturing the membranes might be a step to take, similar to drinking the castor oil. Sometimes the bag is too tight and must be ruptured right at the end to let the baby out. Conversely, sometimes the bag is so loose it doesn't form a good forebag wedge to open the cervix and simply hangs down in the vagina, filling with fluid at each contraction, resulting in no progress for the woman. You might need to call expert advice at this point because there is always the remote danger of cord prolapse when you rupture the membranes.

14. *Oral Stimulation.* A connection between the mouth and cervix has been well established by natural childbirth practitioners. Opening the mouth wide during contractions (even putting the tongue out), proper breathing, kissing, yelling, screaming, talking and tears all can help. Be creative.

15. *Call for help!* Don't resist calling for help if there is continued lack of progress and the mother and baby seem to be deteriorating. Get medical evaluation and don't be afraid to either go along with their suggestions or go back home. Birth is a mystery!

Herbs and supplements you may need to use, as suggested above, include:

| | |
|---|---|
| Blue and Black Cohosh | Celery Seed oil |
| (tea, tincture or tablets) | Castor oil |
| Red Raspberry | Pituitary extract |
| Squaw Vine | Vitamins |
| Blessed Thistle | Minerals — Calcium and |
| Lobelia | Magnesium Orotate, |
| Pennyroyal | Magnesium Oxide powder |
| Valerian Root (tea, tincture) | Protein powder |
| Evening Primrose oil | |

SOURCES ARE:

1. Nan Koehler — Midwife, 13140 Frati Lane, Sebastopol, California 95472, (707) 874-2315 or (707) 829-1131.
2. Katherine Tarr — Midwife, Utah, Author of *Herbs, Helps and Pressure Points*, 780 North 2250 West, Provo, Utah, $4.95.
3. Shelley Sovola Francis, *Acupuncture and Herbs for Obstetrics*, 9110 Hargis St., Los Angeles, California 90034, $6.95.

More Reading Material especially for the woman planning a VBAC.

1. Gayle Peterson, *Birthing Normally; Pregnancy as Healing.*
2. Nancy Wainer Cohen & Lois Estner, *Silent Knife.*
3. Suzanne Arms, *Immaculate Deception.*
4. Constance Bean, *Methods of Childbirth.*
5. Sheila Kitzinger, *Experience of Childbirth.*
6. Alice Miller, *For Your Own Good, Hidden Cruelty In Child Rearing and The Roots of Violence.*
7. Claudia Panuthos, *Transformation Through Birth, A Woman's Guide.*
8. C/Sec Inc., 22 Forest Rd., Framingham, MA 01701, (617) 877-8266 has available an extended bibliography which was prepared by E. C. Shearer for the article, "Preventing Unnecessary Cesareans." C/Sec Inc. also has available publications and information. Write or call them.
9. Nicki Royall, *You Don't Need to Have a Repeat Cesarean."*
10. Diony Young and Charles Mahan, *Unnecessary Cesareans, Ways to Avoid Them.* ICEA Publication.
11. ICEA Cesarean Birth Committee, *Selected Bibliography and Resource Guide.*
12. Stanley E. Sagov et al, *Home Birth, A Practitioner's Guide to Birth Outside the Hospital.* An Aspen Publication.
13. Ina May Gaskin, *Spiritual Midwifery.*
14. Lynn Babtisti Richards, *The VBAC Experience.*

All these books can be easily ordered from ICEA, International Childbirth Education Association, P.O. Box 20048, Minneapolis, Minnesota 55420. They have a great book catalog called "Bookmarks."

Other sources are Birth and Life Bookstore, P.O. Box 70625, Seattle, Washington 98107 and Moon Flower Birthing Supplies, P.O. Box 128, Dept. MT, Louisville, Colorado 80027 or Childbirth Education Supply Center, 10 Sol Drive, Carmel, New York 10512.

# When Labor Starts

*by Katherine Tarr*

As soon as labor has begun the expectant father can offer a prayer and ask a blessing that Heavenly Father will watch over them and their baby and give them any help that may be necessary for a safe experience. You need not be any certain religion to do this. These new little spirits are watched over and helped to be born and a birthing couple can make their birth more special by inviting the spirit of our Heavenly Father to be there.

As soon as labor starts a bath or shower is advisable. If a tub bath is taken, clean out the tub with disinfectant. The area from waist down should be washed carefully (especially where the baby comes out). You can put on clean socks after the bath so your feet won't get dirty and then when you get into bed take them off.

When in labor, the woman should take 800 units of vitamin E and another 800 units every three hours after that until the baby is born. With the help of vitamin E it is observed that even babies that have been compressed in the birth canal for as many as 5 or 6 hours in hard labor come out pink. Without vitamin E many babies have dark purple coloring and have more problems establishing normal breathing. Vitamin E can even make the difference between life and death in a severely stressed baby.

When labor starts, it is advised that a woman drink the following tea (½-1 cup every half hour). To one quart boiling water add ½ cup red raspberry, ¼ cup comfrey, ¼ cup alfalfa, ⅛ cup peppermint (optional) and steep for ½ hour or longer. This mixture has many vitamins and minerals to help enable the body to do it's work effectively. If she is hungry, she can eat nourishing food and drink juices. She should urinate frequently (every hour). A full bladder can slow up the labor and can even injure the bladder.

28

Relaxation is very important. A woman's husband or labor coach should instruct her to go limp like a rag doll and breathe deeply making her tummy rise and fall. This is called abdominal breathing. Observe the kind of breathing you do when you are nearly asleep and try to simulate it. Help her to relax her hands, face, legs, etc. if you see they are tense. Tenseness in the body fights the contractions and intensifies the sensations of "pain." Relaxation helps a woman to handle the contractions easier and have a faster labor.

Another relaxing way of laboring is in a warm bathtub. The bathtub should first be scrubbed well with disinfectant and filled with clean, comfortably warm water. A foam pillow can be used behind the back and under the bottom, if desired. A woman in labor should not be left alone in the tub because occasionally one will dilate very fast in the warm, relaxing water and may have to be lifted out to deliver. Some women get in and out of the tub many times. Respect the woman's wishes and let her do what she wants. A tub bath may not be advisable if the water (amniotic fluid) has broken because there is an increased chance of infection. In this case a warm shower can be substituted and can be very relaxing. Sitting on a chair in the shower may be more comfortable than standing.

## Problems In Labor

If a woman takes good care of herself during pregnancy and her body has received all the mineral and vitamins and exercise it needed there is probably no reason for additional herbal preparations during labor. However, in difficult or painful labors there are a few herbs that can help.

If the labor is sluggish try blue cohosh in capsules or tea. Black/Blue cohosh is an old Indian remedy to make child birth easier. It can help dilate the cervix. If it is false labor, however, blue cohosh will probably stop it. A woman with a history of difficult labors would benefit by taking blue cohosh daily for 3-4 weeks before birth. Some women vomit blue cohosh. If this happens, try something else.

A lobelia enema can cut the intensity of hard contractions to half. It is a relaxant and helps to relax a laboring woman. When she relaxes she hurts less and the uterus can work more efficiently. Use 2 tablespoons tinture of lobelia to one quart of warm water. Use one or two cups in an enema and expel. Put in another one or two cups and hold as long as possible, then expel. The laboring woman should notice a decrease in the intensity of the contractions and should be able to handle them easier. Lobelia can also be taken by mouth in capsules or tea but it must be used in small amounts or it can cause vomiting. If taken internally lobelia should be taken with a little cayenne. Also, the tinture of lobelia can be used by rubbing on the feet or tummy or by putting a few drops (5-10 drops) in the mouth. If lobelia is given too early in labor it can slow down or stop contractions for a while so wait until dilation is a least 6 to 7.

If the labor is very uncomfortable, 4 or 5 calcium lactate tablets (to decrease sensitivity to pain) can be given each time juice or tea is taken. If contractions are weak it may help to lie on your left side. This often helps to increase the intensity of the contractions.

Sometimes when the baby's head is not in the best position labor can be longer. Doing a few pelvic rocks can often correct this and help things move along faster.

# *Pressure Points*

There have been some great results with the following pressure points. After feeling the difference they make, most women won't let you stop.

# When Labor Starts

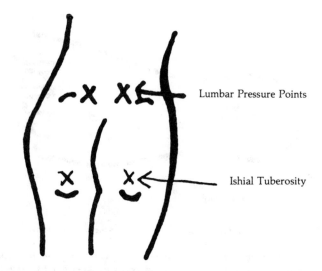

Lumbar Pressure Points

Ishial Tuberosity

The lumbar pressure points are found on the lower back where the straight backbone starts to round out into the bottom. Or, if you know your anatomy — on both sides of the last lumbar vertebrae where the coccyx starts. Try several places in that vicinity and the woman will let you know where it helps best. Some women get quite bossy and tell you "higher" or "harder" or "softer." Just listen to her and you'll find the right spot. Push with two or three fingers during a contraction. These are especially good for "back labor." Husbands quite often tend to push too hard, making it unpleasant. So, if you're a man be gentle.

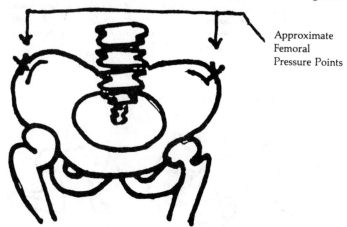

Approximate Femoral Pressure Points

Press femoral pressure points where the hip bones start to curve down in the front. You can press with 2 or 3 fingers or the whole side of your hand. Again, the woman involved will let you know where it helps her the most. Just listen to her.

The idea behind the lumbar and femoral pressure points is that the pressure on the nerves in these areas cut the pain impulses that travel back to the brain and are interpreted as "pain." By pressure you are preventing part of the message from getting back to the brain so the contractions are perceived not the "hurt" as much. It is rewarding to see women in a relaxed, controlled state throughout the labor because of the use of these pressure points.

31

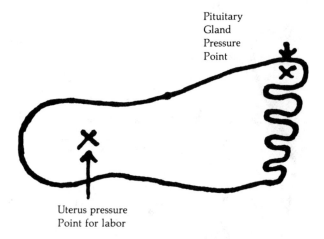

Pituitary
Gland
Pressure
Point

Uterus pressure
Point for labor

*The pituitary pressure point can be used for irregular or ineffective contractions. Massage in a circular pattern.*

*The uterus pressure point on both heels worked deeply with the thumb can help take the edge off of the contractions. This pressure point doesn't seem to be as effective as the others but you can try it to see if it helps. During the contractions you may feel the spot opening and deepening, then closing as the contractions end. After awhile the spot doesn't close anymore (when the woman is about 5 cm. dilated). If the hole feels thicker on one edge it is probably thicker on the cervix on the same side. One heel will go deeply and freely in opening and one will be closed more. The more closed side shows which side the placenta is on. Massaging the tighter side may help the placenta come loose after the baby is born. You may notice a little knot in one of the heels—this is the side the baby is on. So, if the knot is on the right side it would mean that the baby's back is against the right side of the uterus. If the woman has had more than two episiotomies the foot massage usually doesn't help with the contractions because the nerve connections have been cut linking the birth area to the spot in the heel. But you can still feel the changes in the spot on the heel.*

## Positions For Labor And Birth

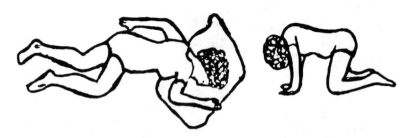

*Relaxation Position*
The weight of the baby rests on
the bed and you can totally relax.

*Hands and knees*
Good for back labor

32

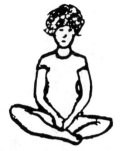
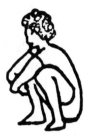
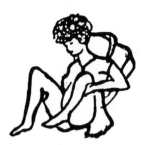

*Taylor Sitting*
Good for watching TV, writing, reading, etc. Use a back support.

*Squatting*
Good for increasing contractions and helping baby down the birth canal.

*Pushing position*

# *The Birth*

If shaking occurs during labor or after delivery a few swallows of cayenne, vinegar, and honey in water (1 tablespoon honey, ¼ teaspoon cayenne in cold water) will warm her up. Also canning jars, empty shampoo bottles, etc. filled with hot tap water and laid along her legs, arms, feet and body will warm her up nicely. A warmed blanket (from clothes dryer or oven) or a heating pad can also be helpful.

As the birth approaches it is important to keep the blood circulating in the perineum area. Sanitary napkins dipped in hot boiled water, then cooled enough not to burn the skin, and put against the perineum area help keep the area circulating with blood so that there will be less chance of tearing. It feels good too. You can also use warm olive oil on the napkins.

As the baby is coming down the birth canal, keep the perineum red or pink by massaging with warm olive oil. Any place that gets white will tear so keep massaging and keep all areas red. Use olive oil on the inside too and pay special attention to the area at the bottom as that is the most common place to tear.

33

You can support under the perineum with your hand on top of a sterile gauze pad or washcloth. Don't hold it together, just support it so the baby's head can ease out. As the baby's head is born support it with your hand so the face doesn't sit in a puddle of amniotic fluid. Gently wipe the face with a clean or sterile washcloth. Check quickly around the neck for the cord. If you feel it, just hook it with your finger and pull it around the baby's head. Check again, some are wrapped more than once. With the next contraction the top shoulder is usually born and then the whole body slips quickly out. If several contractions have passed without a shoulder coming you may have to slip your hand in and try to find one of the baby's armpits. With one or two fingers hooked under the armpit try to rotate the shoulder and pull. Usually this does it.

Reprinted by permission of Katherine Tarr, Provo, Utah, *Herbs, Helps and Pressure Points*, 780 North 2250 West, $4.95

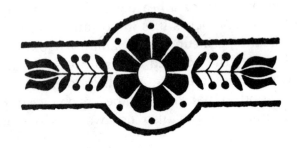

34

## Checklist for a Difficult Labor

- [ ] Food
- [ ] Hydration
- [ ] Ambulation
- [ ] Rest: tincture of valerian root or oil of celery seed
- [ ] Bath or shower
- [ ] Massage/touch
- [ ] Intact membranes causing delay?
- [ ] Emotional support, LOVE!
- [ ] Pelvic presses and/or deep pelvic floor massage
- [ ] Uterine stimulant—black cohosh or ginger, etc.
- [ ] Cervical massage—evening primrose oil
- [ ] Calcium/Magnesium: magnesium oxide powder or magnesium orotate—jitteryness
- [ ] Call for help

35

# Childbirth Resource List

American Academy of Husband Coached Childbirth
— Bradley
P.O. Box 5224, Dept. B
Sherman Oaks, California 91413
Bradley natural childbirth class and teacher training

Association of Childbirth at Home, International
P.O. Box 430
Glendale, California 91209
Childbirth education — the best beginning

American Society for Psycho-Prophylaxis in Obstetrics
(ASPO) Lamaze
1840 Wilson Boulevard, Suite 204
Arlington, Virginia 22201
Childbirth preparation classes, teacher training and certification

Informed Homebirth
P.O. Box 3675
Ann Arbor, Michigan 48106
Workshops for beginning and advanced midwives, herbal
workshops, numerous handouts

International Childbirth Education Association, ICEA,
*Bookmarks*
P.O. Box 20048
Minneapolis, Minnesota 55420, U.S.A.
Catalog issued three times yearly

La Leche League International, LLL
9616 Minneapolis Avenue, Box 1209
Franklin Park, Illinois 60131-8209   (312) 455-7730
International organization dedicated to helping and supporting women breastfeeding their children, Local LLL leaders can provide counseling on an individual basis and in group meetings, newsletter

Jeannine Parvati Baker
Optimum Health Institute
P.O. Box 398
Monroe, Utah 84754, U.S.A.
Hygieia College, Freestone Press, *Spiritual Aspects of Birth and Family Life*

National Assocation of Parents and Professionals
   for Safe Alternatives in Childbirth, NAPSAC
P.O. Box 267
Marble Hill, Missouri 63764   (314) 238-2010
Newsletter with membership, numerous books, resources for educators and professionals

Moonflower Birthing Supply
P.O. Box 128, Dept. MT
Louisville, Colorado 80027
Supplies and books about childbirth and family health issues

Birth
110 El Camino Real
Berkeley, California 94705
Magazine with subscription

Cascade Birthing Supplies Center
P.O. Box 12203
Salem, Oregon 97309
Birthing and medical supplies mail order center, comparable prices and fast service

California Association of Midwives
P.O. Box 420854
Sacramento, California 95842
Newsletter with membership

Mothering
P.O. Box 1690
Sante Fe, New Mexico 87504
Magazine with subscription

The Practicing Midwife
156 Drakes Lane
Summertown, Tennessee 38483
Newsletter with subscription

Growing Parent/Growing Child
22 North Second Street
Lafayette, Indiana 47902
Parenting newsletter with subscription

Birth and Life Bookstore
7001 Alonzo Avenue, N. W.
P.O. Box 70625
Seattle, Washington 98107, U.S.A.
Review newsletter and catalog issued three times a year

CPM — Cesarean Prevention Movement
Summer School — Rm. 203
215 Bassett Street
Syracuse, New York 13210
Newspaper (The Clarion) with membership and chapters

C/Sec
22 Forest Road
Framingham, Massachusetts 01701   (617) 877-8266
Information, publications, resources, and support for parents and professionals on cesarean childbirth, cesarean prevention, and VBAC!

Childbirth Alternatives Quarterly, Whole Birth Catalogue
327 N. Glenmont Drive
Solana Beach, California 92075

The New Nativity
P.O. Box 6223
Leawood, Kansas 66206
Newsletter for do-it-yourself homebirth couples, stressing the sexual aspect of birth such as clitoral stimulation, breast stimulation and dimly-lit seclusion

Midwifery Today
P.O. Box 2672
Eugene, Oregon 97402
Good grassroots newsletter with magazine format

*These excerpts from two pamphlets by the same author will give you an idea of the fine educational material available from The Pennypress. — Nan*

# Cesarean Birth — A Special Delivery

*by Kathy Keolker*

## Introduction

Cesarean birth is becoming more common. While recognizing that it is major surgery with all its inherent risks and concerns, having a cesarean baby can be a fulfilling birthing experience when done with sensitivity and concern for the needs of the family. Until the past few years, cesarean birth was considered a last resort, to be used only when everything else failed, and only after exhaustive attempts to deliver the baby vaginally. With the advent of antibiotics and improved procedures, cesarean birth has become a relatively safe operation. Doctors now use it more often, especially for breech babies and fetal distress. There is a great deal of controversy surrounding the rise in the cesarean birth rate, and the concern is justified due to the physical and emotional impact of childbirth on the family and on society. When parents have planned a family-centered birth, an unanticipated cesarean can be devastating. Any woman contemplating childbirth should educate herself on the issues, options and concerns relating to cesarean birth so that she will understand the pros and cons, enabling her to make informed decisions if faced with the possibility of a cesarean.

The goals of this pamphlet are to: discuss the medical procedures related to cesarean birth; help you plan your own birth experience by choosing options that are important to you and your family; stimulate thought about your own needs and preferences; and encourage you to be informed about the issues.

40

# Summary List Of Options For Cesarean Birth

1. Delivery date determined by spontaneous labor, if possible.
2. To shorten hospital stay, enter hospital the same day as surgery, rather than the day before.
3. Father present for delivery.
4. Necessity for pre-medication; type of anesthesia; types of incision and closure.
5. Modified restraint of the arms, to enable mother to touch baby.
6. Screen lowered at time of birth, or baby lifted above screen.
7. Doctor describe what is happening at birth.
8. Mother may wear glasses or contact lenses.
9. Medication following delivery if mother wishes to be awake.
10. Baby seen and touched before leaving delivery room.
11. Father, mother hold baby after birth.
12. Baby in recovery with parents, if his/her condition permits.
13. Baby breastfed in recovery, condition permitting.
14. Routine admission of baby to Neonatal Intensive Care Nursery waived or shortened, if his/her condition permits.
15. If baby has a long stay in the Neonatal Intensive Care Nursery, parents may visit, hold, and care for baby (to promote bonding of parents and baby).
16. Mother may breastfeed in the nursery, or send in her own milk.
17. Mother may have cesarean roommate, if available.
18. Additional pillows available for comfort of mother.
19. Beltless sanitary napkins (to avoid sanitary belt which irritates incision).

Copies of *Cesarean Birth—A Special Delivery* are available from: The Pennypress, 1100 23rd Avenue East, Seattle Washington 98112. Single copy—$0.50; Bulk orders—$20.00 per 100 (includes postage and handling).

41

# Vaginal Birth After Cesarian

## by Kathy Koelker

The author is a free-lance writer and mother of two sons: the first, born in 1976 by emergency cesarean; the second was born vaginally in 1979.

## RECOMMENDED READING

*Unnecessary Cesareans: Ways To Avoid Them,* Diony Young & Charles Mahan. ICEA, 1980 ($1.50).

*Obstetric Tests & Technology: A Consumer's Guide,* Margot Edwards & Penny Simkin. The Pennypress, 1980 ($1.00).

*Planning Your Baby's Birth,* by Penny Simkin & Carla Reinke. The Pennypress, 1980 ($0.50).

*Cesarean Birth, A Special Delivery,* by Kathy Keolker. The Pennypress, 1979 (Rev. 1981) ($0.50).

Two main references will provide descriptions of the research studies discussed in this pamphlet:

*An Evaluation of Cesarean Section in the United States,* by Helen I. Marieskind, Dr.P.H., U.S. Dept. of Health & Human Services, 1979. (Available at no cost from Clara Schiffer, Program Analyst, Room 723E.3, HHS/Hubert Humphrey Bldg., Washington, D. C. 20201).

*Draft Report of the Task Force on Cesarean Childbirth,* U.S. Dept. of Health & Human Services, 1980. (Available at no cost from Pamela Driscoll, Office of Research Reporting, NICHD, Bldg. 31, Room 2A-32, Bethesda, MD 20205).

# Cesarean Birth — A Special Delivery

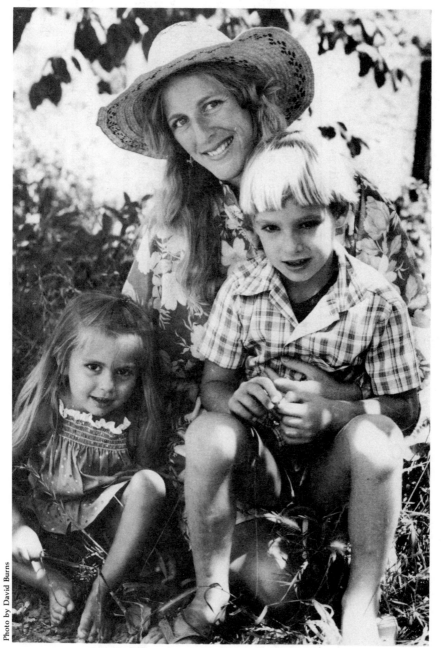

Photo by David Burns

*Wendy Sherman with Arien and Naia (see page 153)*

43

# Preventing Unnecessary Cesareans

*by E. L. Shearer*

| Why C/S Performed | Avoidable Factors | Alternatives |
|---|---|---|
| I. CPD –<br>Failure to progress<br>Prolonged labor<br>Arrest of labor<br>Uterine ineretia<br>Dystocia<br>Failed forceps<br>Failed induction | 1. Lack of patience with normal labor process; misinterpretation of Friedman labor curve. (It's a *mean*, not a *norm*; there is a normal human variation in length of labor. | 1. Trust a woman's body unless clear clinical signs of fetal or maternal distress; stay at home till 5-6 cms; go home if arrive at hospital and < 4 cms. |
| | 2. Recumbent position; lack of mobility in 1st stage. (When woman is upright and ambulatory, 1st stage is shorter, contractions stronger and more efficient, gravity helps, baby enters pelvis at a better angle, mother is more comfortable and feels less pain. Supine position leads to maternal hypotension and reduced uterine blood flow.) | 2. Stay out of bed and *WALK!* Avoid semi-reclining position; no IV unless specifically indicated, then on mobile stand; monitor by auscultation unless electronic fetal monitoring specifically indicated, then alternate EFM with periods of walking. |
| | 3. Exaggerated pushing with prolonged breath-holding in semi-reclining or reclining position. (Squatting increases pelvic diameters, can increase available | 3. Avoid semi-reclining or reclining position for 2nd stage; squat, kneel, stand, or sit on toilet, especially if 2nd stage long or uncomfortable; use these or side-lying position to rotate posterior or |

44

area 20-30%; gravity helps; baby descends at better angle. Hard lengthy pushes result in ineffective pushing out-of-sync with uterus's own bearing down efforts, as well as maternal exhaustion. Pushing with closed glottis, holding legs up, pushing with heels result in tense, tight legs, buttocks, pelvic floor, and vagina, delaying baby's descent and causing more stress on baby's head and mother's soft tissues.)

4. Too hasty use of pitocin after premature rupture of membranes or post-dates; elective induction; artificial rupture of membranes early in labor. (If cervix unready for labor, induction will be in-effective or labor prolonged. Pit can result in contractions too strong, long, and close together, increasing likelihood of use of analgesics or anesthesia and of fetal distress – see below. Pit associated with excessive 3rd stage bleeding and neonatal hyperbilirubenemia. With precautions, risk of infection after rup-tured membranes very small in well-nourished, healthy women.

transverse head. Push only with body's own rhythm; mother avoid holding legs up, pushing with heels, or closing glot-tis; mother's emphasis on opening up and turning into body's signals, not technique.

4. No pit after ruptured membranes unless signs of infection; wait at home for labor (risk of infection and anxiety both lower there); drink lots.

No induction post-dates unless falling estriols or + non-stress or stress test.

No elective induction (banned by FDA).

No artifical rupture of membranes ex-cept late in labor in a few selected cases.

45

| Why C/S Performed | Avoidable Factors | Alternatives |
|---|---|---|
| | Induction solely on the basis of dates runs risk of premature baby if dates wrong; there is a normal human variation in length of gestation. | |
| | Artificial rupture of membranes removes protection for baby's head, can lead to excessive molding; increases likelihood of infection with internal exams, leads to concern over length of labor because of fear of infection.) | |
| | 5. Fasting in labor. (Labor is hard physical work and requires lots of calories to burn. Digestion slows down, in active, labor but continues slowly. 5% glucose solution insufficient to supply energy needs. Times when inhalation anesthesia required are rare; effects on maternal and fetal metabolism and uterine functioning of prolonged fasting not clearly known.) | 5. Eat at will in labor; drink lots. |
| | 6. Narcotics in 1st stage. (Central nervous depressants, can slow uterine functioning, especially if given in latent phase or if labor progressing slowly already.) | 6. No narcotics or epidurals—walking, relaxation, massage, shower or bath, breathing patterns, loving support and encouragement instead. |

46

No epidurals in 1st or 2nd stage. (Slow 1st stage by withdrawing blood from uterus and retarding uterine functioning; slow 2nd stage by eliminating urge to push, weakening abdominal muscles; higher incidence of failure of baby's head to rotate.)

7. Maternal anxiety and fear. (Cause release of catecholamines, including adrenalin, which withdraw blood from internal organs and relax smooth muscle, thus slowing labor down. Release of oxytocin also inhibited by fear, anxiety, and tension.)

7. Increase mother's self-confidence by emphasizing birth as *NORMAL PHYSIOLOGICAL FUNCTION*, not only in childbirth classes and during pregnancy, but from childhood; give extra support in labor; stay home in early labor; improve community options for safe out-of-hospital birth.

II. Fetal distress

1. Misinterpretation of electronic fetal monitoring tracings. (Tracings are difficult to interpret, as some variations are normal; EFM produces many false positives.)

   Reliance on EFM for diagnosis. (According to NIH, EFM is a *screening*, not a *diagnostic*, tool.)

1. Monitor by auscultation unless EFM specifically indicated (according to NIH, no benefit to efm except in high risk cases); confirm diagnosis with fetal scalp sampling before intervening.

2. Reclining position. (Supine position can cause maternal hypotension, reduce

2. Stay upright, out of bed.

47

| Why C/S Performed | Avoidable Factors | Alternatives |
| --- | --- | --- |
| | blood flow to uterus; labor less efficient – see above.) | |
| | 3. Narcotics; epidurals. (Narcotics central nervous system depressants, can depress maternal respiration, cross placenta quickly and can depress fetus, especially if already stressed. Epidurals can lead to maternal hypotension, withdraw blood from the uterus, as well as prolong labor – see above.) | 3. No narcotics or epidurals – see above. |
| | 4. Pitocin. (Pitocin can cause contractions too long, strong, and close together for baby to recover oxygen supply between, especially if already stressed. Increases maternal anxiety and likelihood of use of narcotics or epidurals.) | 4. Use pit rarely and sparingly; turn down or off once labor initiated; allow labor to start on its own; stimulate labor by giving mother a rest, getting her up to walk, relaxing her, or stimulating nipples, instead of pit. |
| | 5. Exaggerated pushing with prolonged breath-holding. (Can reduce oxygen to baby by using up all oxygen with mother's own exertions and retarding blood flow to uterus by building up extreme intrathoracic pressure; supine position leads to maternal hypotension and reduces uterine blood flow.) | 5. Push physiologically with body's own rhythms, in upright or sidelying positions; hold breath no longer than 6-7 seconds.) |

48

6. Hyperventilation. (By several mechanisms, reduces oxygen available to the baby.)

7. Maternal anxiety. (Reduces blood flow to uterus and oxygen available to baby—see above.)

6. Help mother relax upper body, slow or lighten breathing.

7. See above.

III. Breech presentation

Automatic, blanket rules about how to deliver breech babies.

Prenatal exercise to turn baby; external version; X-ray at labor onset; trial of labor; skilled, confident midwife or obstetrician.

IV. Toxemia
Placental abruption (separation)
Placental insufficiency
Pre-term births
Low birth weight

Inadequate nutrition, during intrauterine life, childhood, adolescence, and pregnancy. Use of drugs in pregnancy, prescription, over the counter, and recreational, including alcohol and especially smoking.

Restriction of blood volume and placental size by restricting salt intake or using diuretics.

Education about nutrition and use of drugs in pregnancy—before pregnancy begins, in early pregnancy, and in childbirth classes. *Avoid ALL drugs.* Avoid use of diuretics or restriction of salt; increase protein intake, maintain fluid and salt intake, instead, if fluid retention and high blood pressure becomes problems.

Feed low income pregnant women and growing girls (most low birth weight, pre-term births, perinatal and infant mortality in US occurs to poor and minority women).

49

| Why C/S Performed | Avoidable Factors | Alternatives |
|---|---|---|
| V. Previous C/S | Automatic, once-a-C/S-always-a-C/S rules. Increased risk of maternal death, increased maternal morbidity, increased maternal-infant separation and stress on attachment process, decreased maternal self-esteem all results of C/S. 15% of babies born by elective C/S have respiratory distress. (Risk of dehiscence (separation) of lower segment scar 0.5% with no hemorrhage, shock; risk of maternal or fetal death essentially the same as without scar.) | Labor and vaginal birth unless 1) classical uterin scar (not skin);* 2) new indication for C/S in this pregnancy. Scar may be manually explored after delivery. *Parents may choose to take 1-3% risk of serious rupture with classical scar. If so, should plan to go to hospital in early labor, have IV in place, blood cross-matched and ready, OR and anesthesia alerted, constant labor nursing supervision. With lower segment (transverse) scar, same labor supervision as is appropriate for all labors is sufficient. |

Reprinted with permission from C/Sec Inc., Sesareans/Support, Education and Concern, 22 Forest Road, Framingham, MA 01701. (617) 877-8266. Copyright 1980 E. L. Shearer

50

*This is an articulate, sensible article; a rarity in the scientific literature. — Nan*

# Education For Vaginal Birth After Cesarean

by Elizabeth Conner Shearer, M.Ed., M.P.H.

*ABSTRACT: Childbirth education for parents who elect to attempt a vaginal birth after cesarean (VBAC) has many of the same elements of traditional childbirth education, including the imparting of knowledge and confidence, training in breathing and relaxation techniques, and helping parents to arrange for the most supportive environment and caregivers. Special differences in VBAC parents include the need to mourn the previous loss of an ideal birth, to analyze why they want a VBAC, and to understand the reason for the previous cesarean and realistically assess the chance of recurrence. The fear of uterine rupture or scar separation afflicts both parents and physicians, but has been shown to occur no more frequently than in repeat cesarean. By one analysis the elective repeat cesarean is a higher risk procedure than is a trial of labor. (BIRTH 9:1, Spring 1982)*

In 1980 the National Institute of Health released its full Report[1] and Conference Summary[2,3] of the Consensus Development Conference on Cesarean Birth, which recommended that, "In hospitals with appropriate facilities, services, and staff for prompt emergency cesarean birth, a proper selection of cases should permit a safe trial of labor and vaginal delivery for women who have had a previous low segment transverse cesarean birth." The recent medical literature has several studies of outcomes of vaginal birth after cesarean (VBAC).[4,5,6] This paper presents an approach to childbirth education for parents who plan a trial of labor and hope for a vaginal birth after previous cesareans.

51

# Principles Of Education for VBAC

The first principle in educating parents for a vaginal birth after previous cesareans is that such education is much more *like* preparation for any other birth than it is different. After attending almost 30 VBAC labors, I have learned that the uterus works the same whether it has a scar on it or not. Women may not act the same, doctors may not act the same, but the uterus goes about its work as it always does. Thus, the basic goals of education for a VBAC are the same as for any other birth.

In these classes, there are four important goals. The first is to replace the fear and mystery that surround birth in our culture with knowledge and confidence. Of course, one cannot give specific information about exactly what will happen, because every labor is different. Rather, parents must feel they have enough information and skill to cope with *whatever* the rest of the pregnancy, the birth, and the new parent experience will bring.

The second goal is to provide enough information about the hospital — its options, its restrictions, the risk/benefit considerations of the various technologies that are available so that parents can make decisions about their births. "Taking control" of preparation and planning for birth is so important to parents' feelings of competence, independence, and strength. Hospitals are like any other institution in that they work in overt and subtle, conscious and unconscious ways to make people men and women — dependent, passive, "good patients." Birth, however, is a supremely active and independent act.

The third goal is to help women to get in touch with their bodies, inner resources, and abilities. Learning to trust, cooperate with, and listen to their bodies and their own unique labor patterns is equally as important as "giving up control" to the physical processes.

Many — if not most — prenatal classes are attended by pre-

52

dominately well-educated, middle-class, over-30 parents. The majority are career women, who have planned this birth carefully, they are used to trying very hard to be in control of their lives. It is often hard for them to learn to give up control over labor. Part of the class process is helping these women to accept the pain of birth, to appreciate it as a sign of how strong and well their bodies work, quite different from pain that signals injury or illness. Effective preparation for childbirth includes helping people confront their feelings about pain and strong sensations from the pelvis. It also includes helping them to believe in themselves and their body's ability to function well. One of the most insidious corollaries of the rising cesarean rate if the spread of the belief that many women — some believe *most* women — cannot give birth without medical, technological, usually male, assistance. The next logical step is to believe that the birth process, itself, is somehow inherently dangerous, and therefore bad. Yet, we know that 75 percent of all births will proceed safely, with no more intervention than a watchful eye and a great deal of support.

A fourth goal is to give parents specific tools with which to work in labor. This does not mean a prescription or recipe; labors are like snowflakes — no two are alike. Rather, it means emphasizing that each woman finds ways to make these tools work for herself in her own unique manner.

Of the half-dozen tools which I consider most important, the first is the creation of a supportive environment. I believe the importance of the environment cannot be over emphasized. The mother needs to feel physically, mentally, and emotionally safe, nurtured, and supported, rather than "on guard." In class this means encouraging parents to take very seriously their planning for birth. Where do they want to be? Who do they want to attend them, in terms of professional support? Who do they want around them for support? It is enormously difficult for the father to provide all the mother's support and advocacy during what is a stressful time for him as well. I also encourage parents to stay home until well into

53

active labor, since it is much easier to create a comfortable, supportive environment at home than in any institution.

The second tool is variation of the mother's position. Parents need to understand how standing and walking versus lying down can affect labor, how certain positions help rotate a posterior head, how upright positions, particularly squatting, can facilitate second stage.

Third is calorie and fluid intake during labor. Far from eliminating the risk of aspiration with general anesthesia, total fasting may actually increase the risk by raising the acidity of stomach contents. Fasting may also make it harder for the uterus to work. Labor is a physical process, and burns lots of calories.

The fourth tool is relaxation. I use a number of techniques, including the use of the breath to focus concentration, and to facilitate muscular release. However, I discourage rapid breathing patterns, because I find they demand far too much energy and make dehydration and hyperventilation more likely. Sometimes the energy that goes into controlling breathing patterns is symbolic of the women's desire to control labor. I find that it is almost always counterproductive.

I teach partners the value of touch. In a time of stress, there is something wonderfully soothing and comforting about loving hands, quite apart from touch relaxation skills.[7] Finally, I talk about the use of warm water. Whether in the form of a bath, a shower, or simply hot compresses, warm water is almost magical in helping women relax, feel better, and open up.[8]

## Special Differences in VBAC Parents

All of these tools are for everyone, because they help the mother feel more comfortable and the labor work more efficiently. What is special for people who have had a cesarean before? In my experience, the differences are two. First is the amount of emotional "baggage" women bring to the birth experience. If it is hard for women in our culture to know, trust,

54

and rely on their bodies to give birth, it is even harder when their bodies did *not* "work right" the first time, or the birth did not go according to their expectations. This is just as true for women who have had birth experiences other than cesareans that were not succesful in their own terms — a premature birth, a loss, a baby that was not perfect, or simply a long and difficult labor, particularly if anesthesia was used. It is crucial for both parents to come to terms with their previous birth experience, and to do any left over grieving for their lost expectations and dreams. A healthy baby is every parent's priority, but does *not* equal a healthy experience or a healthy family. Unfinished grief work will come up, unbidden, during a subsequent pregnancy, and women sometimes experience a flashback as they approach labor or enter the hospital.

It is important to explore with parents, "Why do you want a vaginal birth after your cesarean?" What fantasies do you have for this birth? Are you hoping to avoid pain? Do you need to prove something to yourself or to others? What particular fears do you have? Is the mother afraid of letting herself get into very strong labor for fear of the strain on the scar? Is she fearful of a particular intervention that has taken on symbolic meaning for her of the difficulties in her previous labor? Is the father supportive or fearful of a VBAC? How about other family and friends?

It helps both parents if they understand the reasons for their cesarean, and can be crucial for them to get past the point where the cesarean occurred. If the cesarean was for a breech presentation, if she goes into labor with a vertex presentation, she may say, "Now everything will be OK." If she had her cesarean at three centimeters, once she gets to four centimeters she may relax and think, "I can do this now." People who have had a cesarean for so-called "cephalopelvic disproportion (CPD)" have the most difficulty, especially if they reached full dilation or close to it. That fear always looms ahead of them throughout the work of labor. It is important for these women to hear how unscientific "CPD" and "failure to progress" are as diagnoses. All but three women who have come to me having had a cesarean for CPD and then delivered vaginally have delivered a baby as big *or bigger* than their previous "CPD" baby. All "CPD" means today is that *the baby did not get out in the time the doctor thought s/he should.* The vagueness of this diagnosis was discussed in the report of the NIH Consensus Development Task Force on Cesarean Childbirth.[2]

Parents can also be helped by understanding what restrictions and unnecessary interventions in the previous labor may have made it harder for them to make progress. Then they feel there is something they can do to help their body work better this time, such as staying active and out of bed, or changing to a physician who uses less routine intervention.

Gayle Peterson's book *Birthing Normally*,[9] reviewed in the Fall 1981 issue of BFJ, is an important reminder of the strong effect attitudes and beliefs and feelings have on the functioning of the body, as I've suggested above. These influences are generally ignored by physicians. However, there is a danger in putting too much emphasis on how a woman's psychological state affects her birth, possibly amounting to finding yet another way to blame women for what happens to them, to blame the victim, another thing for mothers to feel guilty about. I am quite certain that beliefs and attitudes have led to some cesareans by making it harder for women to let their bodies give birth. Yet, it is hard to believe women have been responsible for the three — to four — fold increase in the cesarean rate over the past 10 to 12 years! Women need to come to an understanding of what part of the responsibility for their first experience lies with them, and what part with their physician.

## *Special Differences In VBAC Doctors*

This brings me to the second difference in the VBAC labor — nervous doctors. If women find it hard to trust their bodies, obstetricians find it all but impossible to trust birth to be a truly normal physiological process, requiring no intervention, most of the time. For VBAC's, many set arbitrary time limits on the length of labor, or require a woman to go into labor by 40 or 41 weeks. Why? Just because she has had a cesarean before—should she be expected to deliver early or have a short labor? If she did not reach at least 5-6 cms. in her first labor, I consider her a primipara for *labor*, even though it is her second child.

Most obstetricians use technology defensively in VBAC labors, in spite of the fact that there is no more justification for routine intervention than in any other labor. If a horizontal scar separates, it does not cause massive hemorrhage, so there is no need for prophylactic IV. The uterus usually continues to contract normally, and an electronic fetal monitor will not pick up a scar separation. In my experience, there is no pain when the scar separates, so a previous cesarean is no reason to deny the use of sedation or anesthesia. There is no reason why women cannot deliver in a labor room or birthing room after a previous cesarean, since there is no evidence that the scar is more likely to give trouble at the last moment. None of these restrictions will help the physician pick up problems with the scar. None are required to manage a separation that does occur. Such restrictions may well make it more likely for a woman to require a repeat cesarean, by limiting her mobility, making her more uncomfortable, and increasing her anxiety, tension, or fear. Even if it means changing doctors after they begin classes, I strongly encourage choosing a physician who is experienced and confident with VBAC's. A supportive doctor cannot give birth for her, but *can* make it easier.

## What If It's Another Cesarean?

Now, what if a woman ends up having a repeat cesarean, after all? This has happened to about 15% of my VBAC couples. Each woman has felt glad she tried to deliver vaginally, anyway. If she had not tried, she would always have

57

wondered, "What if . . . ?" She still has had the satisfaction of knowing that her baby has been born when ready, and that a period of labor has benefited her baby's lungs, readying them for life outside the womb.

## What Is the Risk Of Uterine Rupture In A VBAC?

How "high risk" is a VBAC labor? The fear of scar separation is the justification for all the restrictions mentioned above, as well as most doctors' continued reluctance to attend VBAC labors at all. Many women who have had a previous cesarean also see themselves as being high risk. Certainly it would be simpler if they did not have a scar on their uterus. Nonetheless, all the recent studies have found the incidence of scar separation to be about the same with elective cesareans as after a trial of labor. One cannot compare the separation of a horizontal low segment uterine scar with traumatic rupture of an unscarred uterus or of a classical scar. I have seen two scar separations, both discovered when a cesarean was done after several hours of strong contractions with no progress in labor. In both instances there were no clinical signs, no visible bleeding, no drop in blood pressure, no abdominal tenderness. Blood loss was less than two units, a normal, expected loss for a cesarean.

This impression is confirmed by Shy and colleagues, who used a computerized decision tree analysis to construct hypothetical cohorts of ten thousand women having repeat cesareans and ten thousand having trials of labor.[10] Probabilities of different outcomes were developed from an extensive literature review. They estimated the probability of more maternal *and* more perinatal deaths in the elective cesarean group than among those having trials of labor. According to this analysis, it is the elective repeat cesarean that is high risk for mother and baby, rather than a vaginal birth or trial of labor after previous cesarean.

## REFERENCES

1. US Dept. of Health and Human Services: *Cesarean Childbirth*, Report of a consensus development conference, Sept. 22-24, 1980. Oct. 1981. Available free on request from NIH, Pub. No. 82-2067.

2. US Dept of Health and Human Services: *Cesarean Childbirth*, Conference Summary, 1980. Available free on request from NIH.

3. Shearer EC: NIH consensus development task force on cesarean childbirth: The process and the result. Birth Fam J 8(2):25, 1981.

4. Gibbs CE: Planned vaginal delivery following cesarean section. Clin Obstet Gynecol 23(2):507, 1980.

5. Merrill BS and Gibbs, CE: Planned vaginal delivery following cesarean section. Obstet Gynecol 52(1):50, 1978.

6. Saldana LR et al: Management of pregnancy after cesarean section. Am J Obstet Gynecol 135:555, 1979.

7. Kelin RP et al: A study of father and nurse support during labor. Birth Fam J 8(3):16, 1981.

8. Odent, M: The evolution of obstetrics at Pithiviers. Birth Fam J 8(1):17, 1981.

9. Peterson GH and Mehl L: *Birthing Normally*. Mindbody Press, 1981.

10. Shy KK, LeGufo JP and Karp LE: Evaluation of elective repeat cesarean section as a standard of care: An application of decision analysis. Am J Obstet Gynecol 139(2):123, 1981.

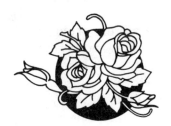

Elizabeth Shearer is a Certified Childbirth Educator, formerly Director of Parent Education of C/SEC, and is in private practice as a birth assistant. She was a member of the NIH Consensus Task Force on Cesarean Childbirth. Address inquiries to the author at 30 Sheafe St., Chestnut Hill, MA 02167.

59

*Here is a copy of the very conservative, but positive, statement of ACOG Committee on Obstetrics: Maternal and Fetal Medicine published in 1982.*

# Guidelines For Vaginal Delivery After A Cesarean Childbirth

Approximately 17 percent of the 3.5 million babies born each year in the United States are delivered by a cesarean birth. At the present time, 25 to 30 percent of these 500,000 operations are repeat cesarean births. Approximately 99 percent of all pregnant women who have had a cesarean birth have subsequent delivery by cesarean section. There has been increasing interest on the part of some physicians and patients in permitting labor and vaginal delivery for pregnant women who have previously had cesarean delivery. A recent NICHD Consensus Conference on Childbirth concluded that vaginal delivery after cesarean childbirth is an option appropriate for consideration.[1]

Specific data on the risk of vaginal birth after a prior low transverse uterine incision are limited but suggest that the risk of maternal mortality from uterine rupture is almost nonexistent and the risk of perinatal death is relatively small.[2] A recent review of the literature from 1951 to 1980 on vaginal delivery subsequent to cesarean birth (28, 742 pregnancies), which included prior classical and low vertical uterine incisions, suggest the incidence of cesarean scar rupture varies from 0.6 to 1.24 percent.[3] When uterine rupture occurred, these studies reported low maternal mortality rates and perinatal mortality rates ranging from 15 to 29 percent. Most reports antedate the availability of modern fetal monitoring, surgical support services, and neonatal intensive care units.

Recent reports demonstrate that a small number of carefully selected patients with low transverse segment uterine incisions experienced an overall potential vaginal delivery rate of 50-60 percent.[2,4,5,6,7,8]* With any uterine scar there appears to be a small but definite risk for rupture in the next pregnancy. There are inadequate data on the risk of labor following more than one previous cesarean birth, irrespective of the type of incision. There is no reliable way to predict the effect of labor on any uterine scar.

* note. These numbers refer to published articles on the subject. When I sent for this statement the references were not included.

# Homebirth Statement

Parents who choose to give birth at home are in essence saying that they are accepting full responsibility for their bodies, their pregnancies and their babies. Responsibility for complications to either the mother or the baby cannot be assigned to the attendant. For most of the birthing population, this responsibility is turned over to the doctor and/or the hospital. If you are in good health, if you eat very well, get physical exercise, have no medical or emotional contradictions to homebirth, then you will, in all probability, be able to have your baby at home safely and with great joy. The decision rests solely with you, the parents. No one else can decide for you or should attempt to influence you, since you are the only persons who are responsible for the welfare of the mother and child. The risks of homebirth should be carefully and fully discussed and understood; they should be weighed against the risks involved in a hospital delivery. Emotional needs and satisfactions should be weighed in relation to risk factors. Fears and insecurities should be openly and frankly acknowledged. Listen to your instincts, trust your 'vibes.' In the final analysis, if you decide that you are going to have your baby at home, having someone else there who has some training and experience with *natural, normal* childbirth is highly recommended. The attendant can observe, offer suggestions and assist *you*. It is *your birth*, it is *your responsibility*. To prepare yourself as well as possible, there are many things you can do. Here are some suggestions. Get excellent prenatal care. Find out what excellent prenatal care means. Educate yourself about excellent nutrition and follow it. Avoid drugs and smoking. Report any medical or emotional problems that may affect the pregnancy. Read as much as you can about birth, about taking care of your body during pregnancy, about health care and related subjects. Go together to childbirth education classes and then practice what you learn. Find an attendant that you have confidence in and that you like. Check his/her training and experience. Set up a complete medical backup alternative with a doctor and hospital in advance in case of last minute complications. See a pediatrician before the birth and arrange for him/her to see the baby as soon as you and the baby feel advisable. There may be other things that you can think of to do. When you have done all that you can, prepare yourselves, relax and have confidence in nature and the power of woman.

61

This statement was prepared by Donna Ha, a midwife from Hawaii,

# Home Birth

*by Nan Koehler*

Why would any woman in her right mind choose a home birth instead of a hospital delivery where all the advances of modern technology are available? This thought runs through the minds of everyone involved with childbirth — everyone except an informed expectant mother. Every pregnant woman who really wants to give birth naturally and experience an intense bonding with her baby must face this choice: hospital or home.

Here is a typical reaction from a woman wanting the kind of birth experience mentioned above when faced with the prospect of a hospital birth. (She'd been told she wasn't a good candidate for a home birth.) "I've thought it over and I've thought it over and I'm afraid to have my baby in the hospital. I'm afraid they're going to take the baby away. I went to visit the hospital and asked the nurse, "Are you going to take my baby away from me?" "Oh no, we're not going to take it. We're just going to take it to weigh it and measure it over in the nursery!" The woman continued expressing her desire to have her baby at home so that she has control over what happens. If she goes to the hospital, she's afraid she will lose control in the impersonality of hospital routine.

Another advantage that many consider quite seriously is the decreased risk of infection at home. The baby is born completely sterile. The first hand that touches it innoculates it with bacteria, therefore it's very important that the mother and father have the first intimate contact with the baby. If the baby is exposed to bacteria to which the mother doesn't have immunity, the baby is in trouble. It's own immune system is immature and as long as the baby is nursing it receives from it's mother antibodies, immune globulins and other factors. That is why hospitals have to follow antiseptic procedures; at home this isn't necessary!

62

Because of the growing interest in home births, there have been a number of studies published for the medical profession, analyses of the comparative degree of safety of home and hospital deliveries. In all publications, midwife-attended home births appear to have a better record, fewer cases of fetal distress and a lower rate of cesarian sections.

The last point, an important consideration for those seeking a home birth, is the desire to experience birth in a religious manner. Most hospitals don't have the time or inclination to help make birthing a spiritual or religious or even a serene experience. At home one can have flowers, candles, music, other children and/or friends. Once the couple has provided for the possibility of a mishap (with good pre-natal care, a good birth attendant and a hospital back-up for emergencies) the birth can become a celebration with family and friends instead of an ordeal among strangers.

Another facet of the spiritual experience is that at home the woman has to come to grips with the pain of labor and her own fear of death. The result is a sense of power, accomplishment and faith in the natural process.

REFERENCES:

Sheila Kitzinger, "The Place of Birth"
Sheila Kitzinger, "Birth At Home"
Lester Hazel, "Commonsense Childbirth"
Marshal Klaus, et, al, "Maternal Infant Bonding"
Lewis Mehl, "Birth & Family Journal", Vol. 2, #4, 1975-76, p. 123
Claude Burnett, et, al, "Jama", Dec. 19, 1980, Vol. 244, #24, p. 2741
Marion Souza, "Childbirth at Home"

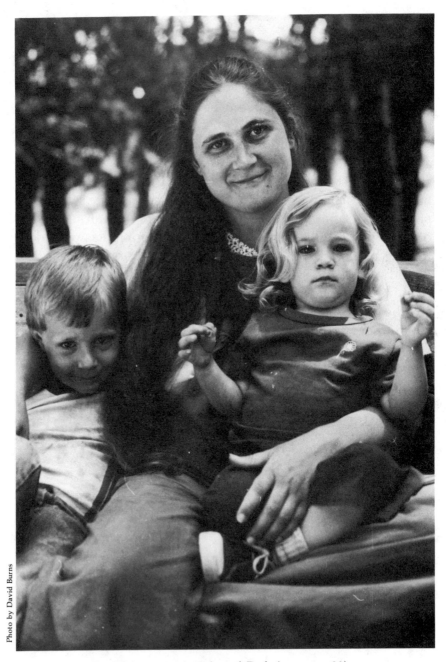

Photo by David Burns

*Kathy Weinper with Zeb and Beth (see page 80)*

64

# Part II

# VBAC Stories

# VBAC At Home

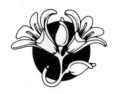

# Leslie and Michael Stanley

## Nan's Story

This woman introduced me to the whole phenomenon of VBAC. She wanted a vaginal birth very badly and came into the office with her mind already made up.

Birth of Jesse, a boy, occurred May 12, 1977, 2:47 p.m.,

We had another woman in labor as well. Leslie had been preparing for this birth for a long time. Her first birth had been a disappointment. She and her husband Mike did not know what was going on and in the end she had bled and was given a cesarean for possible placenta previa. She had a general anesthesia for the whole medical experience, and didn't bond very well with her baby.

This time, her labor began in the early morning between 5:00 a.m. and 6:00 a.m. Leslie phoned me at about 8:00 a.m. By 10:30 a.m. she was 6-7 centimeters dilated, her waters intact, and in good labor. Everything was ready. By about 12:30 p.m., she began to feel like pushing. Her birth was slow but regular and in perfect rhythm with the quiet, sunny spring day. At this point, we got the call from the other woman that her labor was getting intense.

66

At 2:30 p.m., when the head began to show in Leslie's vagina, the other woman in labor also felt like pushing, so I ran off right as little Jesse was born.

As Leslie began her labor, Don (my doctor partner) had set up an elaborate system with the local hospital: to have blood ready for her; and IV set-up all prepared; a vehicle ready in case we had to rush her to the hospital 10 minutes away.

Leslie only complained about feeling pain in her lower uterus once. What was actually hurting her were her round ligaments. I had her roll from side to side a lot. Leslie preferred laboring on her side. She pushed on her hands and knees, kneeling and finally propped up on pillows.

Her birth seemed so easy, so natural compared to how we felt. How scared we felt. It was like walking through a door for all of us. Leslie's birth certainly prepared us for the next. . . .

# Linda and Bill Peters

## Nan's Story

Birth of Mariah, a girl, occurred Tuesday, August 23, 1977,

The second VBAC I witnessed was a whirlwind compared to Leslie's carefully planned delivery. Linda and Bill came to us about a week or so before her due date, stating that they wanted a vaginal birth and that their midwife couldn't help them. They had traveled down from an area north of us. Our response was vague, since they themselves had no definite plans.

Suddenly one morning, a telephone call came that Linda was in labor. They'd driven down the night before with Linda in light labor. By 11:00 a.m. when my partner and a doctor friend went to check her and get some blood, she was 3-4 centimeters dilated, in early labor, all O.K.

67

When I arrived at 3:00 p.m., Bill and Linda were in the backyard smiling and enjoying themselves with their older child and the children of the household they were visiting. She was 6 centimeters, baby in good position, waters intact. I had her drink tea, lay down on her left side and relax. It worked fine. By 5:30 p.m. she was complete and moved inside for the baby's birth. By 6:30 p.m., she was finally grunting. It took her almost two hours to overcome the resistance of her pelvic floor. We broke her waters at about 8:00 p.m. (It was holding back the baby.) In 20 minutes the baby was born in a rush. Linda was squatting, then laying back upright against the wall, then squatting again at the last minute, and the baby exploded out. She tore. Whew! It was a thrill to experience her joy and delight over the baby!

# Linda's Story

Our son Damian was born eight years ago by cesarean section. My hospital experience and my feelings of incompletion with that birth made me realize that I wanted very much to experience a natural birth and that I did not want to experience it in the hospital.

I want to make it clear that I'm eternally grateful to the staff and hospital where Damian was born because I have a healthy eight-year old son, and I'm very clear that had I not gone to the hospital for his birth, I would have had a dead baby. He was breech and the cord prolapsed when I began pushing him out. I knew he was breech and that's why I went to the hospital. But after the birth, throughout my stay at the hospital, I felt totally helpless regarding any decisions made about me, my baby, or our relationship to each other, and I didn't ever want to be in that position again.

Fortunately, I had an aunt that had had a cesarean with her first birth and gave birth to four more babies naturally after that with no problems. So I knew it was possible.

When I became pregnant again, two and a half years after Damian's birth, I began my search: I wanted to find someone who was knowledgeable enough to make me feel confident, someone who was willing to be with me outside of the hospital. Well, that's a tall order, and it sent Bill (my husband) and me on a search over much of northern California. We were living in Paradise, and couldn't find anyone in that area to even do a natural birth in a hospital.

Bill was a carpenter, and his whole crew got a job in Santa Cruz when I was a few months pregnant, so that was the next place we looked. We found a man that attended home births, had a lot of experience and was willing to work with us; but he wanted me to take massive doses of vitamins, and I didn't feel good about that. I figured, though, that if I couldn't find anyone else, I would do it.

We owned some land in Ukiah and planned to move there after Bill's Santa Cruz job was over, so we decided to check there next. I was about four months pregnant at this point. We found two midwives that had organized a birth collective in Ukiah and they were willing to be with me at my birth as long as I was in town near a hospital. Everything went along quite well for the next four months, and it looked as though I had it made when one night, one of the other women in the collective gave birth and began to hemorrhage. The midwives rushed her to the hospital, only to discover that the obstetrician there wouldn't admit her. Apparently, they had decided to quit cooperating with the midwives without giving anyone any notice. The midwives hustled around and found a sympathetic doctor and he admitted the hemorrhaging woman.

Well, this made everyone (myself included) very uneasy. One midwife felt I should find another alternative, and the other said she'd still be at a home birth with me if I wanted one. I still wanted a home birth, but not in Ukiah. We decided to go down to Santa Cruz to see if the vitamin man might consider being at the birth, even though I hadn't been taking all

69

those vitamins. Sadly enough, when we got there, we discovered that he had been arrested for doing home births and was being tried in court. He wasn't able to do anymore home births in Santa Cruz and he eventually left the state.

So, we returned north via Marin County and someone told us about Don Solomon and Nan Koehler while we were in San Rafael. We called them up and they made an appointment to see us right away. I was eight months pregnant, don't forget, and as it turned out, so was Nan!

Don and Nan proceeded to explain to us that they were moving from San Rafael to Occidental and they didn't know if they and their equipment would be in different places, if Nan would be in labor when I was, if she'd have a brand new tiny baby or what. But, they said, if I couldn't find anyone else, I should call them when I went into labor. They gave me a thorough examination, discussed the possibility of my uterus rupturing during labor, gave me some vitamins and sent us on our way back home to Ukiah.

On the 22nd of August, Bill and I and our three year old Damian took off from Ukiah late in the evening, heading for Santa Cruz. We were driving an old flat-bed truck, (which bounced incessantly), because we were going to pick up some oak flooring. Bill was still working in Santa Cruz and we were planning on staying with friends, as we had been doing on and off for months. My "due date" was still two and a half weeks away. When we got as far as Marin County, it was very late and we decided to stop over at a friend's house there. At four in the morning I woke up to contractions, and at eight we called Don and Nan to see if they were still in town.

They were, and Nan was still pregnant. They stayed in contact with us by phone throughout the day until my contractions got more serious.

Up until the time that I went into labor, I never really knew for sure if I had the courage to go through with a normal birth. Even though I knew that a ruptured uterus was rare, even after a cesarean, I was aware of the grizzly possibilities.

70

Bill and I had talked about it and cried about it, but it wasn't until I went into labor that I felt certain and calm resolve about what we were doing. I had prepared myself physically with a wholesome diet, yoga, and exercise. I mediated frequently and sought spiritual guidance from Native American teachers and spiritual practices. So, when Mariah was ready for her birth, so was I.

I spent the day of my labor with Bill, walking around the neighborhood of San Anselmo and wondering at the beauty of it all. I definitely saw life with different eyes than usual. As my contractions became more intense, I quit walking and was content to sit in our friend's garden. Throughout the afternoon, Don and Nan and several friends showed up to join us for the birth. A doptone was placed to my belly and we listened to Mariah's tiny heart beat. My whole labor was effortless until I began pushing. Then I really had to work. As I remember, I pushed for almost three hours, and it seemed like forever before Mariah came flying out. But, there she was, finally, on the outside.

As I write this, Mariah has just walked in, moved a strand of my hair that was out of place, smoothed it back, and given me a kiss and a hug. I look into her little dark eyes and remember the first moment I ever looked into those eyes — now over five years ago. I wonder, would I do it again if I were to have another baby? I just don't know. But I do know that I'm very grateful for the experience I had. My only sorrow is that women don't have more support to choose the manner in which they give birth, particularly if they have had a previous cesarean birth.

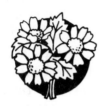

71

# Patricia and Larry Natalini

## Nan's Story

This is the incredible story of the birth of Naomi Ananda on December 23, 1977, at 10:25 p.m. The moon was almost full. She was 7 pounds and 3 ounces.

Patricia's first three births were all by cesarean. She had her first child at a home for unwed mothers at age 16. She wasn't sure why she had had a cesarean and told me that she thought it was due to fetal distress. Her medical records showed that she was diagnosed as having CPD (cephalo-pelvic disporportion). With her second, she made some effort to find a birth attendant who would allow her to attempt a vaginal birth. The general practitioners who agreed to help her couldn't secure proper obstetrical back-up and therefore refused to help her. The third pregnancy took the standard course, with no attempt at a vaginal birth, although she claims that she secretly considered it.

Toward the end of her fourth pregnancy, she learned about the obstetrician I work with and sought him out for help with a vaginal birth. His recommendation to her was to have another cesarean.

Thursday in the office, when all avenues for a safe, normal birth seemed closed to her, I told Patricia I would help her at home if she still really wanted a vaginal birth. (I don't know why I made that offer, rash as it seems to me now. All I can say is that some voice, not mine, spoke.) They were going home to think it over and give me a call if they wanted a home visit in preparation for a home birth.

At 6:30 a.m. the next day, Patricia awoke with contractions. Her husband called me at 8:00 a.m. to tell me that

72

Patricia wanted a home visit and was perhaps in early labor. When I arrived at 10:30 a.m., Patricia was having contractions 5 minutes apart, middling strength, but regular. Her waters were still intact. Patricia breathed with her contractions. A woman friend was there telling her that she ought to go to the hospital. I checked her. She was about 95% effaced and a fingertip dilated. She hadn't eaten yet. All her vital signs were normal. As Linda (our office secretary) and I fixed lunch for her and her three boys, Patricia calmed down in a subtle way. I said I'd stay at her home. Her blood pressure dropped from 140/80 to 125/70. (It was 105/60 in labor!)

By 1:30 p.m., she was still only 1 centimeter, but the baby's head had dropped and was not floating as before. Patricia washed her floors and cleaned the house. We all had tea, and she and her husband and two of the children went walking out in the orchard while I made supper. It was a beautiful winter day. Her contractions began to get more intense. After dinner Patricia took a hot bath. By 6:00 p.m., she was 3 centimeters dilated with the baby's head down and well-flexed. I broke the adhesion fibers which were keeping the cervix from opening. Patricia was completely relaxed. Larry went to do the laundry and while he was gone, the labor became sincere, with 3 minute contractions. At 8:00 p.m., Patricia's waters ruptured spontaneously at 7-8 centimeters dilation. Larry returned with clean laundry to herald transition. All vitals normal. At 9:00 p.m., she was complete and her pushing urge began. We moved from the living room to the bedroom (birthroom). Her pushing was hard work (possibly due to a narrow midpelvis?) The baby was born at 10:30 p.m. with eyes open, trying to breathe. The cord was tight around her neck and I couldn't get it over the baby's head. Rather than dicker with it, I told Patricia to push the baby out fast. She did. She tore inside both her labia, just the mucosa, not the outside skin. It bled a lot. (It scared me, because for a moment I wasn't sure where she was bleeding from!) I made sure that the baby was breathing and stable, then wadded her vagina with gauze pads

73

and waited for my doctor partner to come. (He got lost). Finally, the placenta came at 11:45 p.m. I wasn't nervous until the baby was born. Then, whew! What an affirmation in the power of the spirit, and indominable will, in over-coming all odds. It seemed a miracle to me.

# *Patricia's Story*

Birth is such an incredibly fascinating subject. I'd like to share a bit of my own personal experience with birth. I'm a mother of four. My first three children were born via cesarean section. My fourth, amazingly enough, was born via natural childbirth. I even had her at home!

What a huge contrast! Of course, everyone's experience is different, but for me, having a cesarean was a real nightmare. I found it to be very traumatic psychically, not to mention that it was physically a very painful experience, especially the recovery period. I don't even like to think about it.

My first cesarean was done after I'd been in labor for several hours. There were signs of fetal distress. The baby's head was floating (not engaged in my pelvis), a sign that it was possibly too large to fit through. He turned out to be a nine-pounder. Pretty big baby for a small woman like myself.

With my second pregnancy, I was told by my obstetrician that I would have to have another cesarean. Devastating news! I looked all over to try to find a doctor who would help me have a vaginal birth. I found one who would help me, but since he wasn't an obstetrician, he couldn't do a cesarean if necessary. He couldn't find a single obstetrician in our county to back him up. It never crossed my mind for a second to try it on my own. I was very scared. Being pregnant was very scary. I finally gave up two days before my due date. "O.K., Doc, I give; cut me up." This baby was 8 lbs., 7 oz. My doctor told me that perhaps I could vaginally birth a 5 lb. baby safely. I never forgot that.

74

With my third pregnancy, I put a little bit of energy into finding a doctor who would help me have a vaginal birth. A friend's midwife recommended an obstetrician who was an "excellent surgeon." I was going through a lot of personal problems during this period of my life, and this time I accepted my fate of another cesarean much more passively. The baby was less accepting than I was, though. My labor started a day before my scheduled surgery. I was scared! I was sure that my scar would rupture. I found it much harder to undergo a cesarean being in labor, mostly due to my fear. This child was 8 lbs., 1 oz. They seemed to be getting smaller. Perhaps there was hope for me yet.

Boy, was I frightened when I became pregnant again! The thought of another cesarean was so thoroughly terrifying, and abortion was out of the question. I walked around in dread. Stop the world—I want to get off! That's literally how I felt. I had a secret fantasy that what I really wanted to do was to have a vaginal birth. I was afraid to talk about it to many people because I didn't want to be discouraged by a lot of negative feedback. I so much wanted to have this wonderful experience, if it was at all possible. The few friends that I did share my fantasy with were very supportive and encouraging. My cousin told me the story of a woman she knew who had had three cesareans and then six more children vaginally. That meant that it was actually possible! That story gave me great hope.

I was also determined to have a small, but healthy, baby. I mentally programmed this into my brain. I also watched my weight very carefully. I ate a lot of fresh raw fruits and vegetables, whole grains and fish, and kept away from desserts and fattening foods. I exercised a lot. A pattern had developed with my first pregnancy: I had eaten a horrible diet, gained 50 lbs., and had a large fat baby. With each subsequent pregnancy, I ate a healthier diet, gained less weight and had a smaller baby.

It wasn't until my seventh month of pregnancy that I found

Dr. Donald A. Solomon and Nan Koehler, a doctor/midwife team who did home births. These people were actually willing to help me have a vaginal birth after three cesareans. My dream had come true! My plan was to have the baby in the hospital, obviously the most logical and safe way to go. But things went differently. Let me explain here that I really went through a great deal of inner and outer conflict with this whole thing. Don and Nan were like an external manifestation of this conflict. It went like this:

Don told me he was willing to support me in whatever decision I made, but that he felt that the safest thing would be for me to have another cesarean. Whenever he said that, all my fears would come up really strongly. "Maybe he's right. Perhaps my scar really would rupture. What if my pelvis really is too small? What if I couldn't handle it? Maybe I'm not strong enough. . . ."

Nan, on the other hand, was very positive and gung ho. "You can do it! You can make it happen. It's all in your mind. Just think, this is a rite of passage for you. You'll feel like super woman." And I'd be thinking, "Yeah, She's right!" Nan had me drink raspberry leaf tea, to cause braxton-hicks contractions and strengthen my uterus. Also, she had me massage my uterus with vitamin E. Most importantly, she taught me to visualize my uterus as being strong and resilient, and to visualize the birth the way I wanted it to be. Ah, the power of the mind!

Four days before my due date, my husband Larry and I were told that Don was being monitored at the hospital. (He had just applied for privileges there.) They wouldn't approve of him helping a lady have a vaginal birth after three cesareans. He told me that I could do it anyway, and just not sign the consent for surgery. I just couldn't imagine being in such a vulnerable place and being hassled like that. It was very upsetting news. Larry looked at Nan and asked her if she was available as a midwife. I'm glad he did it, because I didn't quite have the guts to seriously consider a home birth. I didn't actually decide to do it at home until I went into labor two days later.

What an amazing experience! I won't say I wasn't scared. I prayed a lot, which helped. It was so wonderful to be in labor at home with my family and a couple of lady friends. So warm and safe. Our three boys were able to watch their little sister being born! I feel so very blessed to have had this experience. No painful recovery period. No hospital! The baby weighed 7 lbs., 3 oz.; quite a bit smaller than the boys, but bigger than 5 lbs.

My labor was just the way I wanted it to be. Not too long, 14 hours; not too fast. It was real easy until the last 2½ hours. Up until then I was up and about, as Nan had advised, doing what I'd normally do that day — which was to clean the house. I stayed on my feet a lot, my labor being aided by gravity. This was the first pregnancy in which the baby's head actually engaged in my pelvis.

After that, my labor got harder and it was time to lay down and concentrate on my breathing and everything went smoothly. It was so easy! I was high for months afterwards.

I'm grateful to Nan and Don for their support. Especially to Nan. She taught me a great lesson in faith, and I learned that I'm a lot stronger than I think I am.

# Sara Stover

## Nan's Story

The birth of Lilac, a girl, occurred September 18, 1979, 9:29 p.m. She weighed about 7 pounds.

This is another amazing birth story — a personal victory against all odds. Sara's first baby (4½ years ago) was delivered by cesarean. I can't remember if it was because of a surprise breech or simply failure to progress. I do remember that she felt very inhibited during labor and complained bitterly and that after each contraction, there arose from the street below a chorus from the neighborhood children. (She lived in Berkeley at the time.) The birth attendant was passive, knitting, and not offering much labor coaching support.

For privacy and contact with nature, she was camped in the redwoods at a hermitage spot above a small canyon all summer. It was very peaceful there. I was uneasy for two reasons: first, she was 3 miles down a dirt road; secondly, no one lived with her — except her older child.

A neighbor of Sara's telephoned about 8:00 a.m. saying that her waters had broken in the early morning. I told her to come to the office and we'd check her discharge with nitrozine paper. I tried to encourage her to have the baby here. My doctor partner, of course, wanted her to go right over to the hospital. No, she wanted to go home to her own unconventional, but snug, nest. At this point, about noon, the contractions were about 20-50 minutes apart, and strong.

At 6:30 p.m., her neighbor called to say that Sara was in active labor. At 7:30 p.m., they called again saying that she was really doing it. Away we rushed. Upon arrival, three other friends were there supporting her and helping with the older child. She was 4-5 centimeters dilated, in good labor, defecating a lot and having difficulty with the intensity of her labor. It was wonderful to help her relax and do what she needed to do to release the baby. She stuck out her tongue — like a goat, like Picasso's painting, *Geurneca,* and yelled with all her might.

She was complete at about 8:30 p.m., but I urged her to hold off as long as possible with real pushing. The baby came out perfectly. It was hard to keep the baby warm outdoors, but with hot blankets from a dutch oven rigged up over a camp fire, the baby stabilized O.K. Sara squatted over a bowl to deliver the placenta in about 20 minutes. Another magic night!

78

# Shawnee and Jim Colongione

## Nan's Story

The birth of Jacob Ezra, a boy, occurred May 10, 1980, 5:12 p.m. He weighed 8 pounds, 12 ounces.

This is the story of a woman who vacillated wildly between the depths of self-doubt and the heights of great courage. She wanted to experience normal childbirth very much because her first delivery was a source of humiliation for her. She had been alone in a Catholic Hospital in New York City where the nuns somehow made her feel guilty about her response to the pain of labor. (It's always a jolt the first time! How much it can hurt!) With a typical premature-ruptured-membranes-failure-to-progress syndrome, she was sectioned. When she came to us for help, my doctor partner simply refused to participate in helping her with a home birth, so I engaged the help of another midwife.

Shawnee began her labor with mild contractions at 2:00 a.m. By 6:00 a.m., they had grown in intensity and the other midwife called me. (I was again at another delivery.) When I arrived at 7:30 a.m., you can imagine my surprise when I examined Shawnee, who was writhing in pain, and discovered that she was only 2 centimeters dilated, with a thick cervix. Her waters were intact, though; her cervix did respond to massage, and she was having strong contractions every 3 minutes. All her vitals were normal. I massaged her cervix open slowly. Each hour it softened and opened more and more as I stretched it. By 10:30 a.m., she was 5 centimeters dilated with the forewaters at her spines and the baby down to -1 station, with the head flexed. Making progress! The baby felt big.

At 1:30 p.m., Shawnee had a large bowel movement and

79

like pushing. Her forewaters were bulging out, so I ruptured them. This added to the tension, since there was meconium in the waters. It was a real dilemma, because a trip to the hospital, (the sensible thing to do at this point), would have meant another cesarean for Shawnee, which is what she was trying to avoid in the first place. This discussion (and the ruptured membranes) seemed to spur her on. By 2:30 p.m., she was 8 centimeters dilated with a thick anterior lip. She is a DES daughter with a cockscomb cervix. At 3:30 p.m. she was pushing in earnest and I pushed the lip up over the baby's head. Her pushing was slow, but steady. The baby came out and looked fine. No tears. The other midwife and I both suctioned the baby on the perineum very carefully. He was tangled up in his cord. Apgar 5/9. Shawnee cried over and over "It came out of me! It came out of me! We did it! We did it!" Her husband was jubilant, and so were we.

# Kathy and Brad Weinper

## Nan's Story

The birth of Zeb, a boy, occurred on Wednesday, September 17, 1980 at 7:45 p.m. He weighed 8 pounds and 14 ounces.

This is the story of a truly dedicated couple who wanted a home birth, but were unable to overcome the medical hurdles they encountered. Kathy had her first baby by cesarean. The baby was breech, with premature ruptured membranes. Then, another attempt at a vaginal birth with her second child resulted in a cesarean for failure to progress and failure of the

80

head to descend: a classic cause for sectioning a lady. What doctor could resist!

When looking for a good cesarean experience with their third child, they chanced upon my partner, and then upon me.They began considering a vaginal delivery in the hospital and when they began glowing with the prospect of a normal birth, I told them frankly that if they really wanted a normal birth in their circumstance, the only way would be to have their baby at home.

Kathy had contractions all day, but they were mild and 10 minutes apart. She couldn't sleep Tuesday night and called me at about 2:30 a.m. for advice about what was going on. I checked her at 3:30 a.m. and her contractions were irregular, 5-15 minutes apart and mild. Her cervical os was posterior, thick and closed. I told her she wasn't in labor, but her pains hurt her too badly to ignore! I told her that if she couldn't sleep and be normal she should take castor oil. She took 2 ounces of castor oil at 10:00 a.m., then ate a meal, after which she took another 2 ounces of castor oil. She threw all that up and had two bowel movements, but no violent diarrhea. Soon her husband called for me. Kathy wanted my help because the contractions were strong and regular since about 1:00 p.m. At 3:00 p.m. I checked her, thinking she might be in transition. She was 6 centimeters dilated, having good contractions, but with the cervix still thickish and the baby high with bulging forewaters. We went walking between 4:00 p.m. and 5:00 p.m. and then Kathy bathed in hot water to relax. At 6:15 p.m., I checked her again. She was still about 6 centimeters. The cervix was softer and the baby down a little more, but still not engaged. I ruptured her membranes and had her try to push to get the baby to move down some, in the hope that her cervix would dilate better. Her labor got intense. Kathy started yelling and wanting to push at 6:30 p.m. Once again, I urged her to begin slowly with the pushing. Just as the baby was crowning, my doctor partner arrived. He continued the delivery and felt that she was going to tear so he gave her an

81

episiotomy. The baby was out at 7:45 p.m. — all yelling. Ten minutes later, the placenta was out. Home free! Except for the stitching.

# Brad and Kathy Weinper's Second VBAC

## Nan's Story

Beth Rachel was born on April 14, 1982, at 2:30 a.m.      She weighed 7 pounds and 15 ounces.

This time Brad and Kathy didn't bother trying to talk a doctor into helping them at the birth. They secured a back-up for an emergency and pretty much did the whole labor and delivery themselves. The main role I played was in helping her not to tear. And this time everything went absolutely perfectly.

Kathy was up in the early morning (2:00 a.m.) with contractions. She couldn't sleep. Later that day, in the office, she was having mild contractions every 5-7 minutes.

In the early evening she took some castor oil, and by midnight she was in good labor. Her husband telephoned about 12:30 a.m. saying that Kathy was having the baby and had checked herself and thought that she was about 4 centimeters dilated. I arrived at 1:30 a.m. She was 6-7 centimeters dilated, not completely effaced, with the contractions still 5 minutes apart. Her membranes were intact and all vitals normal. She'd been pushing when we arrived, laying on her back, after spending most of her labor on the toilet. I had her lay back on her left side, breathe and not push, etc. She responded with good humor and handled the pain well. By 2:15 a.m., she felt like pushing in earnest. The baby's expulsion was slow and controlled, with minimal tearing (mucosal splits, no perineal tears).

82

The placenta came out perfectly. The only frightening part was two contractions before the baby was born: as the waters broke, there was meconium. I suctioned the baby vigorously, gave it a little oxygen and the baby responded immediately. I stimulated its gag reflex in my over zealousness! (I've seen this done innumerable times in the hospital by vigorous suctioning.)

This birth was a happy experience for the whole family. Kathy's mother was there both times, but she was not as scared this time.

## Kathy's Story

In 1976 I became pregnant for the first time. My ideal had always been to have a home birth. There wasn't a doctor to be found who would help us. I did locate an obstetrician and nurse-midwife who were operating a birth center. We took Bradley childbirth classes and practiced for our birth. My waters broke early in labor, then came some meconium. A visit to the doctor confirmed (by exam and x-ray) a breech, as we had suspected. I had done pelvic tilts since my seventh month to no avail. The doctor and my husband tried to turn her during labor, but that was no help either. (From the minute we entered the hospital, we ceased to have much control over our situation. In the alien world of hospital bureaucracy, the doctor definitely has the upper hand. You haven't much choice, but to believe what he tells you.) My labor was very sporadic. After 24 hours and 7 centimeters dilation, I was sectioned. Brad took our new daughter Chelsea and me home two days later. After that, I read everything I could find about natural birth and VBACs.

My second pregnancy came in 1978. Our doctor did tell us we could try a VBAC, but if it didn't work out he couldn't consent to it again. We prepared for a vaginal birth, with the addition of a class on cesareans so Brad could be with me if the operation was needed. I went into labor. Again, it was slow and sporadic — over 20 hours. I did have some fear of rupturing because all my pains were centered right on my incision. The forewaters had brought about 8 centimeters dilation; the baby's head was at -3 station (very high). The doctor talked with us about rupturing the bag of waters to see if the baby's head would engage. It broke spontaneously; dilation decreased to 6 centimeters, which was expected. It was almost an hour before labor started up again, very slowly. Another hour passed with only a few mild contractions, so the doctor decided on a cesarean. It went well. Brad and I were glad we got to be together for the incredible experience of Bret's birth. I felt a heaviness, though, a sadness at the thought of never being able to have a vaginal birth. I believed that there would be no one to help us if I became pregnant again.

We moved to Santa Rosa in 1979. After our first year here, I became pregnant for the third time. I set out to find a doctor who would let Brad participate in the birth. After finding Don and Nan Solomon, we went to talk with them and learned that they would let us try a VBAC. Then we asked half jokingly if they would help us do it at home. Nan said, "Yes." Don said he didn't really agree, but he'd be there. All things considered, we decided on a home birth. No one could have changed my mind. I did have my fears, mostly of rupturing. I did have my doubts from time to time also; but Brad never let me give up — even with all the insanity that can go through a pregnant women's head.

My first contractions came at about 8:00 a.m. on Thursday. Feeling sure it would be another long labor, I tried to stay busy to speed it up. After dinner that evening, my contractions were quite hard. By bedtime, I was unable to sleep and had to breathe with almost every one. Again, contractions didn't come at a steady, predictable pace. Nan arrived at 4:00 a.m. Wednesday, proceeded to check me and found I had not dilated, although the contractions were quite hard. I found it almost unbelievable, though I suppose part of me was

84

expecting some disappointment. We had no idea how long it would go on like that: hours, days or maybe just stop. I realized that the longer it continued like this with no baby and no real rest, the greater my chances of a cesarean. I asked Nan about taking some castor oil. She told me that I'd need to take about 4 ounces. We talked for a bit and then she went back home. I had only two ounces, so I took that at 9:00 a.m. My sister came by at 11:00 a.m. with two more ounces. I drank it straight.

I checked myself at noon and found I was dilated to about 2 or 3 centimeters. That made me feel much better. Much of my labor was spent in a hot bath; it made me feel more in control. I was so tired that it was hard for me to get up and move around. Brad kept trying to get me to walk around, without much success.

At 4:00 p.m., Nan returned and found that I was dilated to about 5 or 6 centimeters, but the baby was very high. With Brad's help and much to his delight, they got me outside. We walked for about an hour. Then I spent another hour in a hot tub. When Nan checked me again the baby was still very high. She ruptured the water bag and the baby still did not come down. Nan explained that my cervix was soft and loose like jelly, and told me to push gently with the next few contractions to see if I could get the baby to move down. (This should never be done without knowledgeable advice due to the risk of cervical damage.) It worked! The baby moved down, my stomach adjusted and I threw up, (mostly castor oil.) There was no pushing urge with the next few contractions. Then dilation was complete and the urge to push became a reality. No more waiting—I could finally do something! My whole body became part of the process. The baby's head started to appear and disappear. Don arrived as Zebulon's head was crowning. The area around my urethra was burning intensely. I felt like I was going to tear so I asked Don to cut me. He did a small episiotomy and I felt much better. With a few more pushes our baby boy was born. Looking

85

back, it was all like a dream. But the realization is there—we finally make it!

I was due to give birth to our fourth and last child about March 30, 1982. Of course we planned another home birth. In my sixth month, Nan found the baby to be breech. During the next month I tried pelvic tilts, but that was too painful due to a sciatic nerve problem. At my seventh month visit, Nan thought that she should try to turn the baby before she filled me too tightly. There would be time to try again if the baby moved back to breech. So, with a couple of student midwives looking on and monitoring fetal heart tones, Nan turned the baby from the outside. Then she held her in place for a few minutes. I got up and took a walk around the farm for half an hour to get her used to sitting on her head. For over an hour I felt light-headed and a bit strange. I wondered what this little person inside me was experiencing. During our little walk, I knew she was fine. I could see her being caressed and rocked as we walked along. I knew she could hear my voice reassuring and comforting her.

I was awakened at two in the morning, April 13, by the first contractions, 7 minutes apart. By noon, they had stopped. I went to my 2:00 p.m. appointment and told Nan what was happening. She told me to go home and try to rest. Almost as soon as I got in the car contractions began again. By 8:00 p.m. that night, they were real hard. I knew that sleep would be impossible. I checked myself: no dilation. I had to decide if I should wait and see what happens or try to speed things up before I got too tired. I decided to take the dreaded castor oil. This time I put it in the blender with some grape juice and it went down much easier than before.

By 10:00 p.m., I was starting to dilate. I told Brad to go to bed, thinking it would be quite a while. By midnight my labor was getting very intense. I couldn't leave the bathroom, with diarrhea and contractions every minute or two. I was very awake and felt pretty much in control. I decided to push very gently with a couple of the contractions, just to make sure that the baby's head was in my pelvis this time. I had no intention of causing any dilation.

A while later, Brad got up and said that he was going to call Nan. I insisted he shouldn't. He knew better. My mother got up and started getting things organized a bit. Nan arrived at 1:30 a.m. with an apprentice and a visiting midwife from back east. Then came Candace, who had apprenticed with Nan, but was now on her own.

It all seemed to go so quickly; the house was alive. Brad got the kids up and they watched with big eyes. Transition was just about at an end. Now it was time for pushing. Candace massaged my perineum with very warm oil to prevent tearing. I had plenty of coaching and encouragement. The hardest part was trying not to push her head out too fast. When Beth's head was born, things slowed down. When the rest of her body slid out, it became apparent that she was having trouble getting her breathing going. Nan suctioned her with a delee. She didn't like it. Just putting the tube down got her on the right road. A few more minutes and she was doing fine. Things slowly quieted down. Everything was cleaned up. Beth and I lay in bed in the dimly lit room. The feeling was almost festive. I felt like a little kid trying to sleep on Christmas Eve. Listening to everyone talking and laughing in the other room, I kind of wanted to be out there, too; but I was all too cozy and excited in my warm nest.

I am so thankful for all the help I had. My mother was a God-send. During the last part of my pregnancy, I had one cold after another. With very little rest, I felt exhausted. Having given birth seven times herself, my mother conquered some of her fears and took up our invitation to come. She stayed almost a month. With her help, I was strong and healthy by the time I went into labor. She enjoyed the birth, though she was a bit frightened at first. She noted the love and calmness with which it was handled. It was a healing for her in some ways.

If a VBAC is what you want, try to take it to the limit and

do it at home. As you probably know, the moment you set foot in a hospital, the odds are greatly increased that you'll end up with another cesarean. Your home can be the safest, most controllable place for the birth of your child. Hospitals can make you almost as helpless as the baby you went there to birth.

Love and faith to you all!

The birth of Zebulon Abraham born September 17, 1980, 7:45 p.m., 8 lbs. 15 oz., 21½ in. I took 4 oz. of castor oil to speed my home births. I always have long labors.

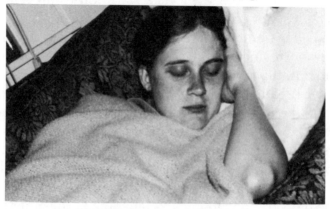

*Early labor, trying to rest.*

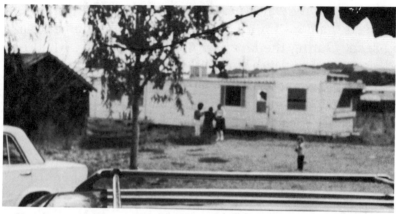

*Returning from long walk.*

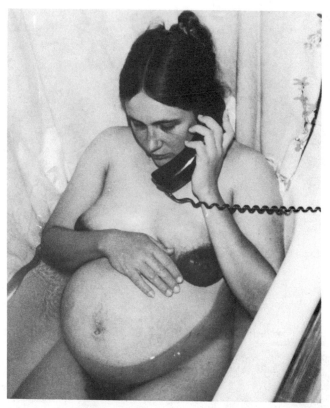

*Spent about half my labor in a hot bath very relaxing.*

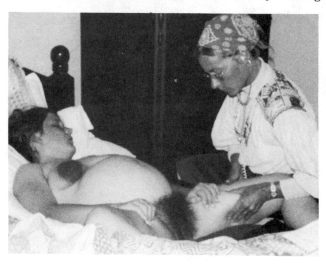

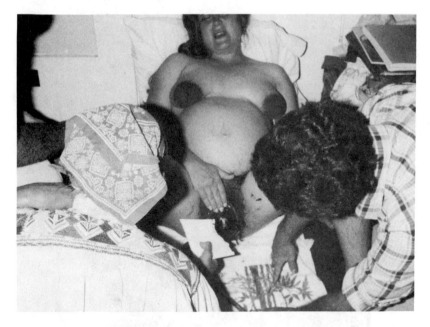

*Crowning trying not to push too hard and fast.*

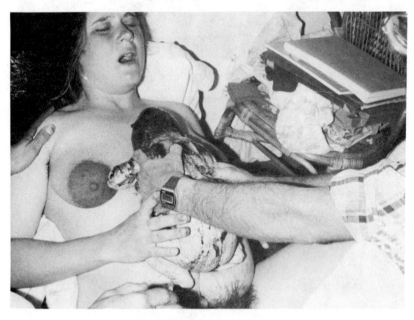

*Blood from a small episiotomy.*

90

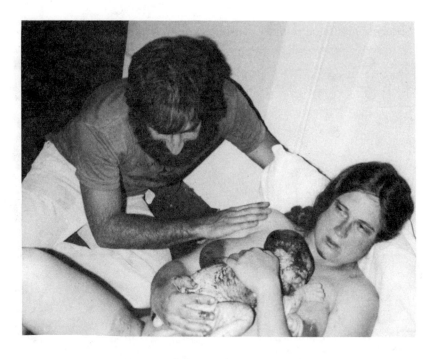

*Cutting of the cord, setting him free.*

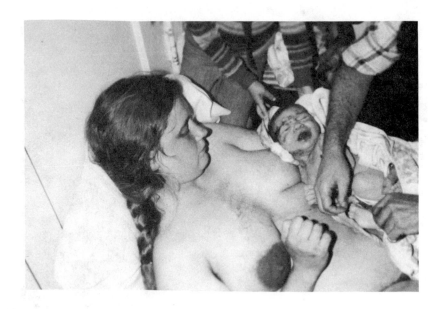

*Educate and have faith in yourself. Hold fast to your dreams.*

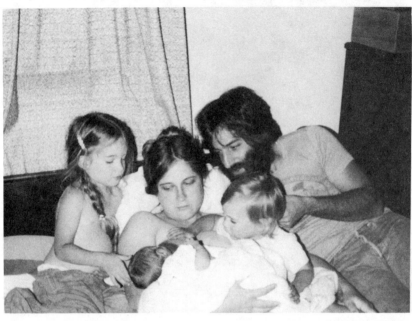

*The birth of Beth Rachel, born April 14, 1982, 2:50 a.m., 7 lbs. 15 oz., 21 in.*

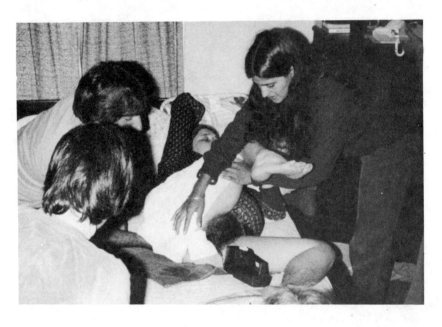

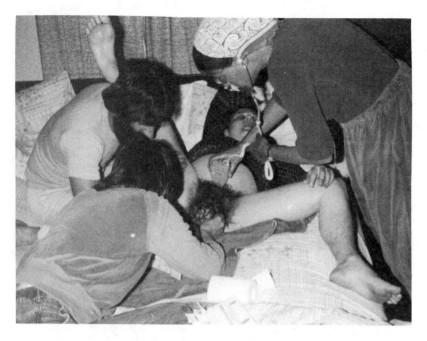

*Warm oil massaged on the perineum. No tearing at all!*

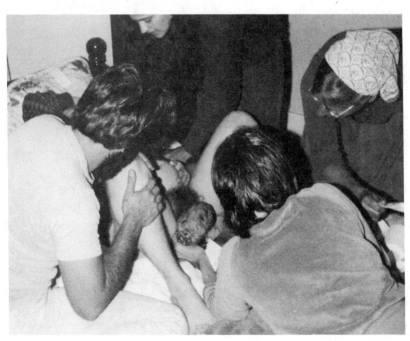

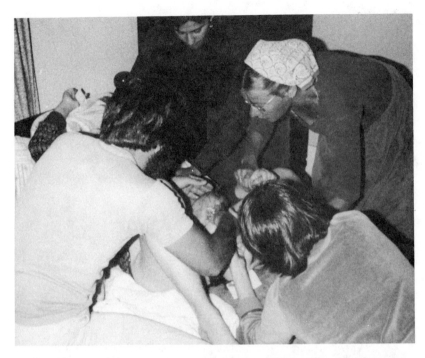

*She had some trouble getting started. Did well after suctioning.*

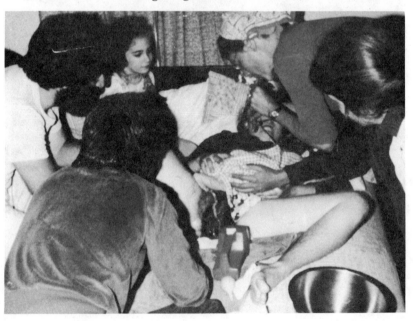

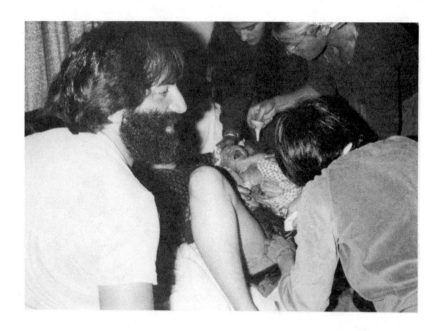

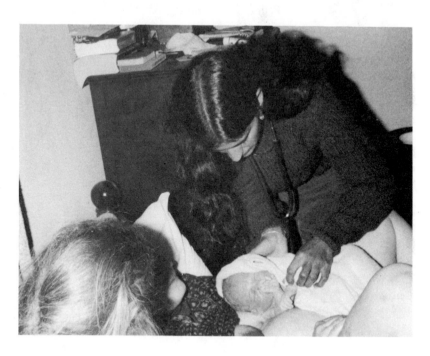

My name is Kathy Weinper. If you'd like to talk, phone (707) 523-0814.

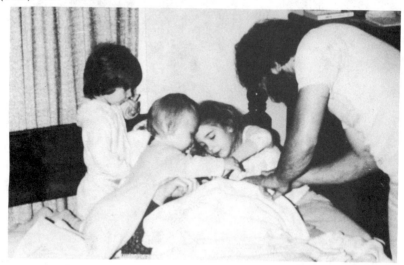

*Where's the new baby?*

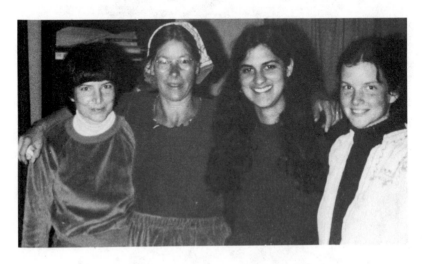

*Much thanks to all our helping hands!*

# Kim Pistey and John Lyhne

## Nan's Story

The birth of Shasta Daisy, a girl, occurred November 13, 1981, 9:41 a.m. She weighed 6 pounds, 14 ounces.

This is a landmark in the personal struggles of Kim and John, who were both still smarting from the drama of their first child's birth. Kim was laboring at home when following a routine vaginal check by her midwife, it was discovered that the baby was breech. The midwife wasn't prepared to help them with a rare presentation and took Kim to the hospital (a sensible thing to do!) But Kim never progressed in her labor after she entered the hospital. Whether she was scared or just wasn't in good labor yet is hard to say. From the way her second birth went, I'd guess she is one of those women who have a long, latent phase of labor.

Kim began having noticeable contractions on Friday. They continued Saturday and Sunday with no dilation. Finally, by Monday evening at 11:00 p.m., she was 2-3 centimeters dilated. Another midwife colleague was attending Kim. We had planned to have both of us there. As it turned out, I was again at another delivery when I got the call that Kim was 7 centimeters and I should hurry over. (I was almost an hour away.) All her vitals were normal and her waters were intact.

Her labor was progressing slowly and I remember Kim was physically strong — her muscles were stiff like a board. She got into a hot bath. Pushing began in earnest about 6:30 a.m. By 7:45 a.m., there was little progress, and when I checked her very carefully to see what was the problem, the baby was posterior. Kim was afraid because her abdomen was hurting in the front. (Maybe because of her full bladder?) Another heavy labor for Kim. From somewhere came her determination and strength, and the baby rotated and was born perfectly with no tears. The placenta was out in 15 minutes.

97

# Kim's Story

My story begins four years ago with the birth of my first daughter. We had arranged a home birth from the start of my pregnancy. Planning as best we knew how, we had read all the books we could find and attended all the classes our midwife offered us. Yet, with my fear of hospitals and birth, we conveniently avoided any information about hospital deliveries, thinking that all would be well and that we wouldn't need it. Therefore, I was toally unprepared when my waters broke and my midwife abruptly determined a breech baby. She then flatly stated that she would only help us in the hospital.

After 45 hours, my labor concluded at the end of a physician's blade. None of the nightmarish contraptions were avoided. I was connected to a fetal monitor and an IV needle with plenty of insensitive nurses around to lengthen my labor and make me more uncomfortable and afraid. Then came the grand finale: an infection on my incision and a very high fever that brought me dangerously close to death. There was the added bonus of being unable to even hold my baby for one long agonizing week after the operation.

Many will argue that the machines and procedures were there for the safety of myself and my baby. Yet, it is my heartfelt belief that it was all those machines that kept me inhibited and made me afraid to carry on with the natural function of my body. Who can truly say? I do believe that if I had been at home I would have been able to deliver vaginally.

When I discovered that I was pregnant for the second time, panic set in. Not because I didn't want the child, but because I thought that the only way the baby could be born was by a gash into my belly. All the physicians that I had talked to informed me that a cesarean was the only safe route to take. Naively, I followed their beliefs until one day a friend introduced me to Dr. Donald Solomon. It was this wonderfully gifted man that gave me new hope that I might yet fulfill my

98

womanliness with a vaginal birth. He was honest and frank, describing all the dangers to me.

Still, these dangers meant nothing to me compared to my fear of the hospital. The realization that I could die in the hospital as well as at home led me to the decision to try at home. At least I would be free of interference. Of course, Don had to refuse to help me at home because of the risk.

It was then that I met Nan, wonderfully confident Nan. She gave me the courage to look into myself to fulfill my ultimate dream. Blessed Nan, who taught me that it was all in my head, that it *was* all up to *me.*

My mantra became the song by Santana called "I'm Winning." I would allow my head and heart only the most positive of thoughts. The negative was there only as an opponent to overcome. My will became that of a sorceress! I was an eagle flying high above all evil.

At birthing time my labor was a normal, well-progressing one. Together with Nan and calming midwife, Carolyn, I breathed and relaxed in the security of my own home. It was transition that became difficult. Ten centimeters dilated with no desire to push, I kept having delirious, exhausted fear that my cesarean scar would burst. Three hours passed. I tried various pushing positions without much progress. Finally, summoning my last ounce of personal power, I remembered the pugilist in me again. My screams were those of a warrior doing combat on the battlefield of life. If I had lost, it would have been death with dignity rather than life with only half my soul.

My four year old daughter stroked the baby's head as it came through the opening. My husband held my legs as they surrendered this new being to the light. As it turned out, the cord was wrapped around her leg. But all ended well with my flower, Shasta Daisy, opening her eyes to find me, instead of the blare of hospital lights.

My after thoughts are simple, summed up in the first few lines of the Dhammapada:

We are what we think
Having become what we thought
Like the wheel that follows the cart-pulling ox
Sorrow follows an evil thought
And joy follows a pure thought
Like a shadow faithfully tailing a man
We are what we think
Having become what we thought.

## John's Story

I came from a family of twelve children and so I had a much calmer perspective on childbirth than did my wife, Kim. In my experience, birth was very common and not filled with fear and mystery. Also, I have had a life-long interest in medicine, and experience in emergency situations.

When I heard that we were to have a birth, I agreed with Kim that we would have it at home with a midwife. We had the great misfortune to meet only two midwives, and then to choose a very inexperienced one over a well-trained woman whose vibes were not as compatible with us.

In the course of the pregnancy, we studied hard and practiced techniques, but Kim's real fear of hospitals, plus my laziness, caused us to skip any preparations for a hospital birth.

In the ninth month, I was sure that the baby was in a breech position. We were assured by our midwife that I was wrong, but lo and behold, it *was* a breech and we rushed to the hospital in early labor. Since I've had good experiences in hospitals, I think that I misjudged the extent of Kim's fears. I tried to help her, but we finally gave in to the doctor, and Kim had a cesarean. I was there in the operating room and saw the birth.

Our daughter was great, but Kim was a shambles. Her body and psyche were both nearly killed in that operating

100

room. She had thought herself a failure since that day. She never came to terms with that failure until last year when once again we were to have another child.

We immediately started preparing for a cesarean birth again. This time we tried all the classes at the hospital of our choice. We went one evening a week to their introduction class and another night to a special class for prospective cesarean births.

It was this class that knifed through our fearful resolve to go the safe route: cesarean. The other couples in the class all looked like scared kids. They were all ready to get cut open without even checking out any alternatives. In our mental mirrors, we suddenly saw ourselves the same way and realized that we had to explore all possible alternatives.

We had the great good fortune to go to see Dr. Don Solomon as our obstetrician. His name kept coming to us from friends. We heard that he was caring and open to birth as the parents and child want it. Even when we thought a cesarean was necessary, he said he would do it in as humane a manner as he could, and we believed him.

As the pregnancy progressed, we went to Don's farm for his class. It was taught by this fabulous woman, Nan Koehler. She is a courageous pioneer, and she and Don both talked to us about the possibility of a vaginal birth. Nan and Don were talking about a natural birth at the hospital, and we agreed. Next, Nan was asking us if we had thought about a home birth.

Don, as a conscientious doctor, warned us of significant dangers that would be increased at a home birth. He also said that he couldn't be there if the birth was at home because of restraints placed on him by his colleagues. Even then, he was open and fair enough to tell us that we should see Nan if we desired.

We gulped and sighed and finally saw Nan. She was enthusiastic right from the start and I saw that Kim and she had a good relationship starting. All of the pent-up sense of past failure and future fear rose up in Kim and she chose the path of nature.

We decided to try a birth at home, with the knowledge that it could still end up at the operating room. Kim wished to battle at home, where she knew the energies and could battle without the fear of medical gadgets and procedures.

The birth itself was perfect, as we knew it would be. Kim fought bravely. She had to. The real fear of a uterine rupture insured that we couldn't just flow through labor. No simple, mellow birth for us. Kim was very scared during the pushing phase of labor. Though she never said so, she was awash with fear and held back on each contraction. This restraint slowed the birth, but it also made the final push easier and so Kim didn't even tear. The baby smiled at us within minutes of birth, and hasn't stopped since. Kim too!

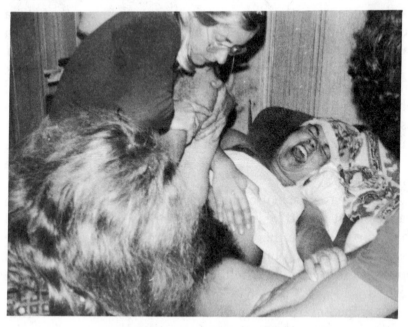

*Kim and birth of Shasta Daisy.*

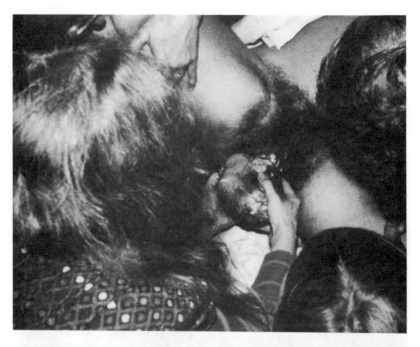

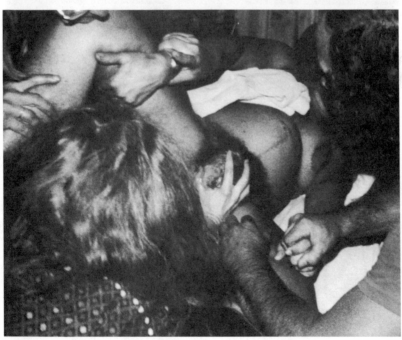

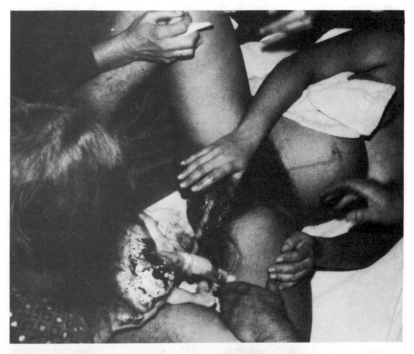

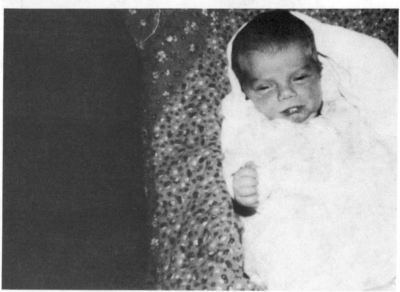

*Shasta Daisy*

# Janine and Greg Ray

## Nan's Story

Janine's story is definitely a vision quest. Every obstacle imaginable had to be overcome in order for her to have a vaginal birth naturally. Her first baby was breech with failure to progress — a complete trauma for her. Her decision to try for a vaginal birth, and then a home birth, came slowly in the course of her prenatal care and preparation for the arrival of her second child, many years later. The support of her husband was invaluable, as is the case in so many of these VBAC stories. His vision and stability were truly what pulled her through in the long run. It was a group effort to support her. Truly a saga! She was late; the baby had been breech again; her mother had been visiting: lots of pressure.

They telephoned about 5:00 or 6:00 p.m., saying that Janine was having contractions. Contractions began after she had witnessed an automobile accident an hour or so earlier. Janine couldn't sleep. They were up all night. They telephoned again around 3:00 a.m. to say that the labor was getting intense. (Once again I was at another delivery and sent my assistant and a midwife student over to check her.) She was about 6 centimeters dilated with medium-poor contractions. They tried to get Janine to walk and squat. Her contractions seemed to be one on top of the other. When I arrived at about 7:00 a.m., she was still 6 centimeters, with a swollen cervix (from not relaxing well). When she laid down, her contractions were 5 minutes apart. The baby was in a posterior presentation, with membranes intact. Her contractions never got any closer together. She hadn't been eating. I gave her a protein drink and some oil of celery seed in water (5 drops to help her relax). Then we went on a "forced march" for an hour outdoors — around 10:00 or 11:00 a.m.

By 1:00 to 2:00 p.m., her progress was still so slow that I

105

was contemplating the need for pitocin and hospitalization, but I couldn't imagine the scenario if we went in at this point, with her slow labor and history of a previous cesarean. (Doesn't look good, does it?) In desperation we smoked some sacrament. We all cried, and like magic Janine opened up. She needed to be touched and rubbed. She wanted contact. We all massaged her—everyone that was there. I never took my hands off her again. She loosened up and was complete with the baby rotated to anterior in two hours! Most of her pushing phase was spent pacing and squatting on the toilet. Her labor pains still weren't that strong. The baby was fine—a beautiful girl. The placenta was delivered with no problems. She bled momentarily from a labial split, but her perineum was intact! Janine was tired and exhausted. We all felt the same. A testimony to the power of natural forces and self-determination.

# Janine's Story

My first daughter, Monique, was born by cesarean section on September 3, 1972. Being young and naive, I knew that women had babies and there was nothing to it. I went to the hospital when contractions were five minutes apart, only to be left in a labor room with a clock to stare at and the sounds of screaming and moaning women to listen to. After several hours of laying on my back, never seeing my doctor, only nurses and interns who checked my dilation periodically, I was told he wouldn't be called until I was at least 8 centimeters dilated. I never got that far. About six hours later, a nurse gave me a shot and I went to sleep, only to awaken to a priest giving me my last rites and asking for a confession. "I didn't do anything wrong; I just came here to have my baby." Wheeled into a bright room, a mask over my face, I was told to count backwards from 100. Hours later, pain, confusion, "Where's my baby?" A nurse calmed me down, told me that I had a 7 pound, 15 ounce daughter, but that I couldn't see her until I was stronger. She was the one who told me that I had had a cesarean and that the baby was breech. Later that evening, Monique was brought to me, but I was too weak to hold her. She looked like a monkey. "Are you sure she's mine?"

My husband and family never wanted to talk much about the fact that I had had a cesarean and I tried to forget it myself. I still didn't quite understand why, and was afraid to ask. About a month after the birth of Monique, I suffered a severe case of peritonitis, due to a burst appendix, undiagnosed until an emergency exploratory was performed. Since then, I have had a fear of hospitals, and an uncertainty about doctors.

Before marrying my second husband, Greg, I went to three gynecologists in Sonoma County to see about having my tubes tied, because I didn't think I could handle having any more children. My Dalkon Shield had to be removed because of the recall and I needed some birth control. Two of the doctors agreed that I should sign a release form for a hysterectomy because a simple laparotomy might not be possible because of the lesions from my cesarean and peritonities. I finally let Family Planning insert a Copper 7 IUD. Some time later I developed symptoms of endometritis, and another doctor convinced me to have my IUD removed, and told me the only cure would be pregnancy or a hysterectomy. I was going to marry Greg in a week and he really wanted children.

Nine years after Monique's birth, I found myself married to Greg, very in love with him, and pregnant. I had decided that I did want another baby, but I was confused, scared, under a lot of stress, and this seemed to be happening too fast. All I knew was that I had to do this birth differently. Many friends and customers of our restaurant highly recommended a doctor, Don Solomon, in Sebastopol. I hoped it would be worth the 45 minute drive.

For my first trip to Dr. Don's office, he wasn't in, and I met his wife, midwife Nan Koehler. Immediately I sought advice for my questions and health problems. I was overweight, constipated, had hemorrhoids, a yeast infection, an outbreak of oral herpes, a bad case of poison oak and a really bad headache. I was in bad shape and it was amazing how Nan was able to put me at ease. We talked for an hour, and I left feeling more confident than I had felt in a long time. She gave me a copy of the handouts entitled *Knowledge is Power* and told me to read as many books as I could. She explained that I would have to learn about vitamins, not take any medication, and become more aware of my own body.

A couple of weeks later I met Dr. Don. Most of my complaints were being handled by then and he recommended some comfrey chlorophyl lotion for my poison oak. We discussed my health history, and agreed that he would let me have a trial of labor "in the hospital."

We started taking Nan and Don's series of natural birth classes and reading everything in sight. We even took the birth classes at Memorial Hospital. The more I learned about home births, the more I became interested. After researching the statistics about vaginal birth after cesarean, and discovering that the major concern was rupture of the uterus, of which there was only a 0.5% chance, I asked Don if he would do a home birth. Don was pretty definite in his answer of "no," and tried to convince me that it would not be a good idea. Nan, on the other hand, said that she would help me, but that I must be very sure of my decision. My pregnancy was going very smoothly. I was very happy and felt very close to Greg. I was watching my weight, eating well, drinking herb teas and feeling fantastic. Greg said that he would support any decision that I made. When I decided on a home birth, I became more relaxed, relieved and confident. Since Dr. Don would not condone a home birth, after my sixth month, I started seeing only Nan.

In my ninth month, the baby turned breech. Since that was the cause of my previous cesarean, we would have to turn the baby, or give up hopes for a home birth. I tried pelvic elevation exercises, with no success. One week before my due date, I tried to turn the baby by laying on my belly, and it worked!

I became very anxious when my December 15, due date came and passed. Feeling restless, and wanting to stay busy, I helped Greg paint our restaurant on December 30 and 31. On the afternoon of December 31, I witnessed a car accident in front of the restaurant, which gave me a sudden adrenalin rush. I started getting contractions 5 minutes apart and had a little bloody show. For 2 hours I kept busy, then returned home and took a hot shower to relax. The contractions slowed to 11 minutes apart, and on Nan's advice I ate a light meal and drank a glass of wine. They became more irregular and I was upset, thinking that this might be false labor. I tried to sleep, but was continually interrupted by contractions. Greg kept timing them, and though irregular, they were getting stronger. At 4:00 a.m. we called Nan, because I had lost my mucous plug. She was at another birth and promised to send someone soon. At 4:50 a.m., when Candace and Carolyn arrived, they determined that I was about 7 centimeters dilated. I was tired and confused, and Candace asked me if I was waiting for Nan, since I was progressing so slowly. Nan and Marilyn arrived at 7:00 a.m., and at 8:15 a.m., Nan broke my bag of waters to help stimulate my labor. During the next 6 hours, I walked outside, squatted with contractions, and pushed to open the cervix. The 4 midwives kept busy taking care of me: giving me protein drinks for energy, black cohosh tea to intensify contractions, herbal cervical massage to help move the anterior lip over the baby's head, hot towels to keep me warm, and with the help of Greg and my brother, Patrick, continual body massage. Around 1:30 p.m., Nan slipped the anterior lip over the baby's head, and discovered a posterior presentation, which meant an even longer and harder back labor. I was completely exhausted by then, and uncentered.

Around 2:00 p.m., I heard Greg and Nan talking about the hospital, and the need for pitocin to intensify contractions, but they knew the hospital would insist on another cesarean. At Nan's suggestion, Greg and I got stoned, and Greg helped me come back into my body. Nan and Greg told me that if I wanted to have this baby at home, I would have to get real serious soon and start pushing. I turned on all fours on the couch in front of the fireplace, and everyone massaged my back and legs as I pushed. The baby rotated to the anterior position and I went into the bathroom and pushed on the toilet, where I felt most comfortable.

Everyone took turns pushing my legs up as I pushed. I vomited on everyone and kept apologizing. The baby crowned on the toilet, and with the head in the birth canal, I walked back to the couch. I could feel the baby moving up and down the birth canal, but Nan and Candace wouldn't let me push it out too fast, so that I wouldn't tear. I moaned and screamed and the head finally pushed through at 6:19 p.m., January 1, 1982.

Greg was behind me holding me up, pushing with me, and giving me confidence to do it. Nan pulled the umbilical cord from around the baby's head, and with the next contraction, the body gushed out. They put the baby on my belly, and while Nan was suctioning the mouth and nose, I noticed the baby was still a little blue. It was an unbelievable feeling to have this tiny body at my breast, looking me right in the eye. We still didn't know if it was a boy or a girl, and we didn't care. It pinked up right away, so we knew it was healthy! Greg finally said, "I can't stand it anymore. Is it a boy or a girl?" Nan said, "Look for yourself," but he couldn't reach the little legs, because he was still holding me up. Someone lifted a leg for us to see, and Greg Said, "It's an Amanda!" She started sucking on my breast right away. The placenta was delivered within the next couple of minutes, and Greg cut the umbilical cord, and then rushed to open a bottle of champagne.

Giving birth to Amanda was the hardest thing I've ever done. Although we were met with unexpected minor complications, we managed to deal with them naturally and at home. The bonding we shared afterwarads brought our family closer together and made us appreciate and love each other so much more.

# *Greg's Story*

Since our attending physician's options were limited by accepted professional opinion, and since hospitals have strict labor ward regulations, we believed that a home delivery was our best shot at a natural childbirth. We were prepared for birth at home or at the hospital, as well as emergency transport if necessary.

It was birth class final time. Janine had labored 20 hours through the night with no sleep, and I'd had only 2 hours of sleep. There was a break in the rainstorm, and I walked to the stream near our house, hoping to break the tension that had built inside of me. The whole thing was going wrong, and I was so frustrated because I felt there was nothing I could do. I cried real deep; it felt good to let go. Returning home I rolled a joint, lit it and stuck it in Janine's mouth. After we shared the joint, I started rushing and tried to set up an emotional link with Janine. At this point, she had passed into transition and had departed to some place where I couldn't find her.

I found myself on the casual/karmic plane of consciousness, a place I had only seen glimpses of before. In that instant, the asking/praying/willing for everything to go right was all that existed to me. Then I sensed Janine's presence there with me, but we weren't alone. The raw spirit of our unborn child was with us. My consciousness then returned to my sobbing body with the knowledge that through hard work, everything would turn out fine.

I opened my eyes, my vision centered on Janine's back, as she knelt on all fours. I saw a shiver of energy shoot up her spine, and I knew she was back in her body. I whispered in her ear that if she wanted to have this baby, she would have to start working *now*, harder than she had ever worked in her life. Boy did she work! After four more hours of pushing, walking, squatting, and anything else that felt good, a head pushed past a stretched (not torn or cut), perineum. Janine and I were both on the couch, she leaning on me, both pushing. Just a few more pushes . . . Hi Amanda! . . . KNOWLEDGE AND *WILL* ARE POWER!

*November 1981, Janine in ninth month.*

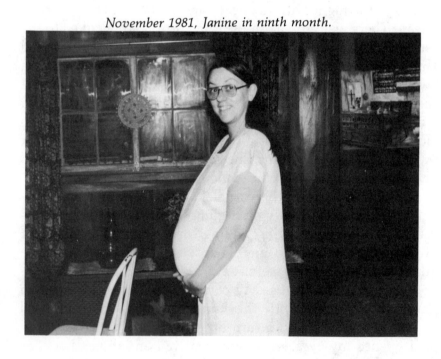

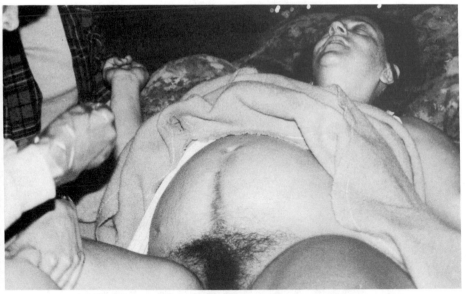

*Midwife examining me — good shot of cesarean scar.*

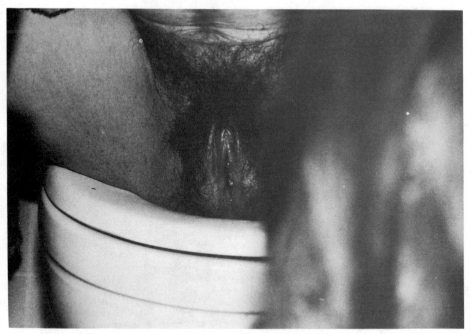

*First showing of the baby on toilet.*

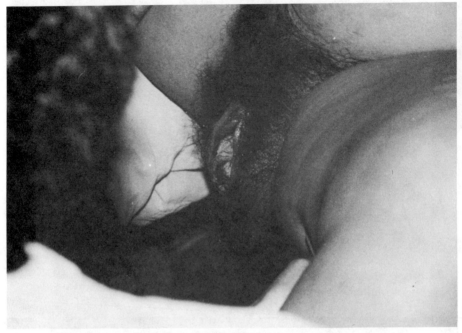

*Later crowning on the couch.*

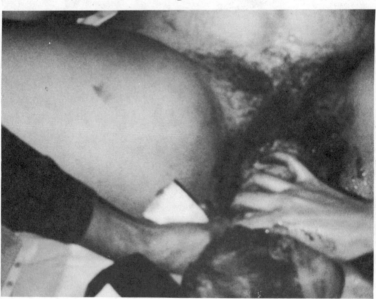

*Birth of Amanda's body.*

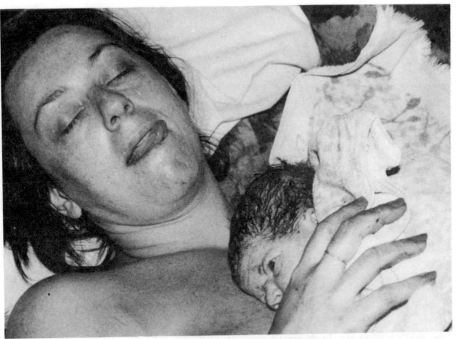

*My first moments with Amanda.*

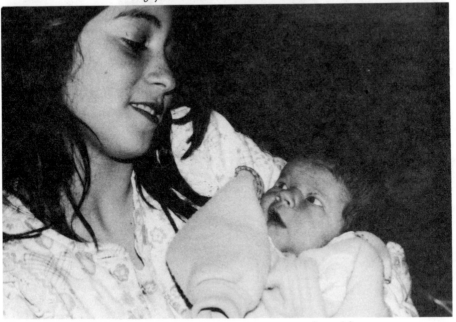

*Amanda with sister Monique — one day old.*

115

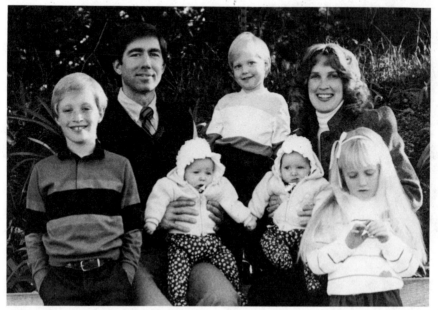

*Ganelle, Jerry, David, Jennifer, Matthew, Sarah, Suzanne Dippé.*

# Ganelle and Jerry Dippe

## Ganelle's Story

Always intrigued by childbirth, after becoming pregnant, it was not uncommon to find me spending hours reading and listening to women's childbirth experiences. During the eighth month of my first pregnancy, I heard of a doctor who attended home births. Quickly we arranged a consultation and decided this was the way for us — a home birth. Our son was born a few short weeks later, leaving us with a satisfied, glowing, fulfilled experience, an experience I would classify as being in harmony with nature, the way God planned for us to birth.

Due to complications, our second child was delivered by emergency cesarean. She was one month premature, and placenta previa was the unfortunate factor that destined this birth experience to be less than we had hoped. Grateful, happy, and relieved to have a healthy beautiful little girl, we were none the less concerned about the alienating hospital procedures. Our separation was traumatic. Today I can still feel the sadness that I felt as I lay in my bed wishing I could see, touch and love this little one with whom we had been through so much together. Many reasons were given during our nine day hospital stay for the many hours apart, and none will ever substantiate these policies. Plain and simple, she needed me and I needed her.

Before becoming pregnant the third time, I again v as driven with an insatiable desire for knowledge. This time my goal was focused on a vaginal birth after a cesarean. I read, as much as was available in books and childbirth publications. However, I found little positive information. After contacting many cesarean support groups, one name kept surfacing:

117

Nancy Cohen. Packing up our family of four, we were off to Massachusetts in May of 1981 for an intensive three day seminar given by Nancy, who was soon to be my mentor. She provided us with many medical journal reprints and studies from other countries, each alluding to the fact that VBAC was possible and in the case of the latter, *standard procedure.* Armed with these reprints, I began to travel from doctor to doctor searching for one who would share my beliefs. Most felt a VBAC was possible with a low transverse uterine incision; however, I had a low vertical uterine incision and this was out of the question. Repeat cesarean was the only answer.

Persistent, I returned again to the doctor and nurse/midwife who attended our home birth. Realizing I was accepting responsibility and was fully aware of the alleged risks, the doctor agreed to a trial of labor in the hospital. Practicing positive birthing techniques, having a loving, supportive midwife and basically taking good care of my body and soul were most important as I now began my third pregnancy.

The nine months passed quickly and finally the due date was at hand. Those last few weeks I confronted some fears I felt had been laid to rest months before. Concern for my well-being, what if this/what if that, ran through my mind in the quietness at night. Frequent talks with my midwife became more important and her experience, as well as her faith in the human body's recuperative and adaptive powers allayed my waning fears. As I looked at the faces of my children, I saw a faith and love that inspired me to trust the Lord, that all would work out for the best. Their faith was so direct and pure, I wanted to emulate this childhood quality. After all, I had done my homework, three and a half years in the making, and had more positive VBAC information than ever before. I conversed with the head of the obstetrics department at Case Western Reserve Medical School. He reported he felt very safe doing low vertical VBACs—more good news. However, as my body was beginning to set the stage for the birth process, I instinctively wanted the perfect physiological "nesting place."

On the morning of March 25, 1982 at 4:30 a.m., my waters began to leak. After an examination by my midwife, I knew I had a long way to go, as the contractions had not yet begun and my cervix was not dilated. The doctor requested we go to the hospital when the contractions began to get strong. Not until 5:00 p.m. did the labor begin, and slowly at that. At 10:00 p.m., I was 2 centimeters dilated and 100% effaced. I was wondering if we could do this birth at home, a goal my husband and I shared. Things began to pick up, contractions getting stronger and we were all wondering if we were or weren't going to the hospital. The midwife talked with the doctor. He reluctantly offered that if we wanted to stay home, he would back us up (a decision he made knowing our strong desires). As if that was what I had been waiting to hear, the birthing progressed from 2 centimeters dilation to delivery in one hour and forty minutes, and we had a new family member in my arms, my secret partner, Matthew Robert Dippé. Incidentally, I had no fears of uterine separation or rupture during this active phase of labor.

No major surgery, no IV, no separation, no tears and no long recovery period—was it worth all the effort to gather the information to do it our way? A thousand times, "Yes!"

I thank the Lord, my loving husband and family, and many friends for all of the support and encouragement. We are so happy to have completed our dream, a low vertical home VBAC. I especially thank my secret partner, Matthew Robert.

## Jerry's Story

Our first child was born at home with a midwife and physician in attendance. The atmosphere was very relaxed and comfortable, which I'm sure made a somewhat difficult birth (occiput posterior) safer and easier. Being in the privacy of our own home with our new baby, allowing for bonding and quiet time together, was GREAT!

119

Naturally, we planned that the birth of our second child would be at home. Unfortunately, a placenta previa necessitated a cesarean section at eight months. We soon found out how totally different and unpleasant a hospital birth was for us. Drugs and surgery, and separation from our child left us totally out of control.

We both wanted to have another child. However, another hospital birth was not desirable. At this point, Ganelle did a lot of research into the possibility of a vaginal delivery after a cesarean section. She read many books, attended birthing seminars and talked with physicians, as well as birthing instructors. Very little information seemed available on VBAC deliveries with a low vertical uterine incision such as Ganelle's.

Ganelle and I talked a lot about all of the pros and cons of a vaginal delivery in the hospital, home delivery and repeat cesarean section delivery. Deep down I always felt Ganelle would be able to have another vaginal delivery and wanted very much for her to be able to birth at home.

Being at home for labor was great. I think that as the day went on the fears of delivery and possible problems diminished. I prayed that the baby would come so fast that we wouldn't be able to get to the hospital in time, and would have to have the baby at home.

As Ganelle's contractions became more intense it seemed more important that the birth be at home. We were both very happy when Matthew was born, and the birth was very fast and easy. How much nicer this home birth was compared to the hospital birth—just close friends and the security of our own home.

It is interesting that since the birth of Matthew, we are seeing so much more information in magazines, television, etc., about VBAC's and cesarean prevention.

120

# Mary and Ken McCoy

## Nan's Story

The birth of Megen, a girl, occurred June 25, 1982 at 11:57 p.m. She weighed 7 pounds, 2 ounces.

My partner, the doctor, said "If Mary McCoy has a vaginal birth, it will be a victory for all your theories." She did it! And any lady out there reading this who is afraid that her pelvis is too small or is the wrong shape, please talk to Mary. My theory is that if the woman can stand the pain and has good labor, the baby will come out. There is no such thing as CPD — cephalopelvic dysproportion. There are difficult births, slow births, dysfunctional labors that can result in trouble, but CPD? I really doubt it. I've seen too many big babies come through small women. The key is having a good labor pattern, which Mary did, and good coping skills, which she developed. My notes on Megen's birth are so short they don't begin to capture all the aspects of this situation. I will try to tell you the whole truth, as I see it. I am laying myself bare for potential criticism, but my desire is for us all to learn, and the only way we can do that is through exploration and fearlessness.

The first time Mary and Ken came to see us they wanted a home birth very much. Mary's baby was breech on the home visit two weeks before the birth. It was too late to do anything about it! My doctor partner wanted them to abandon their home birth plans and go to the hospital. I stayed at home with Mary until she was ready to go into transition. I didn't go with them to the hospital because I had a baby at breast myself at that time. It seemed that everything was going smoothly, except I did know that my partner was concerned about her narrow pubic arch and narrow mid-pelvis. When she got to the hospital, he ruptured her membranes and the baby didn't descend, so he went ahead and sectioned her. Mary was totally

121

unprepared for this experience, and it seemed to reinforce the ambivalence she was experiencing about her new motherhood role. Mary was a school teacher, and was reluctant to give up that job for her new one.

With her second pregnancy, she did stop working and devoted all her energy to her children (inside and out). It was wonderful to see her family flower. I couldn't help talking to her about her desire for a natural home birth. She had several obstacles to overcome: the baby was breech again, and she had had the previous cesarean section. The baby turned to vertex after a week of counseling, meditation and posturing.

When labor arrived, Mary awoke in the night at about 12:30 a.m. with contractions every 4 minutes. She called me at about 1:15 a.m., went back to sleep and awoke again at 4:00 a.m. She was 4½ weeks early by dates, but the baby was obviously big enough to be born, so we all mutually agreed that her dates must be wrong. Luck was on her side that she went into labor early instead of late! By dawn, when my partner went to check her, she was about 3 centimeters dilated, but the contractions spaced out and didn't start up again until about 4:30 p.m. after Mary had taken a nap. By 6:00 p.m. when I arrived, Mary was 9 centimeters dilated, waters intact, the baby's head high and posterior. She half-heartedly began pushing, but was not really pushing in earnest until she passed through a kind of crisis point in her labor. I reminded her that it takes great pain to climb the mountain.

At about 10:00 p.m., Mary said "I just can't do it anymore. I give up. I tried. I'm too tired. I'm sorry Nan. I tried." Her husband was relieved and said "Yes, this is too much. It's time we got sensible," etc. My response was "She is making progress, however slow, and the baby is fine." Besides, in her attempt to go to the hospital, Mary just couldn't get to the door. On her hands and knees she called, "Okay, I'll do it, Nan." She figured out how to work her body to release the baby and she is still in bliss over her triumph!

# Mary's Story

We were fortunate to have a home birth after a cesarean. Seamus, our two-year old, was born at the hospital by cesarean after an attempted home birth. My difficulties began after the surgery: I was not allowed to have anyone in the recovery room with me. (My husband Ken had been with me during the surgery.) I was not given medication because of some mix-up. I was taken screaming to a double occupancy room and left there with strangers. I was still not given any medication. I assumed that everyone was down the hall celebrating with the new baby and I, now that my job was done, was forgotten! It took me several days to express my feelings about this to Ken. I do not remember the first time that I saw Seamus after the birth because of the medication they finally gave me. My recovery in the hospital was slow for all of the above reasons, and because I was located right next to the busy nursery. I was given drugs to sleep and then awakened to feed the baby. I was given pain killers to relieve the pain caused by shots of pain killers. Needless to say, I was glad to get home. I did not feel like myself again for at least two months.

As part of the preparation for this second birth, I had a deep relaxation session with a woman who taught me how to relax and how to communicate with my baby. She urged me to practice during my pregnancy so that I could use the relaxation techniques during my labor. I also saw a psychic healer during my pregnancy. She helped me to free up some energy from my past that might block the full energy I would need for the moment of birth. That experience was very helpful to me in my personal growth because I was able to free myself from some past experiences that had made me angry. I spent time meditating on the things in my past that were good, and I let go of the things that made me angry.

I also spent time communicating with the baby and focused on letting her be herself, separate from me. I tried to release

123

any preconceived ideas I had about her. I also tried not to intellectualize about the baby and her position. I just let my body take over and do what it needed to do to be a mother and to carry the baby in a vertex position. I tried to relax and let my female energy take care of preparing me for the birth. This meant that I had to let go of my more dominant male energy which wanted to take charge and be "in control." As a teacher, I had developed this kind of energy very well.

I quit work in April when I was about 6 months pregnant so that I could relax more, give more time to my son before the birth, and get my head ready to go through with the home birth. My midwife told me it would be a difficult time: I would have to work hard, but if I made up my mind to do it, I could. I read about VBAC births and talked to a woman who had had one. One other thing I did was to try to keep the size and weight of the baby down so that delivery would be easier. (I minimized my consumption of dairy products, which make a big baby.)

In the following weeks, I grappled with the decision: hospital or home? If the baby were breech, we would definitely go to the hospital, try for a vaginal birth and then have a cesarean if necessary. About the seventh month, the baby settled into a vertex position and remained that way until the birth. Ken and I then decided that we would attempt the vaginal birth at home as we had the last time and go to the hospital only if all did not go well.

Five weeks before Megen was due I went into labor, shortly after midnight. I was not prepared for the birth so early, yet in hindsight, I had felt for about three days that I was ready to deliver and would not be able to carry this baby for another month. From midnight until 4:00 a.m., my mother-in-law and I ran through the house washing baby clothes, preparing materials for the birth and timing contractions while Ken slept. (He had a cold and wanted to be rested to deal with the later, heavier stages of labor.) When all was readied, of course, the contractions slowed down! I went back to bed and slept until 6:00 a.m. The contractions were intermittent. When I talked to my midwife, she suggested that I go for a good long walk to get things going again. The doctor was a bit concerned that the baby was only 35 weeks and that we might have difficulty with the baby's breathing. It seemed that the labor was for real, so we went with it, feeling that all would work out fine. The doctor and midwife had guessed that the baby weighed about 6 pounds at this point.

Labor progressed quickly and by 6:00 p.m. I was dilated to 9 centimeters and the midwife came. In another few minutes, I was fully dilated and felt the urge to push. I thought "How easy this has all been! The baby will be here in another hour!" Not so! I pushed for the next 5½ hours and Megen was born 3 minutes before midnight. I thought that I was pushing well and hard for the first two to three hours, but I realized that I didn't *really* push until the last two. I guess I had to learn about that. My pelvic floor was very strong. (I needed to relax it more.) Because my pelvic arch is narrow, the baby was posterior, which caused a lot of back labor and took a long time. At about 9:30 p.m., I decided that I could no longer do it and I wanted to go to the hospital where the pain would stop and I would be done. I tried to get up to go to the car, but the baby had descended into my pelvis so far that I could not walk. My midwife reminded me of all I would go through in the hospital, that my recovery would be longer, and that I had put out so much energy already, all I needed to do was to hold out a while longer.

She also said, "If you want to get up, you have to get down." So when I could not get up off the floor, I decided I would stay at home, give it all I had and give birth to this baby. There was no turning back now. I gave it all I had, which was far more than I even imagined I could do, and with two more hours of labor, Megen was born. I had an episiotomy to speed delivery at the end. The moment I saw Megen and held her in my arms, I knew it was all worth it! I felt such a surge of accomplishment. We did it! We did it!

Throughout the difficult labor, my midwife monitored the baby's heartbeat and so we knew that she was not in distress. If at any time it had become apparent that she was in distress, we would have gone to the hospital. When she was born, she was lovely, relaxed, uttered a few introductory cries, lay on my stomach and then nursed very contentedly.

Our recovery was wonderful, especially compared to the first time. The episiotomy healed well; I was never troubled much by it. My spirits and energy were so good—I felt wonderful the next day. I never experienced those postpartem blues and my daughter and I bonded nicely those first few weeks.

Now that Megen is two months old, I can truly say we made the right decision. I'd do it again and would encourage any woman who is undecided to definitely give VBAC a try. The process of growth I went through preparing for the birth and making the decision to go for it have changed my life for the better.

*In October, 1982, Nancy Wainer Cohen came to Sacramento to give a workshop for couples wanting to attempt a VBAC and to help innaugurate the fledgling Cesarean Prevention Movement organization. People came from all over the West Coast to meet each other and gain support for their unorthodox birthing beliefs. I have included several stories from these couples because the exuberance and confidence of their experiences are an affirmation to the natural process.*

*Here are the words of <u>Ron and Linda Oates</u> announcing the birth of Levi Elijah, December 5, 1982. He weighed 8 lbs. 15 ozs.*

# Linda's Story
## (Her Fourth Baby After Three Cesareans)

We did it! Our Levi was born surrounded by his sisters and brother, and in our own bedroom. Our midwife swooped him up onto my chest as soon as he emerged, and Nathan cut the cord. It was a beautiful beginning! It was an 18-hour labor, and difficult for us at times, but the thought of you during those moments gave me strength and determination.

It was a few weeks after the seminar that we knew for sure that the baby should be born at home. We discontinued our trips to Palo Alto to the OB, and began plans for the home birth with our midwife. The information on VBAC at the seminar was what we had been looking for for the past 8 years and 3 pregnancies. We finally realized what options we had. We cannot begin to express the difference we felt about this birth and our previous cesareans. We were relaxed and confident as the due date approached, knowing there would be no surgery, no drugs, no intervention or separation, and that Ron would be totally involved. We feel such satisfaction.

We thank all of you for your tremendous encouragement and support. The seminar was a real turning point in our lives, and Levi's birth was an experience we will never forget.

We send our love to you all, and to you with upcoming births, our encouragement and our very best hopes for the kind of birth experience that you are looking for.

# Lorin Graham and Doug Spenser

## Nan's Story

This very sensitive and shy couple came to see me in the midst of my busy life in July, 1982 seeking support for a natural birth. I didn't really focus on them until November about a month after they moved to this area to be near me. By that time, Lorin had developed polyhydramnios (which I suspect she had her first pregnancy as well—although it's not mentioned in her records). When she plugged into the medical system for assessment of her condition she was led to believe that their was no hope for a normal baby. (The doctors advice was for her to have a repeat cesarean section and remove the baby no matter what it's status.) After careful deliberations Lorin and Doug decided to wait things out and let Nature take its course. You can imagine the dilemma for me—what to advise them? I could well understand why they wanted to avoid another surgical procedure, especially one with no gift at the end, yet the uncertainty of her condition was definitely beyond my capacity or experience. Their great courage in the face of such a terrible situation encouraged me to support them, no matter what they decided to do. (I had seen a videotape of Shari Daniels in El Paso, Texas helping a Mexican woman deliver a dead fetus only a few months before which gave me some idea of what to expect.) Despite great pressure from the medical establishment, they persisted and below are my notes and memory of their VBAC experience.

Lorin appeared after supper about 6:00 p.m. thinking she was in labor. She'd been having contractions all day and now they were beginning to hurt. I checked her. All vitals were O.K. She was about 3 centimeters dilated and her cervix was very effaced, soft, felt like jello. She took a hot tub with me and my two daughters and went home. After my children were asleep, I visited her again at about 9:00 p.m. and she was now definitely in labor. She went for the prearranged blood work up to see if it was safe to deliver at home (PTT and Platlet Count).

Candice, a midwife assistant, met them at the hospital and returned with them at midnight. Upon return, Lorin felt she'd "shut-down" and her labor didn't seem that strong. I went

128

back to bed (I was 2½ months pregnant) and Candice stayed with them lying down herself.

In an hour and a half, all three came over for another hot tub and Candice wanted me to check Lorin because she was worried about the presentation of the baby. Lorin was 6-7 centimeters with a swollen cervix. I felt the head but it was so high what with all that fluid. There was a good forebag forming. We all decided Lorin should get in the hot tub to dilate more and progress closer to birthing. I helped her change her breath technique and instructed her on how to handle the pain, then went to sleep a little more myself. It was a beautiful moonlight night.

At 3:30 a.m., Lorin was really in good labor again, handling it well. When she was obviously close to delivery, we all went back to the trailer where they lived temporarily. With Lorin on her left side, I, with great trepidation, ruptured her membranes, not knowing really what might happen. A great quantity, at least a quart, of rust colored smelly fluid exploded into the bowl we had under her. Happily, the baby's head came right down. To encourage the baby's head to flex and descend, I had Lorin walk and squat and labor on her hands and knees in a particular sequence that brings the baby down very fast. Within a half hour she felt like pushing. Five pushes the baby was born very easily! Its cord was short and very twisted. The placenta came out immediately afterwards with Lorin squatting over a bowl. No tears! The baby looked darling even with a bloated belly and loose skin. There were peeling patches of skin over the eyes and here and there over the body. An autopsy that morning revealed a normal, well formed 3½ lb. girl. We speculate that the chronic polyhydramnios combined with the short cord allowed the girl to sommersault freely which twisted the cord and compressed the blood vessels eventually killing the baby.

This simple story does not begin to describe the odyssey of this couple. As I stated earlier their courage and resilience are remarkable.

# Lorin's Story

On October 1, 1981, I had a stillborn baby by ceasarean. My baby died during early labor. The cesarean section was planned because the baby was breech, and carried out for no apparent reason (except maybe ignornance on my part). We didn't have an autopsy done, so we didn't know exactly why the baby died.

I wanted to have another baby right away. Doug and I decided to wait at last six months, to give our heads and my body a chance to heal. I conceived a little after six months.

At this time we were living in a tipi in Northern California. We wrote to people all over the U.S. trying to find someone who would help us do a vaginal birth. I had a vertical incision, so no one wanted to attend our birth. We were constantly faced with scare stories, and people trying to discourage us. One doctor told us that no responsible person would attempt a VBAC with a vertical scar!

The breakthrough was when we contacted Nancy Cohen. She gave us names of people in California, which eventually led to Nan. We wrote to Nan, and then drove down and met with her. Nan was willing to attend our birth! We moved to Occidental so we could be closer to Nan. This was during my sixth month of pregnancy. At this time my pregnancy was going well. I felt healthy and confident.

Sometime after we moved, the baby turned breech. A doctor turned the baby to head down. The baby didn't stay for very long. Soon after this, I started having complications. I gained ten pounds in one week. There ended up being fluid in my belly. We had a sonogram done, and it showed that the baby had fluid in her belly. The kidneys and bladder couldn't be seen.

Things got pretty stressful at this point. We were being advised to have a cesarean done, which felt to me like the wrong thing to do. It was really hard listening to my inner voice. Doug and I did a lot of praying. I drank diuretic teas, and did a lot of walking to try to lose all the fluid that was being retained. I immersed myself in trying to heal. Doug and I both felt that we should go with nature and let what was meant to

130

happen, happen.

I started losing fluid. By the time I was at full term, I felt I had lost most of the fluid I had gained. The baby lost fluid also. Around this time, the baby died. We figured out the baby was dead about two weeks after she died. Ever since she got sick, she hadn't been moving very much. Now there was no movement at all. I felt very alone. It was really hard for me to admit that she was dead.

I went into labor on December 27th. All day I was having cramps, which turned painful around 6:00 p.m. or so. Nan checked me, and then I got into her hot tub. It really relaxed me, and made the contractions harder. Around 10:00 p.m., Doug and I went to the hospital to get some blood tests on me done. I was pretty uptight, and my labor slowed down a lot, (I was afraid of having my labor progress and having the baby in the hospital.) Candace (our other midwife) met us at the hospital, and followed us home. My contractions were mild at this point. Everyone went to sleep, and I tried to fall asleep too, but the contractions were getting harder again and I was uncomfortable. I felt pretty complainy. I tossed and turned for around an hour, and then woke Candace up. I was not relaxing, and I was fighting the contractions. I knew that the energy had to change, and felt like the hot tub would help.

We all walked up to Nan's, and she checked me again. I was 6 or 7 centimeters dilated, which was encouraging. I got into the hot tub, and Nan showed me a different way to breathe. I felt a lot better, and my labor really picked up. Hot water does wonders for your body when in labor. I feel that the most important thing about labor is that you have to relax your whole body so that your uterus can do its work. The hot water enabled me to relax my body and not fight the contractions. As soon as I got into the hot tub, the energy changed and my labor progressed.

We went back to the trailer to have the baby. I guess I was in transition when I first got out of the hot tub. I felt like I was mindless — I couldn't even get my socks and shoes on. It felt

131

really good.

The baby's head still hadn't descended. Nan broke the water bag, and the head came right down. I squatted for some contractions, and then got on my hands and knees for some. I felt like pushing then. Candace was going to check me to make sure I was completely dilated, but I had pushed some and the head was already coming down. I pushed for about 15 minutes, and a baby girl came out. I didn't tear at all.

What a relief. I was so happy that everything was over. The birthing went really well. I felt so complete and satisfied. I was sad that the baby died, but happy that her karma was completed. It felt so good to have worked hard to birth her. We had so many obstacles during my pregnancy that seemed to go against a home birth. I felt that we were doing the right thing and stuck it out.

Doing the labor was hard, but not as hard as I imagined it would be. If you can surrender completely, and let your body do it's thing without mind interference, then things really flow and your baby will come out. Your mind can slow things down considerably, if you let it. I was amazed at my power of endurance. Once I accepted the pain, I had a great time.

The last three months of pregnancy were a very hard experience for me. By listening to my inner voice and having faith in my beliefs, everything turned out good. It was a big lesson for me.

# Doug's Story

In January of 1981, Lorin became pregnant and we were very happy about the whole thing. We had a normal early pregnancy. Our prenatal care was with a conservative doctor who had delivered me long ago. We mistakenly thought that he would support us in our decision to have a midwife deliver the baby at home.

During the 5th month of pregnancy, we moved to an apple farm where the farmer employed a large scale spray program using the toxic chemicals Sevin and 2,4,-D, which contains Dioxin. Our home was surrounded by sprayed orchard and Lorin took long walks among the trees for health.

In her 6th month, Lorin started retaining fluid and became borderline toxic. The baby was lying breech. Our midwife didn't feel comfortable delivering a breech, and our doctor recommended a cesarean. We knew no one who would turn the baby, and other doctors recommended a section, backed up by scare stories about the horrors of a vaginal breech. Lorin did the pelvic tilt to turn the baby, but to no avail. As the due date approached we became very worried. We didn't understand that we could refuse a cesarean.

On September 28th, Lorin lost her mucus plug. Our midwife came and thought she heard a faint heartbeat. The next night the labor got harder. Lorin was awake all night. In the morning there was a small meconium stain. We went to the doctor who scheduled a section and told us to go to the hospital immediately. When I asked him to attempt a vaginal breech, he refused to discuss it. We went home scared and angry.

We called our midwife. She agreed to meet us at the hospital. We drove to the hospital in the pouring rain. The sky was dark and grey. At the hospital, they wouldn't allow our midwife in the labor room. Our doctor scolded us for being late.

Lorin was prepped for a section. When they listened for a heartbeat there was none to be heard. We went downstairs to have a sonogram done. No heartbeat. We went back upstairs, then back downstairs for another sonogram. Still no heartbeat. Our doctor said that "We might be in trouble" and recommended a cesarean. We felt very scared, confused and out of control. We agreed to a cesarean.

Lorin went to surgery. I went for a very sad walk with our midwife. The doctor did a vertical incision on Lorin's uterus and delivered a perfectly formed, red haired little girl, weighing just over four pounds. She had a short cord.

133

I saw Lorin in her hospital room. She was very high on Demerol. The first thing she said was that while under anesthesia she heard them say "still-born." We were all crying a lot. A nurse brought the baby in. Lorin looked at her, but didn't hold her or bond with her.

After 2 days Lorin came home. We did some legal work and arranged to have the baby buried on our land. We buried her under two large maple trees, and named her Harvest Rain. After the funeral, I felt terrible. Lorin recovered well, and in 5 weeks we moved to California. We both felt very empty. We were both very angry at the hospital and our doctor. The day we left was very hard and full of tears.

The winter turned out to be very hard. I was sad and angry. Every day I would find something to get upset at. My moods were very hard on our marriage. After six months, we decided to make another baby. We had a very good wholistic M.D. doing our prenatal care, but he felt he couldn't risk delivering a baby vaginally when the mother had a vertical scar on her uterus. We wrote all over the country and for months found no one to help us do a VBAC. Finally, in the fifth month, we drove to Sonoma County to talk with Nan. She agreed to help us if Lorin would take excellent care of herself and be willing to work very hard. Six weeks later we moved to Sonoma County.

Sometime in her 7th month, Lorin gained ten pounds in one week. Her belly was full of fluid. We thought nothing major was wrong, but did a sonogram to be sure. The radiologist came to us and explained that the sonogram showed fluid around the baby's liver. He said that the baby's chance of being normal were very slim. I felt my throat drop to my stomach.

We took the sad news and drove to Nan's. The sky had turned dark and grey. It was pouring down rain. It was thirteen months after Harvest's birth/death. It gave an erie feeling.

Don suggested that we go to Mt. Zion in San Francisco for a more extensive sonogram. The sonogram showed that the

134

baby's abdominal cavity was full of fluid. It also showed immature lungs and no kidneys or stomach. The doctors concluded that we had a very malformed baby and that we should "terminate the pregnancy for maternal safety." She pointed out that the baby could continue to swell, putting Lorin in danger. She recommended a cesarean section since Lorin had a vertical incision on her uterus. She told us not to attempt a home birth. She mentioned that if the baby did survive a section, it would go immediately to the neo-natal intensive care where the excess fluid would be drained and possibly a total blood transfusion done.

We left the hospital and drove home. At this point, we were faced with a hard decision to make. We faced sectioning another dead baby or worse, possibly having the baby's only living hours filled with pain, tubes and bright lights, and again not being able to bond. The medical people were pressuring us to get a cesarean as soon as possible. Nan was getting a lot of pressure on her end. We wanted to go with nature. We felt that if the baby couldn't survive a vaginal birth, so be it. On the other hand, we felt like bad parents for not doing everything we could to try to save the baby. We finally decided to go with our insides and wait for Lorin to go into labor. Nan stood behind us, despite the risks involved for her.

Next we tried to stimulate labor. First with castor oil, then with evening primrose oil. Neither worked. In the meantime, Lorin started drinking diuretic herb teas. In a period of about 2½ weeks, the swelling in Lorin's belly reduced and she lost the ten pounds of fluid she gained. Then we waited for labor to begin.

On December 27th, I came home from work and found Lorin just finishing up cleaning the house. She was looking for other things to do. She stopped long enough to say that she was going to have the baby tonight. We ate dinner and around 7:00 p.m. the labor started getting stronger. Nan came and checked Lorin and said she was dilating. Around 9:00

135

p.m., we drove to Santa Rosa to have blood tests done for a rare condition where a dead baby in utero can cause the mother's blood not to coagulate properly. On the way, the labor pain started moving to Lorin's back. We both expressed fears of having the labor progress rapidly and the birth happening at the hospital, which neither of us wanted. At the hospital, the labor slowed down. Candice and our doctor met us at the hospital and we did the tests. They showed proper coagulation. Candice, Lorin and I went home.

When we got home around 11:00 p.m., Candice and I went to sleep. Around 2:00 a.m., Lorin woke us up saying the pains were uncomfortable, and she wanted to go sit in the hot tub. We walked up to Nan's and woke her up. She checked Lorin and found her more dilated, but the baby still had not descended. Nan showed Lorin how to breathe to stay relaxed during the contractions. We decided to have Lorin sit in the hot tub until she dilated more and then rupture the water bag. So, we went to the hot tub. We sat quietly in the clear, cool December night. The sky was full of stars. The almost full moon moved across the sky. The crisp air brushed our faces. The only sound was our own breathing, deer moving through the brush, and Lorin breathing with contractions.

Around 4:00 p.m., the moon started to go down. Lorin was in transition. She got out of the hot tub, and we started to walk to the house. Lorin was so high that she couldn't get her shoes on without help.

After we got settled at the house, Nan broke the water bag. She then had Lorin do five contractions walking and standing. This helped the baby to engage. Next Lorin did five contractions on her hands and knees. During the height of the contractions, Nan pressed on Lorin's sacrum to spread the bones.

Lorin then returned to laying on her side, with her leg being supported by Nan. As the baby started to crown, Candice rubbed warm oil on Lorin's perinium. Six or seven contractions later, out came a baby girl, perfectly formed except for a short, twisted cord. Lorin lay panting as a holy energy filled the room. I was near tears looking at this new little being. We sat playing with her little fingers and toes, oohing and ahing. Lorin held her for a long time. I went outside just in time for a beautiful red winter sunrise low in the eastern sky.

After breakfast, we wrapped baby up and took her to Santa Rosa for an autopsy. The autopsy showed a perfectly developed girl with all her organs mature and intact. I felt great relief for the whole day. The next day, I felt emotionally terrible, signaling the start of the mourning period. We buried baby in a grave behind our house after a short ceremony. Now when I stand by her grave I feel deep sadness and grateful feelings that everything went as it did.

### Postscript to Lorin and Doug's Story

Instead of waiting 5 years to conceive again, as I advised them, Lorin became pregnant only 3 months after her second baby's death. Needless to say we all dithered about that for some time, but they decided to try again. (Living on the farm with me, I could keep close tabs on Lorin this time.) Shortly after her second month I found a monograph on polyhydramnios which said that the largest percent of cases had no obvious cause and under the heading of possible factors (right on top of the list) was malnutrition. So that was the tactic I took with Lorin this time to sheperd her toward a normal baby. She had carrot juice several times a week, greens every day, protein supplement and farm eggs and milk. I only wish I had started earlier pressuring her in that direction.

I wish I could say it all ended happily. As with all of life, our destiny usually isn't that clear cut. After much study and very careful preparation Lorin arrived at her due date— January 2. All was quiet! When a whole month went by with the baby constantly rearranging itself, (breech, then transverse, then head down with Lorin becoming an expert at self-palpation and changing her baby's position), we decided

137

it was time for castor oil. They wanted to give birth as privately as possible and I, myself, had a new baby to care for so they opted to do it alone, with only my senior apprentice in attendance. I thought there might be trouble with the cord again, what with all that movement, so I lent them my doptone to monitor the baby carefully. Her labor progressed normally throughout the night of February 3-4, when at dawn almost completely dilated her waters broke. Instead of the head descending into her vagina out swooshed the cord and a little hand and arm! Nothing to do but have another C-section! Can you believe! Approximately 9:30 a.m., Jediah was born, 10½ lbs., with a lot of long blond hair. There is more to this story and if you are interested you can contact Lorin Graham, 13140 Frati Lane, Sebastopol, CA 95472.

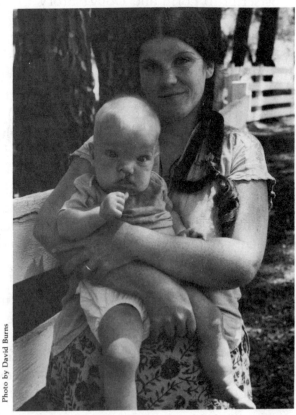

Photo by David Burns

*Lorin Graham and Jediah*

138

# Linda and Dennis Johnson
## (Another Couple from the Sacramento VBAC Conference)

A new hand
in ours . . .

*Name:* Alex James
*Arrived:* March 4, 1983
*Weight:* 9 lbs. 6 oz.
*Parents:* Dennis & Linda
*Sisters:* Allison & Amanda

The Handiwork of God

Dear Friends,

Alex was born at home after about nine hours of labor. It was really pretty quick and easy! (Hard to believe.) The last couple of hours were tough, but he was born so fast at the end, Dennis and I were in shock. I was supported during my labor by my midwife (her mother had three VBACs) and three wonderful friends (Mary K, Jenni and Ann). The hospitals here do not acknowledge the need for labor support. I see that support as being the major reason for my successful labor.

I changed doctors one and a half weeks before my due date. (My midwife was living about four hours away in the Bay

139

Area and I felt the need to have all the bases covered.) My new doctor was cooperative and confident, and worked with me to plan for a positive hospital experience. His support was important to us yet we knew he wouldn't "freak out" when the baby happened to slip out at home.

As the time for the birth drew near, I felt such great inner peace it's hard to describe. All would go well and it did. There was never a lack of progress or support or love around me as I labored to birth Alex. The constant presence of positive "vibes" made all this happen. To those of you planning your VBACs, I say — surround yourself with people who love you and believe in you, and "go for it!"

—I love you all! *Linda*

P.S. Treat yourself to an herbal bath afterwards! (I'd be happy to send you the recipe.)

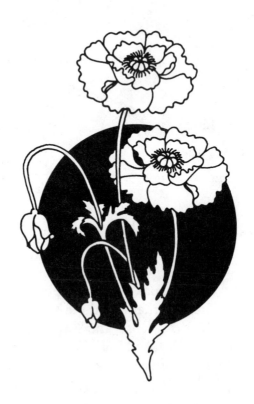

*Sometimes things don't go exactly right. I want to include a story here of a VBAC which could have resulted in a disaster for the mother had there not been medical support. At a birth, there is always a close brush with death. It's a fact that one has to come to terms with if the desired end is a natural birth. Happily, Mother Nature doesn't make many mistakes so that the brush with death is usually only a remote possiblity.*

# Ama Wickham

## Ama's Story

I am laying in bed at my friends house in the hills outside of Garberville where I finally ended up deciding it was the best and only place to give birth—not in a motel, not in a hospital, no place but home. Kim's house is like home to me. I have lived in these hills the last three years—so here he was born. I have written the whole birth story down, but have to type it up and xerox it and I will send it to you.

This is just a brief account to let you know I had him naturally with a lot of labor and pain—extreme relief when that head finally came out and no sensation at all of it being in the birth canal. I was so numb at that point, it wasn't until they put a mirror down and showed me the point of his molded head that I realized he was really there. I held my hand on his head to push him out, at the insistance of my midwife (the same one who was at my first c-section), which helped. Warren was with me and I am so glad he was there, as well as two midwives, Kim and her boyfriend.

After he came out crying and healthy, so much blood gushed out that Lorraine realized I must be retaining the placenta. I was rushed to the hospital in an ambulance with no blood pressure and two IVs of saline solution in each arm and oxygen, which they gave me over a three day period, in addition to three units of blood.

141

I am recuperating at Kim's house now and being cooked and cared for by her and another friend, Sherri, as Warren had to get home and take care of his life too. I'm going home in two weeks to my new home in the Siskiyou's.

This boy has brought extreme peace, love and joy to my life and also allowed me to let go of the pain and confusion of my first cesarean birth. I remembered many things you said during labor and thank you for your guidance and encouragement.

—April 23, 1983

# Lily's Story

I wanted to write and tell you of Ama's (Patty Wickhan) birthing. I don't know if Lorraine called you, so I will write. Thank you for helping her try to find an alternative in your area. We are glad she came home and decided to stay here, and Lorraine and I agreed to help her give birth.

After two days and nights of "rehearsal," Ama finally went into active labor at about 12:30 p.m., April 23 (one month past dates). A friend checked her and she was 4 cenimeters dilated. Lorraine got out there (3 miles down the road past Heartwood) at 6:00 p.m. and she was 8 centimeters, head -1. I got there at 7:00 p.m., the water bag was bulging out of her, so we broke it at 8:00 p.m. Head settled a little, posterior still. She was up and down all night (blizzard, snow and rain night!), labor would stop and go. Enema, massage, squatting, resting, talking, etc.

Anterior lip finally really left at about 4:00 a.m. (4-24) and she started pushing. Meconium in the water and slightly unstable heart tones and a tired Ama made Lorraine and I concerned, but Ama was determined to stay home. We had her stand and squat (supported) for all pushing and the head finally started coming down. (She has a narrow mid-pelvis.) Up until second stage, her labor had not been real strong, easy to deal with rushes and not a lot of pain. Second stage was

142

hard for her, but she worked well with it.

Baby boy was born at 6:00 a.m., (gest. age – 43 weeks). The cord was wrapped loosely around neck and body. He started up fine. A boy was what she had dreamed of and the father was the one she hoped too (a black man, not at the birth).

Immediately after he was born, Ama started pouring blood all over the floor (she had been trickling a little during labor – cervix?). Lying her down and herbs kept it to a minimum, but she kept bleeding and no placenta. Lorraine reached up and found it firmly attached inside. All the usual tricks (even Pit) and prayers didn't make it come loose and Ama lost a lot of blood.

The ambulance met us on the road at 8:00 a.m. (IV set up, etc.) and we took her to Bill at Garb Hospital. He removed the very large, very calcified placenta in the emergency room without medication (I held her down and sang to her); and she received two units of blood, tons of Pit and Meth, and a few stitches.

Ama is fine now, recovering well and thankful to be here. She is so high about having had a home VBAC and says she would do it all again. She says she wished she had eaten lighter during her pregnancy and had a smaller baby (she gained 38 pounds and the baby was 9½ pounds but she has a beautiful, huge baby, very calm and bonded.

# Elizabeth (Liz) and Mike Griffin

## Liz's Story

We had a great birth with Cory, our third child. We had had two sections with our first two children: with each we'd tried for natural deliveries, the first at home.

When I became pregnant with Cory, I went back to my same doctor who'd sectioned me with my second (Kaiser Permanate). He absolutely said I required a third section after two sections, even though he'd suggested attempting a VBAC with my second. Two cesareans made all the difference. I was panicked. He, at least, agreed to letting me go into labor first and, if I came in complete, he'd go ahead and deliver vaginally. But he insisted I not wait at home but come in immediately. I think he was reading my mind.

For a month or two I brewed over what to do. Mike, my husband, did not want me to be dishonest with the doctor. I knew of only two private doctors who would let me attempt a VBAC after two c-sections. So Mike got busy on the phone and finally, after much hassle, our policy was switched from Kaiser to private insurance coverage. This was a great relief to me to be able to choose any doctor.

My cousin, a mother of five (the latest two additions having been born at home), recommended Nan. I was very hesitant to do anything. She dialed the number for me and told me to just talk with her. We soon went for a visit and talked more.

Nan was very knowledgeable and had a wealth of information to share. She had a very positive attitude. It was just the encouragement I needed to get going. Gradually I started to follow Nan's "positive birth plan." I took many vitamins (something I've never been able to do consistently). I was swimming twice a week at the "Y" in a pre-natal class. I tried

144

to walk as much as possible and forced myself to squat while working in the garden. My husband and I even visited a psychic. We also attended classes at Rainbow's End. One great book was the *Silent Knife*. Reading about other VBACs really encouraged Mike and me.

In the last few weeks before he was due, I began taking primrose oil capsules which help to soften the cervix. I also took pituitary extract tablets and drank teas all suggested by Nan. I was feeling really good and getting very big. The baby remained real high right up until labor was under way. The primrose must have done something because two weeks prior to my due day, I was beginning to efface. It had taken three days of labor to get that far with my first child. This was a real plus for us.

We had decided on a team of four midwives and attempting the birth at home. Don was to be our back-up, should we need to go to the hospital. We made the decision to stay home at the end of our pregnancy. Earlier we'd intended on going to the hospital in the later stages of labor. I was very happy to be staying home so our children (3½ and 22 months) could be a part of the birth and not be separated at this important time. We didn't bother to tell friends or relatives of our plans, of course. We needed only positive input.

The closer to my due date we got the more Braxton-Hicks I experienced. On my due date, they were regular for long periods of time. Both my other two labors had begun in a similar manner. I knew it could be soon. Mike and the midwives assured me it was only false labor and to ignore it. That night when contractions started up again, I did just that. We ate dinner and put the kids to bed. Mike went to bed also; he was due at work at 3 a.m. At about 9:00, I decided to call Caroline (one of the midwives) to check her work schedule for the next couple days. She suggested I have someone come when Mike was to leave. We live 30 minutes from town. My sister was the only person who didn't have kids to bring along. So I asked her. We had already planned for her to be in charge of our kids.

She arrived at 2:30 as Mike was on his way. My contractions had been increasing gradually in strength. They were three minutes apart as they had been all evening. I relaxed comfortably on the couch with them unable to actually sleep. I took some magnesium oratate tablets which helped me relax further. I was very tired, having been up early that day and having walked a lot also. The increasing discomfort of the contractions I blamed on fatigue, thinking I was still in early labor. Sis rubbed my back for me and that felt wonderful.

About 4 a.m., I rushed to the toilet feeling lots of pressure. As I sat down, my bag of waters burst all over the room. It was a great relief but then I spotted the greenish tint of the fluid. Both my other children had had mecomium in the ambiotic fluid too. I was worried it might mean going to the hospital, but when we called Caroline she wasn't worried as long as we could hear the heart tones. She decided to come, though I warned her it was probably still early.

Fifteen minutes after we hung up, I felt that incredible urge to push that I'd always wondered about. The contractions were no longer painful but the urge to push was very strong. Now I knew why women yell and grunt. The sounds just come forth!

My sister received a crash course on panting. "Don't let me push!" I'd yell after each contraction, and she didn't.

We quickly called Marilyn, another midwife closer to our house than Caroline. We had to put the phone down to deal with a contraction; when we picked it up again, she was already gone. She heard familiar sounds, I guess. We were very anxious for them to arrive. I wanted to know if I could push or was this some crazy labor where I was having such urges in early labor. My kids were awake now and giggling from their spectator seats on the couch.

Yeh! The midwives arrived. I was almost complete! Several more contractions and Caroline slipped the anterior lip over Cory's head. Marilyn had called Mike at work — telling him if he wanted to see his baby born, he'd better hurry. Everyone

146

was busy and smiling. I couldn't believe I was already in second stage, and neither could Mike when he arrived. I was on my hands and knees most of the time, while Mike rubbed me all over. Everyone was cheering me on. "He's past your tail bone," Zoe said. Next he was at my peranium. Madrone supplied hot olive oil compresses and I could feel his little head and see it in the mirror. Soon it was out, followed quickly by shoulders and body. All nine and a half pounds born with my peranium intact. Thanks to Mike for his faithful massage nightly.

Cory was born at 7:19 a.m. We couldn't believe it as we held our beautiful new son. Everything had seemed to go so quickly and easily. Our prayers had truly been answered today. Soon the landlord and his wife were at the door. He'd been feeding the calves and heard me, summoning his wife who assured him the baby was coming soon (mother of five). The midwives were wonderful. They were right there for us and knew their business well. What a difference it was!

Thanks to everyone, especially Nan, for setting us in the right direction and uniting us with the midwives who could take her place while she was home with her new baby, Sarah.

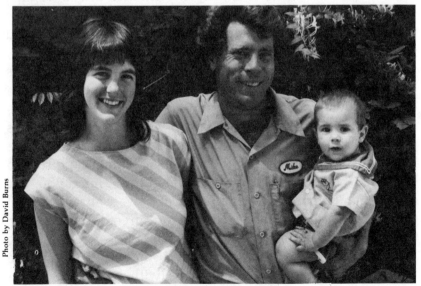

*Photo by David Burns*

*Liz and Mike Griffin and Cory*

147

# Mike's Story

When our son, Cory Michael, was born, it would have to rate as the most amazing moment of my life. The actual birth can be told in a few sentences, it was so quick and easy. My wife had been having Braxton-Hicks for quite some time (2 weeks, a month?) so when her due date came we weren't expecting anything. Patrick, our first child, now 3½, was something of a strike against us, because we had thought Liz's false labor had been the real thing, so we stopped eating and drinking, and started breathing Saturday morning at 2:00 a.m., so by Sunday at 6:00 p.m. we were fairly discouraged. Liz's waters did break at 5:00 a.m Monday, and the doctor was discouraged that we (Elizabeth) had not slept, so he recommended that we go to the hospital for a relaxant (6:00 a.m. Monday, decision was made) and some sleep, so we went. Liz got her shot, went to sleep, and when she woke up had a fever (Liz 102, baby 104). When the doctor found out, he prepared her for surgery and delivered Patrick by c-section at approximately 8:30 p.m. Monday.

When Liz became pregnant the second time, I told her it was time to do things the way my mother did (5 vaginal births), so we went to Kaiser. There only one of three doctors would agree to a VBAC, under the condition that we would go to San Francisco (Kaiser-Central) for this delivery. Silly us, we never even faced the fact that we'd have to drive 70 miles to meet a stranger and have our baby in a different hospital, one we'd never even seen!

When Liz went into labor (Friday at 4:00 a.m., even less prep this time) we went to Kaiser offices, the doctor said, "Yes, you're in labor," and then "Well, it's time to go to San Francisco." Liz had her clothes for Santa Rosa, mind you, but not for San Francisco. She started crying; we realized what all this meant, and fortunately, the doctor "offered" to send us to Community Hospital.

At noon, we were at Community, being told that since the fetal monitors read "baby in distress" (with every contraction

148

the baby's pulse would slow), we needed to operate immediately. So Jessica was born at 2:37 p.m., with the cord between her head and the birth canal, by a staff straight out of M.A.S.H.

It's funny, though, because every midwife we met in association with our third child's birth asked if the doctor or anyone there had Liz get up and walk around for a few minutes, even walk just around the table (this might jiggle the baby, causing the cord to free up). They also spoke against the value of checking a baby's pulse when the mother was flat on her back.

When Liz became pregnant the third time, it was back to Kaiser, and by two months into the pregnancy my wife was really down, as we now had two c-sections against us and were looking at a third (they'll do a VBAC after two cesareans in San Jose, but they're not that liberal here in Santa Rosa. Liz decided she wanted another kind of health/delivery plan, and made me go through the rig-a-ma-role of changing health plans at work so she could go to a doctor she wanted to see, one who would work with us.

Liz's cousin had recommended Nan Koehler and Dr. Solomon as the people to see, I guess to the point of dialing the phone and handing it to her one day as they sat in Chris's kitchen talking (we still hadn't left Kaiser at that point. After visiting Rainbow's End, meeting Nan and Don (who gave her the most thorough examination she'd ever had), and reading Nan's manuscript (this book) and handouts, Liz decided these were the people she wanted to deal with.

We began to prepare for the birth in the manner they recommended (daily walks, birth classes, watching our food, vitamin E, water intake, relaxation exercises, and some psychological self-examination for factors that might have contributed to the first two cesareans), keeping especially close contact with Nan and the midwives. As the day approached, we began to feel better and better about the birth — what a confidence knowledge brings! In fact, we became so

149

confident that I joined Liz, Nan, Marilyn and Madrone in the belief that we could have this baby at home, at our own place, rather than under the lights in some hospital.

August 3rd was our due date, and Liz felt she was starting labor. However, Carolyn (who had agreed to help us, as Nan could not be in attendance) had warned us that it could be a long labor, as Liz didn't seem to progress rapidly. Therefore, I went to work as usual, and at lunch Liz said her labor had stopped (more Braxton-Hicks?).

Marilyn and Madrone, Nan's apprentices, were visiting that day for a pre-birth visit and an exercise I will explain later, and they left about 4:00 p.m., convinced, as I was, it was false labor. After dinner, Liz went out to the garden, and her contractions strengthened, so we were wondering. I went to bed at 8:00 p.m., as I go to work at 3:00 a.m., and Liz paced and slept on the couch, because she said she was more comfortable there. Twice during the night she got me up to rub her back, but she said she was sleeping some too, so I went to work at 2:30 a.m., when her sister came out so Liz wouldn't be left alone.

At 4:00 a.m. her labor got to be uncomfortable, which we had been told to consider the beginnings of labor. Immediately after this, she felt the urge to go to the bathroom, her waters broke there, and she began transition. Liz called Carolyn who left immediately, as did Zoe (a fourth midwife who had joined us to round out our team, for maximum experience), along with Marilyn and Madrone.

When Carolyn got there around 5:15, she was almost completely dilated and at 6:00 I got a call at work — "You'd better get home if you want to see this." When I got home at 6:50 a.m., Liz was on the toilet, disheveled but very happy. I squatted against the bathroom wall, and she sat in my lap, so I could hold her and work her pelvis apart with my hands. After a few minutes we moved to our bedroom, where the midwives parted Liz's labia so I could see the top of Cory's head. What a rush!

Moving along side Liz, I rubbed her any way I could, playing with her nipples, doing anything I could to please her. Carolyn and Zoe asked if Liz wanted to see the head. We looked up and it was already out! A gentle, twisting motion, timed with the contractions, and Cory was born at 7:19 a.m., only three and one half hours after labor started.

Victory was ours, a perfect baby!

In retrospect, I would have to say, and I'm sure Liz would agree, that if we conceive again we shall take the same path to bring the baby into the world. It has been, again, the high point of my life, married or single, to have this happen this way, so quickly and easily. And it has raised our mental, spiritual and physical relationship to a higher level. We feel more complete in each other.

If you look at our birth story, the actual birth is not that much, much more being said about the preparation and the circumstances that led up to it. This is the way I feel: that there is a direct relationship between the amount of preparation and the experience itself. It is actually an inverse relationship—the more you want it, seek it out, try to understand what is happening, the easier the actual act becomes. If I had to put it in one word, it would be to make your wife comfortable, to do what suits her.

I had always felt we were capable of the experience we had. It's like we were robbed, and robbed ourselves the first two times. You can see what happened without sufficient preparation (Patrick—only a Lamaze course, Jessica—no prep) versus when I tried to do what my wife wanted. Not that it was easy. We had enough bad times and hard moments, even with me trying to please her, but she was patient with me because she knew I was trying. Also, we had a goal that became more tangible as we worked together.

She still hid some things, for instance, when, on her due date, she went for a long walk with Marilyn and Madrone, and yelled her heart out in a ceremony with them, because Nan felt that she should use the relationship between the mouth and cervix (see why she hid it from me?) to free up some of my wife's inhibitions about expressing herself, about letting things go enough to dilate easily, and with a minimum of effort.

It was only after Cory was born, and she had dilated so quickly and easily, and I had seen this for myself, that I could whole-heartedly accept some of the more esoteric facts and believe so fully, in this alternative way of giving birth, together.

Do whatever suits you best, home or hospital, but don't let anyone decide anything for you. The midwives always presented everything as a choice, recognizing our own power to set up our own birth, and as Dr. Solomon said when we told him we weren't going to the hospital (he didn't approve), "Well, you'll probably have a better experience for it."

I can't say enough about doing your own research—it was only by going to birth class every week, and reading, talking to people, asking questions and following those questions up that we learned about the research paper from Mississippi. It described women who became pregnant again after being sectioned the first time and were put in three categories—repeat c-section, started the VBAC path and quit, and VBAC's, and how the VBAC group, as a whole, experienced the least amount of difficulties. About the hospital in Ireland that has done VBAC's since World War II, 2,700 approximately and how only 8 women had to go into surgery (including minor surgery). Their rules—no anesthesia in labor and no artificially stimulting the labor. About the women who had five c-sections, was going to the hospital for the sixth, and had the baby in the car (VBAC's are possible! This happened to a friend of a friend).

And the unsung heroine's are the midwives. At all times we felt our experience was their experience, not an 8:00 to 5:00 shift they were putting in.

Marilyn, Madrone, Carolyn, Zoe and Nan—Thank you again.

# VBAC *In the Hospital*

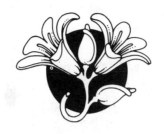

# Birth Story

by Wendy Sherman

*Every birth is an experience of a lifetime. But if you have ever experienced a traumatic birthing, then a calm, joyous, natural birth takes on the sheen of victory. It was with an overwhelming sense of victory, joy, and love that I watched my baby girl come into the world with the same majesty and magic that has accompanied birth since the dawn of humanity. As natural as birth is, it had taken a lot of effort for me and my daughter to share the beauty and bliss of a natural birthing. And because it was made possible for us, in part, by the knowledge that others had done VBACs before us, I want to pass on to others the lessons and experiences that led us to our triumphant VBAC birth.*

*Naia's birth story really begins with that of her brother, Arien Jesse, who was born 3-1/4 years before Naia's grand entrance into the world. . . .*

## Part I: Arien's Birth Story

For many years before Arien's conception, I had wanted to have a child. I had prepared for motherhood, years in advance, through regular fasting, a nourishing vegetarian diet,

153

daily yoga, and through studies in Cross Cultural Child Development. A credentialed teacher, I loved working with children, and looked forward to having my first baby with eager, romantic anticipation.

My husband and I were teaching school in Jamaica when we decided it was time to begin our family. I was a bit concerned about the lack of childbirth information and classes, and was not entirely confident in the local midwife who would assist us with the home birth we both wanted, but, nonetheless, I was ecstatic to be pregnant, full with my long-awaited child.

Throughout our pregnancy I continued a nourishing diet, adding fish since we lived by the ocean. With daily yoga, walks of 1-2 miles, and swims in the warm Carribean, I felt I was in the best possible shape for giving birth. Still, occasionally, doubts would break through my veil of "positive thinking" so, towards the end of my pregnancy, I went to an OB/GYN in Montego Bay just to make sure my regular visits to the midwife clinics hadn't overlooked anything. I was surprised when the doctor told me that the baby was quite large and might give me problems in birthing. But I didn't want to alter our plans for a home birth and go all the way to Montego Bay to birth just because of the baby's size. I knew my pelvis was adequate. And, in a way, I was reassured that the baby was big since I had been having dreams where the baby was quite tiny and would slip out before any help could arrive.

Those dreams should have given me a clue to my subconscious fears: *I was feeling unprepared!*

Labor began at 3:00 a.m. on February 7th, 1978. I was thrilled! I knew from the books I'd read that I should go back to sleep, but I was too excited to do that. I did manage to wait until dawn, however, to send for the midwife. She arrived at 9, crisp and brisk, saying "we'll have that baby out by noon!" It sounded so easy! Contractions continued to be fairly mild, even when they got closer together, and I beamed "This is

154

easy!" more than once. But by sunset the midwife began to get discouraged. Accustomed to the rapid birthings of Jamaican women, and anxious to go home, she urged me to push. I didn't feel like pushing, but made a pretense of it to make the midwife happy. She gave me thyme tea and asked me if I'd eaten enough okra (traditional Jamaican food for pregnant women) during my pregnancy. My husband and I got the uneasy feeling that all was not well. By midnight we agreed to go to the hospital, an hour away down a rough bumpy road.

By the time we got to the hospital, I was feeling fairly panicked. I was led into a group labor room and neither my husband nor my sister were allowed to be with me. Pitocin was administered, and contractions came too hard and fast for me to manage with breathing. The nurses joked about the white woman who couldn't give birth. I became even more panicked. My waters were broken, and were dark with meconium. A doctor examined me, said that the baby was entering the birth canal with my cervical lip between his head and my pubic bone. An emergency cesarean was ordered. At that point, I was glad to be relieved of this nightmarish experience. I was frightened, both for my own life and for that of my baby, and I prayed as they wheeled me into the operating room and everything began to go black.

The next thing I remember is being wheeled out of the operating room and being told "You have a big, fat, baby boy!". They tell me that I smiled, and I know I was relieved and happy that he was well, that it all hadn't been in vain. I wanted to see him, to hold him, but was too much under the anesthesia to be able to talk. I was cold, and couldn't even ask for a blanket. Every baby cry I heard I feared was that of my son, and I longed to have him with me. It was several hours before I came out of the anesthesia enough to be able to stop a passing nurse and beg her for my baby. It seemed to take forever for her to bring him to me! But, once he arrived, he didn't leave my side throughout our 7-day stay in the hospital.

I learned to nurse Arien "football" style, propped on pillows

155

by my side. He was groggy for more than a day, and didn't ever learn to nurse well (to this day he is a "dabbler" when it comes to eating), but it is just as well that he didn't nurse those first few days, as I was receiving antibiotics intravenously and he would have received large doses of them through my milk. After a few days I insisted that the IV be taken out because it was extremely painful and hampered my ability, which was minimal enough, to hold my little son.

Actually, he wasn't so little! He as 9½ pounds, and 22" long at birth! And, despite his initial grogginess, he was strong, healthy, gorgeous, and alert — I couldn't have been a prouder Mama! It took me a long time, however, to get out my birth announcements. It finally dawned on me that, despite my rationalizations to the contrary, I felt like a failure at birthing, and felt remorse that my son had had to endure a traumatic birthing. (To this day Arien often approaches life with a "this is hard" attitude, and I've wondered if it reflects his difficult birth experience.) Indeed, the scars from Arien's birth went much deeper than the one down my belly. I vowed that, if and when I did have another child, I wouldn't put either of us through such a harrowing experience.

And so when I became pregnant with my second child, I wanted to do my best to give to us both the calm, conscious, joyous birth that I had so hoped to share with Arien Jesse. I knew that it would be a challenge. But then, everything about my second child's appearance in my life held challenges — and also hope.

## Part II: Naia's Birth Story

As was her older brother, Naia was conceived on a tropical island (this time on Maui, Hawaii). But here the similarities between the two pregnancies end.

I knew right away that I wanted to try a natural birth again this time. But in my search to find an OB/GYN to support me

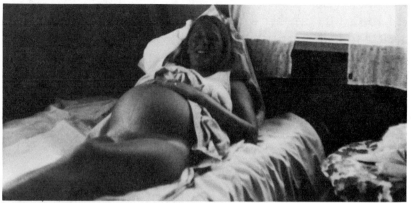

*Wendy and Arien*

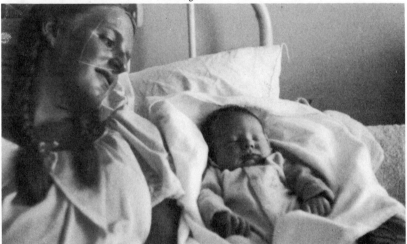

in this, I came across strong opposition. "Once a cesarean, always a cesarean" was the rule of every OB doctor on the island. Over and over again I was told that it would simply be too dangerous to try a VBAC birth, that there was a high risk of rupturing along the old cesarean scar and that, if that were to occur, I could die within 20 minutes and the baby would likely die too. I was told, by several doctors, "It's much better to have a planned cesarean than to try a natural birth and end up with an emergency cesarean — and that's if you don't rupture and die before the cesarean can be done." One doctor told me that he was planning on doing a cesarean on a woman whose first child had been cesarean but her second vaginal, because

157

he hadn't attended her second birth. Most of the doctors told me it would be dangerous for me to labor at all, and that I should simply pick a day near my due date at which time they would gladly plan on doing a cesarean for me.

It all sounded so cold and mechanical. What about the dangers of cesarean birth? None of the doctors felt that there were true dangers involved. What about the pain I knew it to entail? And what about the baby? Couldn't the baby at least choose the day, if not the time, it was to be born? I felt it should be able to do so.

In the waiting room of the top OB doctor on the island, I met a young woman, near term, who was planning her second scheduled cesarean in a few days. She said it had never occurred to her to try to have a natural birth; that her first-born had been born naturally, without problems, but her second had been breech, so cesarean. She simply accepted that, although this baby wasn't breech, she should follow the rule "once a cesarean, always a cesarean." I couldn't agree with her. Somewhere inside myself, I knew that a natural birth was possible, and that it wasn't as dangerous as the doctors made it sound. I felt that the doctors were operating out of fear and convenience and, although I had some fears of my own, my Inner Knowing was beginning to make its presence felt.

The Islands provided well for us. I ate lightly, mostly off the land, on fresh fruit and vegetables, fresh eggs, and lots of sweet potato root and leaves (traditional Hawaiian food for pregnant women). I made a daily tea of the lemon grass and gotu cola that grew wild around my island home. I wanted very much to remain on Maui for the birth of this island-spirit child. I even considered trying a home birth again, and the most skilled midwife on the island agreed to help me. My family physician also agreed to help me if I absolutely insisted on staying. He told me that VBAC births had long been accepted in Europe, and he encouraged me to try, though he said he felt I should be in more experienced hands. My friends feared for my well-being, and I had to constantly face feelings of doubt. I knew that, for the birth to be safe and uncomplicated, I had to feel absolutely clear and calm about it, which meant facing subconscious as well as conscious fears.

I realized that it was more important that I give to my child, as well as to myself, the greatest chance of having a successful birth than it was to remain in Hawaii. So I packed up my belongings, gave up my beloved island home, and returned to California just 3 weeks before the baby was due to arrive.

I had lived in Sonoma County, California, before going to Jamaica. During that time I had met Nan Koehler, teaching herbology and natural birthing at wholistic healing retreats. I knew that she and her husband, Don Solomon, (an OB/GYN), had helped several women to have successful VBAC births. I had visited family and friends in California over Christmas, and had gone to see Nan and Don at that time. They had given me hope as well as practical suggestions for having a VBAC birth. They had said they would be willing to help me with my birth if I would return to California in time to prepare for it. In attempting to remain on Maui for the birth I hadn't given myself as much time as would have been ideal, but I dove in full-force those last 3 weeks of the pregnancy!

It turned out that Don and Nan would be on vacation during my due time, but I was able to take several of the classes they offered, and benefited greatly from their counsel before they left. In Nan's class, I learned techniques for relaxation, came to know what to expect at each stage of labor and how I might want to deal with it, saw films of relaxed birthings, and began to gain confidence as well as information. Nan introduced me to other women who had had VBAC births, and I was encouraged by their victories. As I learned more about VBAC births, learned more about birth in general, my fears began to lift. The more I spoke with other women who had faced their own fears and DONE IT, the more I came to believe that I could do it too. The statistics were in my favor. My cesarean scar tissue wasn't in as much danger of tearing as the doctors on Maui had implied.

159

Many of the women who had had VBAC births with Nan's help had done so at home because doctors wouldn't let them do it in the hospital, or because they had enough faith to do it at home. I was gaining in faith with each passing day, but I wasn't sure if my cervix "worked," and I didn't want to do another last-minute rush to the hospital. I wanted to have a calm, well-planned, prepared, hospital—but NATURAL—birth. It was feeling, more and more, as if that would become a reality!

One of Nan's suggestions to me, to encourage my cervix to "work," was tea of prostaglandin-stimulating herbs such as sarsaparilla, licorice, fenugreek, and gotu cola. I was excited and encouraged, since I had been drinking fresh gotu cola tea throughout my pregnancy. Nan also suggested, as a substitute for her presence at the birth, a highly competent and confident midwife named Carolyn.

Carolyn had never done VBAC birth before, but she had home-birthed two of her own breech babies, and wasn't afraid of the challenge. I attended classes with her in addition to those with Nan, practicing breathing techniques and giving to my support-system of friends a chance to learn how to be of assistance.

The doctor who Don recommended was a wonderful choice, too. The first time I went into his office, I asked his receptionist-wife about the possibility of trying a VBAC birth and she replied "Of course it's possible: my first child was born by cesarean, and I had three more naturally afterwards!"—Hooray! I was finally in the RIGHT doctor's office. I finally had the support that I needed to truly believe that I could have the safe, natural birth I so wanted for my baby!

To prepare myself for a calm, prepared birth in the hospital, I went on a tour of the hospital and attended one of their "natural birthing" classes. I told the class, as we went through our introductions, that I had had a cesarean but was planning on a natural birth this time. The other pregnant mothers/couples cheered, but the instructor said "But Ms. Sherman, that's not usually done. We do have classes on cesarean birth, however, which you might want to attend." I didn't attend them, and I didn't attend another of the hospital's natural birth classes either. I knew I didn't need doubt. I knew that, more than anything else, I had to believe that I could have a natural birth. I knew that I had to believe in the power of the mind as well as the body, and in the power of prayer. These beliefs had been challenged all through this pregnancy. Yet I had faced my fears, had done what I could do to minimize them through preparation, had confidence in both my doctor and my midwife and, most important, had come to have confidence in myself! Glory Be!

The last few days of our pregnancy were precious to me. I enjoyed my ballooning belly and the relationship that had grown so rich between me and the little one within me. I had learned a lot from this little being. I felt her strength and innate wisdom. It seemed that she nurtured me as I nurtured her, and focusing on her had never failed to calm and center me during the trying times of our pregnancy. We had been through a lot together, but I knew that we had been learning together all along.

The day before her birth, I finally felt ready to let go of the special relationship we had been sharing, and begin the new one that birth would bring. I wanted to surround myself with roses, and stopped to pick some. (I found out later that the fragrance of roses is supposed to be specific for birthing, aiding in relaxation.) That night, I wrote out directions for my friends and the hospital staff: everything from the recipe for an electrolyte-balanced laborade (see *Mothering* magazine, Winter 1980) to "what to do if a cesarean does become necessary." I wanted as little hospital interference as possible: no drugs, no monitors, no shaving, no episiotomy. If a cesarean were to be necessary, I wanted to be awake for it and, in any event, I wanted the baby left with me at all times and not taken away for washing, weighing, etc. I went over the list with my friends, put plastic sheets on the bed, and went to sleep.

As with Arien's birth, labor began at 3:00 a.m. But this time I simply smiled, said a silent greeting to the little one-to-come, said a prayer, and went back to sleep. I awoke at 6 when the bag of waters began to leak, fixed a pot of relaxing tea, and wrote in my journal until 8, when I awoke my friends and phoned the midwife. My friends made up the laborade and took care of Arien when contractions got harder and closer together. I walked as much as I could, effleuraging (lightly massaging) my belly. My sister arrived, bringing with her soft music, white candles, and incense. She massaged my hips and thighs when contractions placed pressure on them, and it never failed to soothe. I don't remember it as being painful, but I do remember saying, a couple of times, "wow!", and acknowledging the power and intensity of the experience.

During contractions I breathed as deeply as I could, counting the number of breaths and retaining them as long as I could. I had learned Lamaze breathing, but because of my yoga training, deep breathing (more the Bradley method) came more naturally to me. As I inhaled, I often envisioned a flower opening, a visualization that I feel aided in dilating my cerix and certainly aided in relaxation.

When Carolyn arrived, I was surprised to discover that I was only about 4 cm dilated. She felt it would take all day and, as she had a college exam to take, and I was feeling very calm and comfortable, I told her to go ahead and take it. We agreed to meet at the hospital later. Shortly after she left, however, the doctor phoned to tell me to get to the hospital right away. I told him I didn't want any hospital interference and he replied "O.K. but just get here! Now!"

We arrived at the hospital at noon: white candles, music, and all. The nurses were a bit unnerved by it, but proceeded to go about their usual routine, short of what I'd specified not to do. And at that point, I didn't care. I was in another realm, totally involved, relaxed, and unconcerned about what went on around me. Still breathing as deeply as I could during contractions, hearing soft music between contractions, and taking drops of Bach's "rescue remedy" occasionally, I experienced the intensity of giving birth, but didn't notice it as painful.

I often communicated mentally, and sometimes verbally, with the baby, and every now and then prayed for strength and guidance, especially from Mother Mary. The hospital was a Catholic one, and in the corner of the labor room was a statue of a monk or Jesuit priest. At one point I glanced up at the statue and it was transformed into the image of Mother Mary, reaching out her arms towards me, bright light all around. I felt comforted, safe, and secure, sure of protection and guidance.

When my body said "push!" I was thrilled: here was the feeling that I never got to experience with the birth of my son. It is a powerful experience! I only had to "blow-breathe" through a few contractions while the doctor pushed back my cervical lip, then it was "all forces go!" and I knew why they call birthing "labor"! It's hard work pushing out a baby! I was lucky, I guess, because I had a few minutes rest between pushing contractions. I asked the doctor if it was normal and he replied "No, but it's normal for you" and he explained Bach Flower Remedies to the nurses. A sense of calmness prevailed.

With each contraction I could see more and more of my baby's head, and I didn't even notice that I'd been pushing for more than an hour before a shock of wet black hair appeared. It was a miraculous appearance in my eyes, and I marveled at it in the mirror, not at all prepared for the next, more glorious miracle, when my baby's head appeared between my legs. Her face slightly bluish, with a dainty nose, fat cherub cheeks, and eyes wide open, she looked like a fat little angel coming forth from my very own body! I still can see it in my mind's eye and still feel the sense of profound awe, reverance, and love that flooded through me at that time. One more push, and her tiny body slid out. I reached down to receive my newborn daughter, whispering "Welcome, little one!" as I wiped mucous from her tiny nose and mouth. She looked at me with the clear eyes of an ancient sage, that seemed to say "We did it!". She snuggled against my breast, nursed a little bit, then fell serenely asleep. It was 2:30 p.m., less than 12 hours from the first faint stirrings of labor. I hadn't even noticed that I'd torn considerably, and even as the tear healed, it seemed insignificant compared to having to heal from a long abdominal incision!

I felt a tremendous sense of accomplishment, felt quite proud of myself and of the team that Naia and I—and all who had helped us—had been. Working together we had won, had won a triumphant victory.

Postscript: March 19, 1985 I finally had a home birth experience. My third child. Brendan Sean-Michael, was born at home. Nan and Dr. Steevers assisted. Again my sister Maloah was there. She played her zither until my contractions became strong, then put on her zither tape so that she could massage my hips and legs as she'd done during my labor with Naia. This time contractions were more painful than I had remembered them being from Naia's birth, but I envisioned myself standing waist-deep in a tropical stream and did deep breathing as I had done before. Labor went even more quickly this time, beginning at 9 p.m. with leaking waters and faint contractions. Contractions didn't get intense until 1:30 a.m. and Brendan was born at 5:30 a.m. He was so calm when he was born that I was afraid that something was wrong with him! But he was just serene, having made his grand entrance into this world amid the sound of zither music and the love of his family. My mother was there, holding the mirror so that I could, once again, thrill to the sight of my child coming forth into the world. My mother still talks about this, her first birth experience (other than birthing her own 6 children, only one of which she remembers watching being born—me!). My mother feels especially close to Brendan because of this early bonding. For me, it was as if I had come full-circle: from the nightmarish 5:30 a.m. c-section birth of my son Arien to the blissful 5:30 a.m. home birth of Brendan. Thank you, Nan, Dr. Steevers, and Arien, Naia, and Brendan.

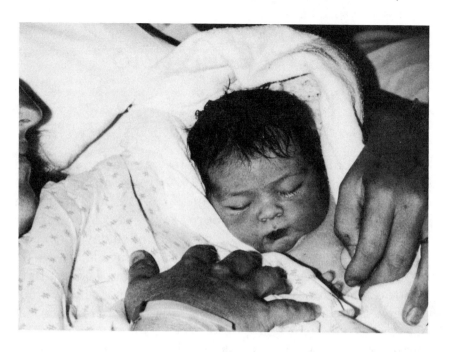

*Wendy and Naia*

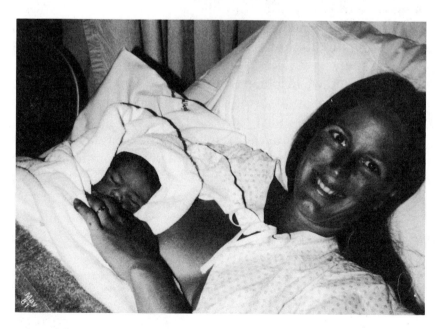

# Lori Delgado

## Lori's Story

My first daughter Angela was born via cesarean section in Novato, California on April 25, 1979. I was notified of the surgery at 5:00 p.m. She was born at 6:13 p.m. I had seen Angela minutes after she was born. I was awake to hear her first cry. However, our eyes didn't meet until a day and a half later. She didn't start breastfeeding until 9 days later.

When I was pregnant again three years later, I wasn't having too much fun expecting a repeat performance. My midwives, Nancy Bardacke and Tekoa King of San Francisco, let me know that I was going to be taken care of at this second birth. Still, I was feeling sick inside. I wasn't believing in myself at all. Now, I wish that I had, because 9 months is a long time to worry about nothing.

My second daughter Samantha was born in the hospital vaginally, after 14 hours of labor on July 29, 1982. After 24 pushes, she was curled up on top of me. Our eyes met at the same time and we held hands. She started sucking right away. She gazed at me and I gazed at her for two hours or so. I was so excited that I couldn't sleep all night.

We went home from the hospital on the next day, 18 hours after her birth. The second birth was a breeze compared to the first. Something like a mosquito bite compared to a bear munching on your abdomen.

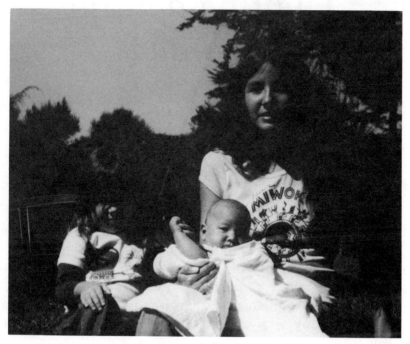

*Lori and daughters*

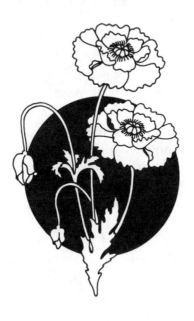

# Cynthia and Jay Redman

## Cynthia's Story

My first son, Alex, was delivered by cesarean, a breech baby. My mother had delivered three babies by cesarean and I grew up thinking that you had to have your belly cut open in order to have a baby. I had also had a miscarriage three months prior to Alex's conception, leaving me fearful and positive that my body could not carry a baby full term. There had to be something terribly wrong with me. These combined factors made my pregnancy a terrified time in many ways. I was extremely frightened and unsure, and I feel this element of fear led to my cesarean more than the actual position of the baby.

From the beginning, after the initial disappointment and feelings of failure, I was fortunate to have the support of several women who had had cesareans. I didn't harbor bad feelings about myself and the birth too terribly long, although I vowed that "next time I was going to do it the *right* way."

I conceived Emmett the very month we decided to become pregnant again and that made me feel strong and capable. From the beginning, I knew that I had to gather together all the lessons that I had learned from Alex's birth and hold firmly to them. I knew it would take extreme conscious effort on my part not to go over the edge to fear again. I was much calmer this time. Often I felt that this was because the last birth had been (in its way) so bad, nothing that could happen would be any worse. Also, the miracle of having a whole, beautiful son already gave me a lot of strength.

We repeated Bradley childbirth classes, and I took it all very seriously this time. I knew what I had to do. I listened intensely, did my homework, practiced. I knew that, for me, it

168

_Cynthia Redman and Cory_

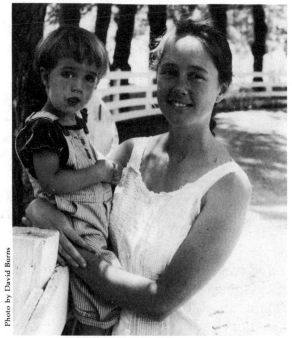

Photo by David Burns

would not be easy to have a natural birth, but would be something that I would have to work hard at achieving. It was a very serious thing for me: fighting the fear. Whenever I would start to get frightened, I would consciously try to feel the life and strength of the baby within and this would help. I also tried to be in an accepting state of mind, and not be attached to any preconceived ideas of perfect birth. I tried to see birth as the natural at-home act that it is meant to be. I learned to anticipate with excitement, instead of fear. This obviously worked for me. Emmett's birth was perfect, and perfectly natural, taken right from the birth script I had written in childbirth class.

I had irregular contractions Monday night, four days before my due date. Contractions were not very heavy, and ended at dawn (as with my last labor). I started losing my mucus plug Tuesday. Tuesday night, more contractions, I wanted to go to the hospital. Jay said "Cindy, you're not ready," but we called Leslie Helmick (a friend and Bradley instructor who had agreed to attend the birth) and went to her

169

house Wednesday morning. She checked me — no dilation. Oh well! Wednesday night, more contractions, heavier this time. We took a long walk, a hot bath, a glass of wine — anything to either bring it all on or make it stop. The contractions continued as before, ever present, but going nowhere. On Thursday, my due date, I saw Dr. Steever at my regular weekly appointment. He said that I must have had my dates wrong. The baby was still way up high and not very big. "This could go on for weeks," he said, "See you next week." I was getting pretty depressed and discouraged and tired, and not getting much sleep at night. By Friday night, I had had it. The contractions were the heaviest of all. I was determined to get the baby to come down.

I went out and walked and walked around in circles in the dark and fog, stopping to squat with contractions. I wanted to go to the hospital. I was in tears, sobbing. Jay said "No. The contractions are not close or constant enough. If you go to the hospital, they will give you a c-section." I was ready to kill him. I cried some more and then I finally learned how to sleep between contractions. Boy, they felt so heavy, but in a way I was learning to live with them. I felt like the pain had always been part of my life.

On Saturday at dawn, the contractions stopped again. I had really had enough! I talked to Leslie on the phone. She conferred with Joan Lashbrook and told me that they thought that I was trying to have another cesarean. Hmmm. I think that made me mad. I tried to take a nap but the pains wouldn't stop. Jay called Leslie. She told him to wash his hands, cut his fingernails and check me. He checked me and felt what seemed to be the bag of waters bulging. The second he touched it, everything accelerataed. I threw up. Off we went to the hospital.

I was calm and lucid. We prayed and meditated. I thought "I can handle this. I am unafraid." Leslie met us at the elevator. We were whisked into the alternative birth room, a quiet, comfortable, cheerful, sunny room. I was seven centimeters dilated, and by the time the doctor got there, it was almost time to push. (No time for internal fetal monitor, standard procedure for previous cesareans!) Pushing felt fabulous, my dreams come true. I didn't seem to experience transition. At one point, the heart tones dropped slightly, so Dr. Steever ruptured my membranes, gave me an episiotomy, and out fell Emmett. He was put directly to my belly and the cord was cut after it stopped pulsating. The baby's feet were gently massaged to get him going. He was blue but picked up right away. He cried a little, nursed right away, and fell asleep in my arms.

Jay and I and the baby were left alone. We were so elated and high. It had all been so easy and calm and loose. I have an ease with Emmett that I didn't have with my first baby. Again, the element of fear was not present this time around.

*Here is another testimonial from the Sacramento VBAC conference I told you about earlier where a potential trauma becomes a victory for the woman because the experience affirmed her own ability to birth a baby—even prematurely.*

# Dianne Martell-Williams

## Dianne's Story

I'm writing to all the good friends I met at Nancy and Claudia's VBAC seminar because I know you'll understand and listen and help me heal from my miscarriage.

My story actually begins before the VBAC seminar in mid-September when I was 8 weeks pregnant. It was Clint's 2nd birthday. We were having a fun birthday celebration and, in the midst of all this merriment, I began spotting. Panic! This didn't happen the last time! It can't be normal! An anxious call to my doctor was greeted with the secretary's assurances that "This was very common, nothing to worry about at this point." (How easy for her to say, — It's not her baby!) Friday evening, my husband out of town, the spotting turned bright red and I felt some cramping. My doctor's partner explained the symptoms to watch for, but felt all was still O.K. I knew better. My baby was dying and no one would listen. I remember just sitting on the couch and crying that night. When I woke up the next morning, I no longer felt pregnant. The first symptom that always tells me I'm pregnant other than missing a period is, strangely enough, post nasal drip! It was gone that morning. But because the amount of spotting was so minimal I convinced myself everything was O.K. I mean, if a woman miscarries, she knows it, right? All that blood and tissue and placenta? So everything must be O.K.

About a week after returning home from the VBAC seminar, I knew I couldn't fool myself any longer. I did a home pregnancy test which was very definitely negative. I saw my doctor the following afternoon. Another test done in the office was — alas, negative, and an exam revealed a 6 week size uterus in a 12 week pregnant woman. We discussed my options — a D&C or a wait and see attitude. Perhaps my period will start. I really cried on the way home. Reality had really hit again and there was no denying it this time. After a week of waiting, working hard and participating to the max in my aerobics class, I got very depressed because nothing happened. I talked to my doctor and discussed the D&C. He would let me be awake. It's only a twenty minute procedure, and I could go home two hours later. So I scheduled an office visit for the 11th of November, and the D&C for the morning of the 12th.

That first week of November was just hell. My thoughts went from rationalizing the necessity of the D&C in making everything "O.K.," to hating my body because it wouldn't cooperate. The worse time was at night when the distractions of caring for a two year old were gone and I was alone with my thoughts. During one of my nightly second visits to the kitchen for a cup of tea, I ran across a few pages in Nan Koehler's manuscript on herbal abortion. She talked about using herbs to abort an unwanted pregnancy by not allowing the fetus to implant and by telling your body this isn't an appropriate time to be pregnant. "Could this help a woman miscarry?" I wondered.

So Sunday morning I finally got a call through to Nan. She said my condition was known as a "missed abortion." The baby stops growing, but for some reason the body still thinks it should be pregnant. Maybe, part of the placenta is still living or perhaps the pituitary gland hasn't gotten the message somehow to produce the right hormones to allow the body to abort. She assured me I couldn't hurt myself with an herbal abortion. She recommended taking some evening primrose oil capsules to soften the cervix and then sipping the herbal teas throughout the day. I obtained the herbs from the co-op and began with the capsules that afternoon at 3:00 p.m. I mixed pennyroyal, tansy, black cohosh, scullcap, and squawvine and brewed a quart of tea. (I'm an avid tea drinker so the tea part was easy!)

I woke that night at midnight to use the bathroom and was shocked to see I was spotting. "I'll be damned, I don't believe this!!" I went downstairs and had another cup of tea and remember feeling almost overwhelmed with a sense of power. I fell asleep feeling some mild cramping. Monday morning the spotting was brown again. Tears and depression again. Why won't you let go?? I went to my exercise class. We had a new instructor who did 25 minutes of the hour class with non-stop, jump up and down, hard aerobics! I lasted the whole hour and was ready to drop when it was over. But no more spotting. That night was the worst. Another 2:00 a.m. cup of tea (regular tea — no herbs since that morning) accompanied with lots of tears. I wrote a letter to my sister-in-law who had miscarried a few months ago. I thought, "Why me?" Why, Dianne, are you unable to terminate any pregnancy by any means other than a surgeons knife? First the cesarean and now a D & C. I felt so inadequate. So alone.

Tuesday morning I decided I needed to really clean my house. I started in the kitchen. "Oh, I've got to clean this oven. – Its awful." As I began doing it I thought, "What's the matter with you? You're actually cleaning the oven, – That only happens in dire emergencies!" Could this be a "nesting instinct?" An hour later I started spotting again – bright red. I went to my husband's business and decided to rearrange the furniture in the office and really clean it up. Now I had some definite cramps and flow like a period. (Good Diane, don't sit down!)

That evening I cleaned the bathroom, made some supper for Tim and finally got Clint to take a nap at 5:00 p.m. The cramps were feeling more like contractions. I called Tim at work and asked him to please get home! We ate a quiet supper together. I ate very lightly. Now I was definitely uncomfortable and in pain, but loving it. I kept moving from the couch, to the toilet. Then Clint woke up and wanted to nurse. I *very* reluctantly agreed, but after 5 minutes asked if he'd had enough. He very nicely cooperated!

By 7:30 p.m, the contractions were coming one after another with little or no rest in between. I went upstairs and Tim finally succeeded at distracting Clint with some books and a TV program. I lay in bed, sweating profusely, trying to breathe slowly, and relaxed. I did O.K. I did O.K. for about 45 minutes without a coach. Oh the pain, the bleeding and nausea and diarrhea! Finally, I couldn't take any more and called to Tim to give me a pain killer left over from my c-section two years ago. He found them. I asked what the expiration was on them – 11/82. "Good, give me one!" I hobbled back to bed. He and Clint went back downstairs. I was so cold. In a few minutes, I could feel the drug. I no longer felt such intense contractions.

"Oh this darn cold and runny nose, what timing." Then I sneezed twice and felt the placenta pass. "Oh my God, Tim!" I was on the toilet when he got upstairs. "Honey I did it. I'm sure

174

its the whole placenta. The contractions have stopped." "Please find a glass jar, wash it an bring it to me." "You're kidding!"

"No, I must do this." I know the doctor will want to see it. Maybe we'll be able to find out why this baby died.

Of all things he brings me a pickle jar! It really helped break the tension. I just laughed and laughed. I picked the placenta up and placed it in the jar. I had seen it and I had touched it and now I could say good-bye. I felt so much relief, and I relaxed. My body was my friend again, my very best friend.

I called my doctor that night, and he agreed that I had probably passed the complete placenta. He wanted to see me first thing in the morning. He took one look at the placenta and said, "You did it. It's complete." I felt so powerful. I had had two months to grieve for my baby, and now I had let go.

I said, "You know, I must know what's inside that placenta."

He said, "You will. We'll have a pathologist examine it. We should know in about a week."

After discussing the routine precautions and talking about my feelings and emotions, (he initiated it, believe it or not), I mentioned using the herbs. To my utter disbelief, he said, "Well herbs are not hocus pocus. They are like crude drugs and they probably did help you start contractions." Now that it is all over I feel mostly relieved, a little depressed, and *definitely* tired, but mostly relieved.

I know this has been a sad story for all of you to read, but please know that the ending is a happy one. I have learned and grown so much and really wanted to share it with all of you. A million thank yous to Nan for her knowledge and support, and to Nancy for her wonderful letter of support and encouragement. It really helped to write this letter. Thanks to all of you for listening.

*Here is a sequel to the story of Dianne and Tim which came recently in the mail. February, 1984.*

It's been quite a while since I've written but I know you'd enjoy sharing our good news! Yes, we can finally proclaim,

175

"We did it!" What's even more exciting is we did in the peaceful, joyful surroundings of our home! But let me start the story at the beginning.

We became pregnant in May and began searching for a health care provider and hospital. Tim was very skeptical of the home birth idea because we live 30-40 minutes from the closest hospital and midwives cannot attend VBAC's at home in Arizona. I did find a certified nurse midwife who had attended about 12 successful VBAC's in a Phoenix hospital. Naturally, hospital policy posed all sorts of requirements and restrictions — no birthing room, IV, monitors, examination of the scar, MD on premises during labor and delivery. She was the only midwife attending VBAC's (legally) so I decided this was my best alternative. During the course of my prenatal care, I discussed, at length, my unwillingness to accept any intervention. We agreed I would sign a release form in order to facilitate this once at the hospital. It was obvious during the last month or so of pregnancy that Marilyn (the CNM) was growing tired of my constant questions and debate.

Luckily, in October, when we began Bradley classes, I was given the name of a lay midwife who was interested in being a labor advocate for us. We met 3-4 times before the birth and decided it would probably be a good idea to be prepared for the baby to arrive en-route to the hospital as I would be laboring at home and then driving one hour plus to the hospital in Phoenix. We borrowed a friends camper and put it on our truck. I prepared all the sheets, towels and blankets and ordered some basic supplies to have on hand. My lay-midwife said she'd bring her suitcase of equipment including oxygen. I felt somewhat relieved that there was a possibility I wouldn't have to fight it out at the hospital.

One Sunday, my midwife and her family came over for dinner and to meet Tim. I shared a letter Nancy (Cohen) had written to me with my widwife and it really stirred some discussion and thought. There were two points Nancy made that impressed us: 1) it's unfair to move a laboring woman and 2) we were setting ourselves up as victims again. That night she and I decided we could do it at home. Tim was still concerned but agreed to take things one step at a time. The following morning at 4:30 a.m. labor began! (At my last prenatal visit I was 2-3 cm, 80% effaced and 0 to plus 1 station, so I knew it could be anytime.) My midwife (mine brought another along to help) arrived at 11:00 a.m. and found I was 5-6 cm. I was really excited to be progressing so quickly. I sat in front of the fire, took a warm bath, laid on the couch—just enjoyed the freedom of doing what felt good for me. I was 10 cm by about 2:30 p.m. and began pushing. It really hurt to push and I hated every minute. I could never get comfortable—we tried the toilet, all fours, semi-sitting. We finally ended up semi-sitting. Clint, our three year old, was next to me holding a mirror so I could see the baby's head. After an hour of stretching, grunting, moaning and swearing, Alex's head was finally out. I couldn't believe it! He was covered with vernix and had lots of dark hair. We waited three minutes for the next contraction and then out came his body. He was placed immediately on my stomach and remained there for several hours until I gave him to Tim so I could shower. I remember during the pushing saying over and over "I just want this to be over; I've had enough." Refering not only to the pain and the birth, but also to the pregnancy. It was such a stress-filled pregnancy, planning and negotiating for the VBAC. I also remember loving the hot compresses. Everytime she removed one to replace it with a warmer one I'd scream "put that back." I also remember Clint saying, "Mom, now can you read me a book?" right after Alex was born! It's so fun to laugh about this now! Alex didn't want to nurse until about an hour after he was born, though I kept encouraging it as the placenta was taking its time coming out! Finally, when I lifted my hips to get a clean pad under me—out it came.

Even as I write this letter, it's hard to believe it all happened at home! I always knew I could give birth vaginally so long as I was in a place where I felt comfortable and safe and surrounded by truly caring people (not strangers!). I feel so indebted to my midwives for their willingness to take the risks they did to allow us such a beautiful birth, and to Tim for letting me have this baby at home, the way I wanted all along. I love all of you . . .

177

# Melinda and Ron Curry

## Melinda's Story

Eileen Elizabeth was born on January 28. She's a big (8 lbs. 13 oz. at birth), healthy baby. Unfortunately, I had my second cesarean. Let me share our story and feelings with you.

After the wonderful seminar in Sacramento, we went on the search for a home birth attendant. Arizona law prohibits anyone from attending a previous cesarean mother at home, and even unlicensed lay midwives won't touch such a case. We found a midwife who was comfortable with the idea of coming to our house during labor to check progress and going with us to the hospital as a labor support person. We kept the doctor we had seen—the one with the highest VBAC rate and best non-interventive reputation in Tucson.

I must say I was never completely happy with our situation, but felt as though things could work out in spite of it all. I worried a lot and went over every "what if . . ." possibility I could think of. Ron and I were beginning to look forward to the days ahead when we could sit back and concentrate on family life and not worry about the big day.

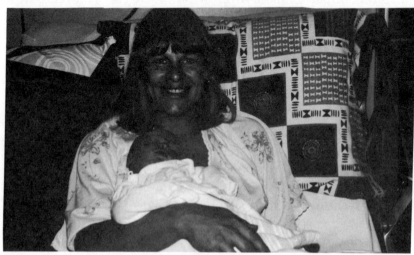

*Melinda and Eileen*

178

We took Bradley classes and found the series very informative. I ate well and exercised. We read and talked a lot. I even ordered and studied the page proofs of Nancy's upcoming book, *Silent Knife*. It's great — be sure to get a copy when it's out!

Two days past the due date, the full moon came out, the barometric pressure went down with a rainstorm, and I went into labor. Contractions began at ten minutes apart in the late afternoon. Our midwife came over just after midnight, and we didn't go to the hospital until daylight. Checked in at 5 cm. dilation. After an initial hubub, "previous cesarean," the hospital atmosphere was calm and surprisingly helpful and cooperative. We had a super labor room nurse who was at our side almost constantly in a supportive, loving way. After an hour and a half I was 6 cm. dilated — and stayed that way for four hours. The baby was posterior, the head was still "way up there," and the cervix was "getting swollen." That was "the problem." Our doctor had told us before that no progress in hard labor after several hours was a sign of a problem, but I didn't believe it and didn't really think that would happen to me and my body anyway!

I knew then that we couldn't win this one. We had side-stepped "procedure" on several counts: no IV, no fetal monitor, no hospital gown, not going to hospital at start of labor. In some eyes (like ACOG and our doctor's partner) I wasn't even a good VBAC candidate with that damn CPD on my record. I know these things don't preclude a successful VBAC at all, but in this community everyone is still pretty backwards as far as VBAC is concerned. I had an epidural, and the cesarean went smoothly. Ron was at my side (he wasn't permitted in the room for Patrick's birth) and was the first person to notice and say, "It's a girl!"

I won't tell you how "wonderful" it all was, but there was no fear, no hate, and no bitterness on my part. Ron and I feel as though we did everything we could to have a safe VBAC in Tucson. The worst part about writing this letter is knowing

179

how bad you will feel for us. We feel bad about our being the other side of success, but we aren't as devastated as we thought we would be. We have a gorgeous baby daughter who greatly eases any pain. And she sleeps more than the 8 hours/day our first baby slept, so there is some justice in this world! We also think that our experience may help future VBAC hopefuls in that some of our demands may become routine and make the difference for success for someone else. We feel satisfied that we gave it our best effort, and we'll never regret the emotion and hours we put into it. We still plan to encourage other people to give VBAC their whole-hearted effort.

We send our thanks to all of you for your good wishes and support — especially to Diane Martell-Williams up in Tempe who spent lots of time on the phone with me. And for those of you who anticipate a VBAC — DO IT!" This VBAC movement will make a difference!

# Sandra and Hiroshi Sato

## Sandra's Story

It's an hour's journey from my home in Fairfield-Suisun (CA.) to Nan Koehler's in Sebastopol. The scenery of this fabled wine-growing region changes remarkably. The frequent journeys through "The Valley of the Moon" for prenatal care provided ample time for dreaming.

I daydreamed about my Cesarean Deliverance (VBAC) — How it would involve a home birth, immediate contact and breast feeding with the baby. How I would have power and control over my life in contrast to my previous cesarean delivery.

180

*Erica Ayami Sato born June 2, 1983*

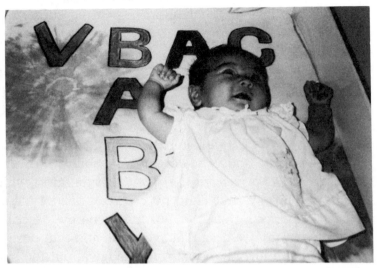

Well, I didn't get my "gold medal" but I did qualify for the bronze and I finished my marathon. Let me tell you what happened and what I learned from the birth of my beautiful baby girl, Erica Ayami.

I labored long and hard. The pain was incredible. I must have pushed for a "world record" time. Through it all, I felt the sunshine presence of an incredible amount of faith and support. It came from within and from my support persons and my husband. One flew in from Colorado, one drove from another county, one was local, one was my courageous husband. All having completely different backgrounds, they formed one of the most unusual and effective synergisms of support. I feel tremendously enriched by having experienced the faith and support of this synergism. It came from Nan Koehler who, while not physically present due to her pregnancy and the distance, labored long and hard to prepare me for the birth. I remember discussing the "cpd" diagnosis, the indication for a cesarean delivery, with Nan and her immortal statement, "Medicine is not based upon science. The pelvis moves, you know." I remember her remarkable pledge to refuse payment should she not succeed in helping me toward Cesarean Deliverance. What a marked contrast to the doc-

181

tors, who demanded that I allow them to injure my body and take away my power through more expensive surgery for their convenience and profit.

Support also came from Nancy Wainer Cohen, Claudia Panthos, and my fellow classmates in my Positive Birthing seminar, who showed me the scientific evidence and gave me emotional support to have complete confidence in the safety of a VBAC.

Support came from Gayle Peterson, who introduced me to the knowledge of the body's healing powers and the power of intuition. Having experienced the negative synergism which resulted in having my first child by cesarean delivery, I am more than convinced that the positive synergy described above resulted in my Cesarean Deliverance, and that positive energy was much more than just "knowledge about methods of preventing a cesarean."

Difficult as the birth turned out to be, it gave me the chance for complete emotional and physical healing. Emotionally I feel whole again. It is as if the creative process that started with my son's labor, so cruelly terminated by the surgeon's knife penetrating my body for the c-section, was finally completed with my daughter Erica's VBAC birth. I was no longer the owner of a cesarean-damaged uterus. The thrill of my life was to successfully conceal from the medical people at the birth and throughout my nine days of postpartum care in two hospitals (without having to tell a single falsehood) the fact that I had had a previous cesarean. It was as if the scar had disappeared!

But alas, I didn't completely learn the lesson of my first child's cesarean delivery: Trust your body; trust your intuitions; do not seek assistance unless there is a clear external indication of trouble which necessitates obstetrical interference.

In retrospect, I know that I was placing my life in jeopardy by asking for help from the medical system. I should not have let down my guard, etc., when I entered the hospital. I knew there were alternatives, such as visualization. Had I realized the seriousness, I would have been able to effect a rotation. Also, I would have pursued the prospect of medical help at home (episiotomy) with greater vigor. And last of all, I really believe that had I done nothing and continued to have faith, Erica might have been born spontaneously. But I gave up hope when I heard intervention was on the way, although my attendents did tell me to keep on trying.

This one lapse of faith proved dangerous. After pushing for a record number of hours (while the baby's heart rate remained strong — a depressed heart rate being the previously agreed upon "clear" signal of trouble, which would necessitate obstetric interference) and with the appearance of moderate meconium and the baby continuing to be in the posterior position, I was informed that Nan was trying to make arrangements for a woman doctor to come to my house to do an episiotomy, to facilitate rotation of the head. I gave up all hope of rotating the baby myself and awaited obstetric interference. As she was some distance away, the doctor wanted me to get quicker help.

I then decided to ask Dr. "Friendly" for assistance. It seemed like a simple job. I'd be out of the hospital in hours. Low forceps would be used and an episiotomy would be performed. He was waiting in the emergency room area of "Friendly General Hospital" when I arrived. By 11:40 p.m., I was settled, with my husband present, flat on my back in the labor room, while two attendants followed in a separate car and another completed admission paperwork. The nurse brought out a fetal monitor. I asked her if she was planning to use it; she said no. She took the baby's heart rate and I was concerned about the slightly depressed heart rate (110 — noted for the first time). She administered $O_2$. My attendants arrived and got me off my back. From 11:40 p.m. until 12:05 a.m. when she took me to the delivery room, the nurse was in and out. She never took another heart rate. The whole operation appeared very casual, considering the depressed heart rate. The doctor discussed the birth, agreed to allow all my at-

183

tendants to be present, and told me I wouldn't require anesthesia for the forceps if I "could stand his hand in there."

Finally at 12:05 a.m., at least 25 minutes after the 110 heart rate was noted, I was taken to the delivery room. I dreaded the stirrups but there was no use in arguing, especially considering the necessity to use forceps. At least I placed my legs there under my own power, as the nurse had me crawl without assistance from the labor bed on to the table. I heard the doctor saying they couldn't get a pediatrician in time.** At about 12:10 a.m., with everyone in place and with me feeling a sense of personal power and dignity despite my perceived need for assistance, we proceeded to wait for the doctor's assistance so I could give birth.

Without a word of warning, much less my consent, I felt the excruciating sting of a needle: the administration of anesthetic, which I thought was a local. I found out afterword it was a pudential block. It was fortunate I didn't know that then, as it would have destroyed my feeling of elation, but I remember wondering later why I never felt the birth itself. I had thought a pressure episiotomy would be done. I went into another contraction, and was again surprised by a second needle. My midwife calmed me, faced with a fait accompli. I regained my sense of composure.

Then instead of proceeding, the doctor insisted I had feces in my vagina and that he felt a rectal-vaginal fistula. I didn't believe it — my attendants denied any knowledge of it — but he was a doctor and it's hard to make a mistake about feces. (Looking back, it seems incredible that feces would still be spilling out of the vagina after several hours of pushing, even if a large fistula were present.) At any rate, while he was considering this problem, at about 12:24 a.m. my midwife asked the nurse if she could borrow the fetascope to check my baby's heart rate, which had last been checked over 40 minutes earlier. The nurse responded by taking the heart rate herself. She announced it had gone down to under 100 and was faint and falling.

Dr. Friend then asked, "Have you ever had an episiotomy?"

*Zoe (midwife) with Sandra and Erica.*

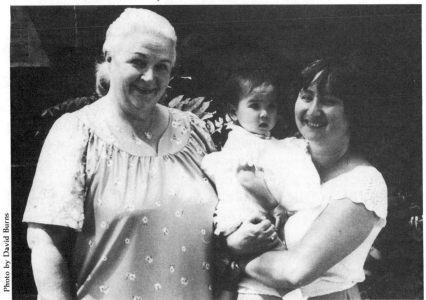

I said, "No." "Well, you're going to get one now," he stated. And with that, he did a large left lateral episiotomy (to avoid the fistula, a decision that proved right for the wrong reason, as I know I would have had a third degree tear had he done a mideslateral episiotomy). A quick forcep rotation and she just fell out. Erica was born at 12:25 a.m.

After all those hours of pain, I didn't feel her emerging from my body due to the pudential block. I was deprived of this feeling, which caused me pain. The pudential block was administered while Erica was being asphyxiated (as indicated by the heart rate), and wore off before I was sutured. I was surprised to hear the doctor say, "The cord's not pulsating." Erica was immediately taken to a table out of my sight to be resuscitated. I did not see her lifeless body or blue color. I only heard that she was a girl and I was elated. I thought she was being suctioned for meconium. Then they announced the apgar score: 1-3. My attendants stated she would be kept three days to a week. I was concerned but determined to work out a way of having bonding into this experience. I relied on intuition and believed she would be fine. While she was resuscitated, I was left unattended to bleed from the episiotomy. I lost more blood than from the c-section for my first child.

185

I was sutured and unnecessarily catherized and given a 3.5 gram prophylactic dosage of ampicilin for the prevention of infection due to the fistula. I just wanted to get out of the delivery room and see my baby in the nursery, so I let them have their way and quietly submitted to the doctor's treatment.

Dr. Friend told a bunch of scare stories. She had brain damage, cerebral palsy, etc. I relied on my intuition and told him I believed she would be fine. (Of course, I had never seen her limp condition.) This faith was in sharp contrast to my cesarean delivery, when my greatest fear was of having a brain-damaged baby. Then I had allowed my body to be cut open and my baby amputated from me, on the unsubstantiated pretense of possible brain damage. But Erica was breathing on her own and in no apparent distress.

Time passed quickly; my husband and attendants left. I remained in the hospital on the assumption that I would be able to have contact with my baby. At 4 a.m. I first asked to see her. I was told I would not be able to see her until 6 a.m. due to my fever. It was 100 degrees, up from 98.6 on admission, most probably due to the blood loss and dehydration. The fever was down to normal in a few hours. I also had an elevated white count, normal following a difficult birth, which was further "proof" of an infection. I believed Dr. Friend and settled for a glimpse from the nursery window on the way to my room at 4 a.m. (I was kept in recover longer than necessary by the doctor.)

Had the doctor leveled with me and told me that I would not be allowed to see my baby in the nursery or even from the window, I could have exercised my option to go elswhere much earlier. He had offered to transfer Erica to the intensive care nursery at "Alternative Birth Center" Hospital in the City. But he was too selfishly worried about himself to consider my needs, and so out of touch with bonding that he and the nursing staff perceived my initial request to see my baby as an "inappropriate affect." On the basis of the elevated temperature and white count and the supposed fistula, the doctor placed me in contact isolation. For the hospital staff's convenience, I was kept in strict isolation. I was later told that because I was incontinent of my vaginal secretions, I could not leave the room even to see my baby through the nursery window!

But from 6 a.m. until 9 a.m. I called the nurses asking to see my baby. At 9 a.m. I was informed of the contact isolation. I argued and asked to go elsewhere. Then I was told that my baby would be transferred to "Alternative Birth Center" Hospital. Although the ambulance personnel had her stabilized in an incubator down the hall from me for two hours, I was not allowed to see her until she was out of legal custody of "Friendly General Hospital" and on her way out the door. At 10 p.m., almost ten hours after my baby was transferred, the doctor finally returned to examine me, but would not release me even for ambulance transfer, and I had to sign out "against medical advice." The medical records state "patient is out of touch with the principles and practices of appropriate health care. Wants to breast feed baby."

At "ABC Hospital" I was treated well, despite the unusual nature of my admission there, and the fact that the medical records from "Friendly Hospital" made it look like I was grossly negligent in obtaining care for my baby. We had 24 hour access to her. I started breast feeding, and in four days she was examined by a top-notch specialist and determined to be completely normal. She was sent to room in with me 24 hours a day. My husband could visit all the time and even stayed overnight. My faith and intuition proved justified!

As for me, there were serious problems. The day of my arrival at "ABC Hospital" I was taken for surgical repair of the fistula. They had an IV in me were conducting an examination prior to surgery when they found no evidence of a fistula — and proceeded to congratulate me!

I did develop an infection of the episiotomy and bladder, which did not respond to initial antibiotic treatment. I was given a second antibiotic, and two units of blood were transfused. The episiotomy broke open and took several months to heal completely.

Nine days after the birth I was released and soon regained my health. I don't know what I would have done without the loving support of Nan and my attendants during my hospitalization and postpartum. They called, visited, and even provided the blood transfusions. One attendant gave; another's husband gave.

187

At one year of age, Erica proved advanced, having crawled at five months and walked well at nine months. Neither "Dr. Friend" nor "Friendly General Hospital" will account for their actions (only part of the story is told here), blaming the home birth. I had not intended to take action, giving them the benefit of the doubt. But since they behaved this way, I intend to fight back. I have asked for a state investigation. I intend to straighten things out!

Every home VBAC is a victory for personal power over mindless technology (and technicians), regardless of the outcome, and as such, is a part of the movement to save the earth!

# Nancy and Peter Coughlan

## Nancy's Story

The process of preparing for the birth of our second child began immediately after our first birth. Our first daughter, Michelle, we had planned to birth at home. Instead, we had a cesarean section in the hospital. The events that brought this about were many. I had the typical cesarean scenario with premature rupture of the membranes, baby's head never engaging, slow progress halting at 4 cm, and so with my temperature rising and my energy waning my husband and I agreed to a c-section. I was diagnosed by a consulting physician as having CPD. My own obstetrician, Dr. Solomon, was not so sure. Neither was I. I knew how I handled the labor and I felt that there were too many psychological and emotional factors that had affected the process. I doubted that it was totally a physical problem. It took me awhile to reconcile my feelings of failure. The saving grace was being awake for the cesarean birth and bonding with my daughter. The total love and wonder my husband, Peter, and I experienced was so positive that it outweighed all other emotions.

As we approached our decision to have another child, I knew I did not want a repeat experience. I took a clear look at what I experienced as dissatisfying in our first birth: a poor shared labor experience and support system, tenseness and an inability to relax and go with the labor. We wanted a vaginal birth. Our reasons for desiring a vaginal birth were many. We feel the natural process is always the best. We wanted the best for our baby and feel that the process of labor, birth, and bonding is very important for the health and well-being of an infant. I needed, for my own integrity, a sense of completion with my first birth. My husband and I wanted to work together better this time and to share a labor with full commitment. Dr. Solomon said there was every possibility of a vaginal birth, but that we must know that it could also be a repeat c-section. We decided to commit ourselves to preparing for a vaginal birth. We knew that it would take strong intention and preparation and that there was no guarantee—it still could be cesarean.

I began a program of regular vigorous physical exercise, vitamins, and herbal teas. I read everything I could, talked to everyone I knew, and then did whatever made sense to me. I looked at my doubts and insecurities and saw what old and negative thought tapes were still playing that would be unproductive. I looked at my mother's negative birth experience and how that viewpoint had been passed to me. I saw my own inability to trust my body's capacity for birthing, and I saw my fears of pain and my tendency to want to be saved from it. I practiced relaxation, visualization, and self-hypnosis. My husband, who had done self-hypnosis in the past, prepared a tape for me that I listened to daily. In the tape, he would bring me into a relaxed state and visualize a totally normal, natural birth experience in detail, from pregnancy through birth. He included key words and phrases to induce relaxation and gave me affirmations regarding my body's ability to birth and to trust the natual process. We took birth classes from our midwife and visited the hospital to assure a supportive environment.

About my thirtieth week, we found that the baby was breech. I was truly taken aback. Up until then, both of my pregnancies had been very healthy and normal. I began to worry. I didn't know if I was prepared to attempt a vaginal breech birth. Every day for a month, I laid on a slant board to turn the baby with no result. I confronted the possibility that I had created a breech baby so that I wouldn't have to go through labor. It was the truth of this that led me to a deeper commitment to a vaginal birth. I applied myself more seriously to preparing. The baby turned and I was on top of the world. I knew I could do it.

As our due date drew near, we felt prepared and excited. We felt we had done everything we could to prepare, and we looked forward to the labor and birth. I felt very positive and clearly felt it would be a vaginal birth. My only lingering doubt was my ability to handle the pain.

At my Thursday checkup, my doctor said that I was 90% effaced, my cervix was tipped forward, the baby was lower and I was basically ready. On Saturday evening, I experienced some very mild, fairly regular contractions for three hours or so. They promptly disappeared after a warm bath. As we worked in the garden on Sunday evening, the contractions began again. After a bath they slowed for a while and then picked up. At 9:00 p.m., I felt sure it was beginning. I called the midwife because we wanted her there fairly early on in labor for support. We had not called our midwife soon enough on our first birth for her to guide my handling of the contractions before I became tired and tense. Our midwife said she was ready to come at any time, and to call again when we were ready for her. I wanted to try to sleep, but sleep was impossible. We called her back and she arrived about 11:00 p.m. By midnight or so, contractions were five minutes apart and strong. I was handling them well and my husband's support was impeccable. I truly felt relaxed and could feel myself opening up. I kept my goals in mind and visualized a progressing labor. Ellen checked and found me a tight 3 cm. After a long bath, I was up to 4 cm. I remember feeling slightly disappointed as I felt I had really opened up far more than that. Ellen reminded me that the first five are the slowest and once at five she was sure I would really go. Hours later, I was still at four, but a very stretchy soft four, and Ellen felt good about the progress. By then, contractions took all my concentration and my husband's relaxation talks. The contractions were every three minutes. I said I was ready to go to the hospital. I didn't feel that I could remain relaxed enough to make the 45 minute car ride, if I waited much longer.

It was just mildly disrupting to check in and get accustomed to the hospital environment. One of my cues on the birthing tape was to deepen my sense of relaxation upon arriving at the hospital. I felt that the birth would be imminent. I was sure my labor would progress rapidly and that I would have my baby just after daybreak.

But things were going slowly. I had not progressed past five cm after five-six hours of very strong, regular labor. I felt the sun shining through the window. The clock neared 8:00 a.m. Don said that the baby was still high and that my bag of waters, not the baby's head, was on my cervix. He and Ellen agreed that if the waters were broken, the baby's head would drop and dilation would progress. My husband and I agreed. I still felt confident, although I felt some fear about the contractions intensifyng beyond what I could handle. They assured me that it was time to get on with it before I became too tired. I knew I had to go on and couldn't stay forever at a comfortable level of labor (not that it wasn't intense) and expect to give birth.

I felt the difference in contractions immediately after the waters were broken. Don assured me that the head was moving down and now we'd see what would happen. Then I felt something new. I felt a pushing sensation. It began mildly and

191

strengthened with each contraction. Ellen said it was probably the feeling of the baby's head pushing on the cervix. But the sensation kept increasing until I was having fullblown pushing contractions 60-90 seconds long and two to three minutes apart. Don encouraged me to breathe through them so that my cervix would not be irritated with the premature pushing. They kept getting heavier. Don encouraged me to think positive and showed Peter and Ellen how he wanted them to direct my breathing. The contractions became so strong that my whole world became my husband's voice and his breath. All there was in the world was this incredibly overpowering physical sensation of pushing and my husband's voice and breath to guide me through. Vaginal checks became almost unbearable. I became very bitchy. I blew until I could no longer blow and then I'd make huge grunting yells until I could blow again. Don suggested a mild muscle relaxant to help me to breathe through the contractions so that I could continue to dilate. After a couple of hours of this, the next vaginal check showed an irritated cervix at a tight four cm. The talk turned to cesarean. I was in another world. I was sure I was doing my best and that it should be working. But it wasn't and it took me awhile to see it and agree to the c-section. I knew I just couldn't continue on with the pushing contractions, they were so powerful and intense and yet weren't doing anything. It was another hour before I was taken to surgery.

I can still vividly recall the contractions subsiding as the epidural anesthesia took affect. I was very glad to be awake and to have my husband there with me. As the cesarean was not totally painless, my husband and I breathed through the surgical birthing. It caught me off guard, but I kind of liked it. I was still working — still an active part of birthing my baby. And then she was there. I couldn't wait to hold her to me. We had done it. We had birthed our baby. The lonely hour spent in recovery by myself was the only let down. I was ecstatic; in love with my baby and my husband. The time ticked by

*Nancy Coughlan, Michelle, and Julia*

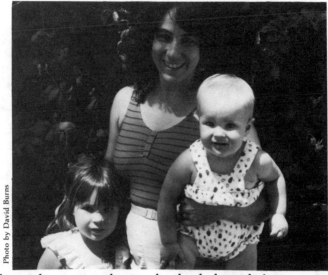

Photo by David Burns

slowly with no one there who had shared the moments.

Once we were all together, our world was whole and at peace. Julia Rose was beautiful and healthy. We were in love, and we had labored hard for our child. She was a big baby for me (I'm under 5 feet) 21" long, 7 lbs. and 13 oz., and posterior. Julia roomed in with me and never left my side. This, I feel, is essential for cesarean births. Without my baby there, I was a patient recovering from surgery. With her, I had given birth and she gave me strength and purpose. She nursed me back to health.

I am very satisfied with my birth experience. It was the next step for me, and I feel complete. I really experienced my labor and was supported through it. Nan was an endless source of information and emotional support. Her strength and conviction gave me confidence and power. Don served us wonderfully as our obstetrician and gave us even more as a birth attendant and support person. He gave us more than 100% of himself to help us in having our birth the way we wanted it. I gave the birth everything I had, and my husband gave his total love and support. What more can there be? Whether the cesarean was necessary could be debated endlessly. To me, what is important was the intention, the commitment, the process of birth, and the satisfaction, health, and well-being of all of us. To these points we had succeeded.

193

*Zoe (midwife), Sandra and Erica, with Nan and daughters Shayna and Sarah.*

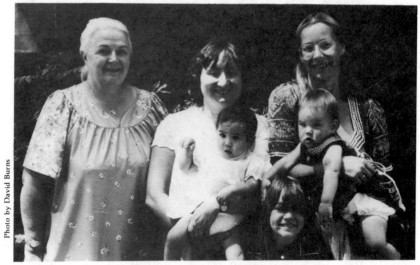

Photo by David Burns

# Conclusion for the VBAC Stories

*by Nan Koehler*

It's been almost two years since I began gathering these stories. My perspective has shifted and crystalized somewhat because during this time, I've also had another baby (my fifth) and couldn't attend births because of poor health. This enforced time of introspection with refocus on classes and prenatal care has given me an opportunity to articulate what I've learned intuitively by helping women have VBACs.

In helping a woman give birth, one looks for and maximizes two basic principles: first is to help her establish a good labor pattern — strong regular contractions which are close together. This is done through diet, exercise, proper hydration, vitamin and mineral supplements, rest and, of course, education to alleviate fear. Second is to teach or encourage her to use as

194

many styles of coping as possible. In good labor, if the woman can bear the pain, the baby will be born. Pain brings the baby. The intense pain is nature's way of insuring that we bond with our baby. It seems to me that we have to go through physical and psychic pain/changes to produce children.

In giving prenatal care, what one looks for are the double messages. The "I feel fine" when she has dark circles under her eyes. These help us know if the woman might have trouble birthing and/or if she did have trouble, where the problem might have originated. Gayle Peterson has elaborated on this theme in the book *Birthing Normally*. What I want to write about is a subtler reality which has helped me understand why some women have trouble giving birth. One certainly can't tell from the outside who will have difficulty. Sometimes the healthy big-hipped woman ends up with a c-section while an unhealthy small-hipped woman has a short labor with no problems.

Many, many words have been written on a concept that might explain this phenomenon — I will try to summarize it on one page! First, it is most important to understand and accept as real the idea of karma. For every action, there is a reaction. For every kind deed done or kind word spoken, a kindness returns, or something good returns. This good might not be in the way one expects, but it does come back. The same is true for evil or cruel deeds. For example, thoughtlessly yelling at our children results in failures elsewhere. Let's say that a woman's karmic destiny is to have trouble in birth. This might not be the woman's personal karma; it may be her mother's or her baby's, or her husband's which she unconsciously acts out. Who knows where it comes from! The fact is, it's there. Here is where the idea of Samskaras, at least as I understand it, helps us to understand karma.

It is as if we are all liquid crystals able to move about in energy fields which overlap and influence each other. The energy fields of the atoms that make up our bodies were

195

gathered by our mother, and hers by her mother and so on. These energy fields have a certain power because of their history. For example, if your mother ate poorly, you won't be really healthy and if you in turn don't eat well (to make up for your Mom's failure) your daughter will be even less healthy and so on. This principle can be applied on all levels, psychic as well as physical.

Then, secondly, how does one undo this karmic destiny? It is very easy to answer in words, but very difficult to accomplish. PAIN, CRYING, FREAKING OUT, in short, SUFFERING (deep emotional experiences of ourselves) burns away the karma. Gandhi and Jesus taught this. The pain we feel is actually an in-tunement with our primal selves. Luckily, when a woman is pregnant, she has the gift of hormones and fatigue to reveal to her emotional states or feelings she never dreamed she had. (Usually we try to avoid those intense feelings!) Trouble comes when we try to deny those feelings. "Hello, dear," she says as her husband walks in the door, when what she's really feeling is "Boohoo, HELP me." She is probably experiencing a time of low blood sugar and she needs to eat. Nevertheless, the way in which we emote fatigue will reveal to us our weaknesses—our parental programming which can lead to compulsive behavior.

These compulsions are what can lead to c-sections! The body knows at all times what to do: when to eat, when to sleep, when to work, what to eat, etc. Only the "shouldn't and shoulds" (from our cerebrum) sensor our instinctive self. Most of the time, this is very appropriate, but *not when giving birth*. Without being too crazy or frightening our mates too much, we can allow ourselves to emote by letting our feelings come to the surface, while part of ourselves stands by and says "Hey, look at that," "I'm really angry" or "I'm really happy;" realizing that no one *made* us feel that way. That was simply the response our body chose, and where that's established, who knows. Just watching, witnessing what's happening, takes the power and the overwhelming energy of those feelings away so that we can make calm assessments of our situation. "Really, Doctor, I'm in a lot of pain, but I like being on all fours on the floor." (Not many woman dare to get off the bed in a hospital setting even when their body wisdom tells them to. Yet it's been well documented that the pelvic dimensions enlarge when the woman is on her hands and knees. Many women with a posterior baby are sectioned when a simple change of position would have helped them give birth vaginally.)

This transformation in consciousness has happened for all the women in these VBAC stories—even those who were sectioned again. Remember, not everyone is traumatized by being sectioned, and the goal for birth, viewed as a Rite of Passage, is female empowerment and transformation resulting in proper bonding with the baby. This experience can happen for any woman as long as she feels as though the route of delivery was *her* choice and afterwards she has adequate support for a long period of isolation with the baby.

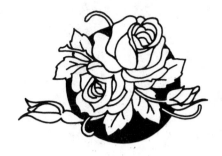

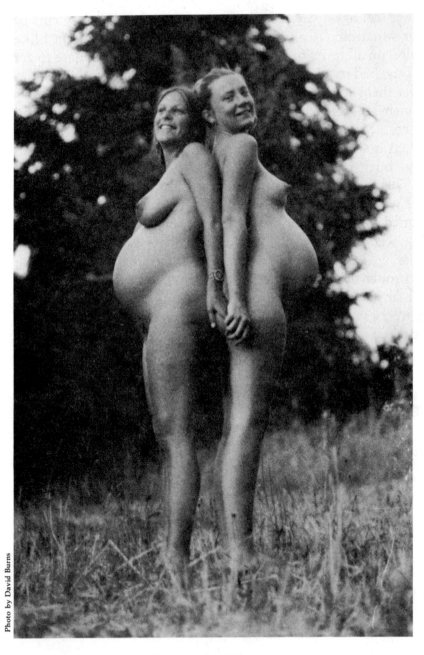

Photo by David Burns

*Chandra and Cher*

198

# Part III

# *Preparing the Body*

# Reading List For Pregnancy

There are hundreds of books available which discuss pregnancy and childbirth, and the full time job of parenting. This is a list of many of the most current or the better ones available. Whether you are choosing to give birth in a hospital or at home, reading is one of the best ways in which you can prepare yourself for the birth and the changes in your life which will follow. Keep in mind while reading that in order to become intelligent consumers of medical care, we must know what we want and need, what our rights are, and how to get exactly what we want. Being well educated about pregnancy, labor, birth, and parenting, we are better able to assume responsibility, share in the decision making that affects our bodies and babies, and enjoy to the fullest our growing families.

## PRENATAL NUTRITION, FETAL DEVELOPMENT

*Wise Woman Herbal for the Childbearing Year.* Susan Weed.
*Preparing for Motherhood, Nature's Way.* Paul Bragg.
*Meditations for the Expectant Mother.* Helen Brennerman.
*Confessions of a Sneaky Organic Cook.* Jane Kinderlehrer.
*Are You Confused?* Paavo Airola.
*Diet for a Small Planet.* Frances Lappe.
*A Child is Born.* Nilsson and Infelman-Sundberg.
*Better Food for Better Babies.* Gena Larson.
*From Conception to Birth.* Rugh and Shettles.
*In the Beginning—Your Child's Brain Before Birth.* M. and L. Rosen.
*Life Before Birth.* Ashley Montague.
*Nourishing Your Unborn Child.* Phyllis Williams.
*Nutrition Against Disease.* Roger Williams.
*The First Nine Months of Life.* G. L. Flanagan.
*The Malnourished Mind.* Elie Shenour.
*Exercises for True Natural Childbirth.* Rhondha Hartman.
*Macrobiotic Pregnancy.* Alice Feinberg.
*Pregnancy as Healing.* Lewis Mehl and Gayle Peterson.
*Pregnant Feelings.* Rahima Baldwin and Terra Palmarini.
*Prenatal Yoga and Natural Birth.* Jeannine Parvati Baker.

## HOSPITAL BIRTH AND SIMILAR ISSUES
*Birth Without Violence.* Fredrick LeBoyer.
*Forced Labor, Maternity Care in the U.S.* Nancy S. Shaw.
*Immaculate Deception.* Suzanne Arms.
*The Cultural Warping of Childbirth.* Doris Haire.
*Understanding Childbirth in America.* Sally Ong.
*Woman's Doctor.* William Sweeney.
*Maternal Attachment and Mothering Disorders.* Marshall Klaus.
*A Woman in Residence.* Michelle Harrison, M.D.
*Entering the World, the De-medicalization of Childbirth.* Michael Odent.

## PATIENT'S RIGHTS
*Talk Back to Your Doctor.* Arthur Levin
*The Rights of Hospital Patients.* George Annas.
*Have It Your Way.* Vicki Walton.
*Birth Reborn.* Michael Odent.

## HOME BIRTH
*Homebirth.* Gilgoff.
*Hearts Open Wide.* Wellish.
*Birth.* Raven Lang.
*Birth Goes Home.* Lester Hazell.
*Childbirth at Home.* Marion Souza.
*Childbirth is Ecstasy.* Walzer/Cohen.
*Emergency Childbirth.* Gregory White.
*Home Oriented Maternity Experience.* H.O.M.E.
*The Home Birth Book.* Charlotte and Fred Ward.
*Two Births.* Brown and Lessor.
*Spiritual Midwifery.* Ina May and The Farm Midwives.
*Ettinghausen Method, Homebirth At It's Best.* Nial Ettinghausen.
*Birth and the Dialogue of Love.* Marilyn Moran.

## BREASTFEEDING, IMPRINTING, AND FEEDING SOLIDS
*Abreast of the Times.* Richard Applebaum.
*Breastfeeding and Natural Child Spacing.* Sheila Kippley.
*Making Your Own Baby Foods.* Mary and James Turner.
*Nursing Your Baby.* Karen Pryor.
*Please Breastfeed Your Baby.* Alice Gerard.
*Preparation For Breastfeeding.* Donna and Roger Ewy.
*The Complete Book of Breastfeeding.* Eiger and Olds.
*The Rights of Infants.* Margaret Ribble (old, but still useful).
*The Womanly Art of Breastfeeding.* La Leche League.
*Touching.* Ashley Montague.
*White Paper on Infant Feeding Practices.* The Center for Science in the
   Public Interest.
*The Tender Gift.* Dana Raphael.
*The Family Bed.* Tine Thevenin.
*Maternal Emotions.* Niles Newton.

201

## OTHER BOOKS ON PREGNANCY, LABOR, BIRTH, AND POSTPARTUM

*The New Childbirth.* Erna Wright.
*A Season to be Born.* Suzanne Arms.
*Birth.* David Meltzer.
*Natural Childbirth and the Family.* Helen Wessel.
*Birth.* Caterine Milinaire.
*Childbirth Without Fear.* Grantly Dick-Read.
*Commonsense Childbirth.* Lester Hazell.
*Husband Coached Childbirth.* Robert Bradley (Bradley Method).
*Methods of Childbirth.* Constance Bean.
*Our Bodies, Ourselves.* Boston Women's Health Collective.
*Pregnancy, Birth and the Newborn Baby.* Boston Children's Med. Center.
*Pregnancy, the Psychological Experience.* Arthur and Libby Colman.
*Prenatal Yoga.* Jeannine Medvin.
*The Experience of Childbirth.* Sheila Kitzinger.
*Whatnow? A Handbook for New Parents.* Rozdilsky and Banat.
*Why Natural Childbirth?* Deborah Tanzer.
*Exercises for True Natural Childbirth.* R. Hartman (Bradley Method).
*Essential Exercises for the Childbearing Years.* Elizabeth Noble.
*Joyous Childbirth.* Gold and Gold.
*Special Delivery.* Rahima Baldwin.
*Secret Life of the Unborn Child.* Verny & Kelly.
*Whole Birth Catalog.* Ed. by Janet Ashford.
*Ideal Birth.* Sondra Ram.
*The Healing Power of Birth.* Rima Star.
*The Art of Breathing.* Frederick LeBoyer.

## LAMAZE METHOD — there are numerous Lamaze books, some are:

*A Birth in the Family.* Elizabeth Bing.
*Awake and Aware.* Irwin Chabon.
*Painless Childbirth.* Lamaze.
*Preparation for Childbirth.* Donna and Roger Ewy.
*Thank You, Dr. Lamaze.* Marjorie Karmel.
*Six Practical Lessons for An Easier Childbirth.* Elizabeth Bing.
*Childbirth Without Pain.* P. Vellay.

## CHILDREARING AND CHILDHOOD NUTRITION

*The Magical Child.* Joseph Chilton Pierce.
*The Feeling Child.* Arthur Janov.
*Your Vegetarian Baby.* Retundi.
*Nature's Children.* Juliet De Baircali Levy.

202

*Education and Marriage.* Hasrat Inat Khan. Vol. 3.
*Whole Parent, Whole Child.* Polly Berrien Berends.
*Loving Hands.* Fredrick LeBoyer.
*Water Babies.* Sidenbladh.
*Children of the Dawn.* Joshua Halpern.
*The Book of the Mother.* Shivalia (Children's Liberation Front).
*To Love A Baby.* Sandy Jones.
*The Continuum Concept.* Jean Liedloff.
*Herbal Pathfinders.* Conrow & Hecksel.
*Food For Thought.* Maureen Minchin.
*The Baby Massage Book.* Tina Heinl.
*Child's Body.* The Diagram Group.
*The Roots of Love.* Helene S. Arnstein.
*Childhood Illness.* Jack G. Shiller, M.D.
*Feed Your Kid Right & Changing Your Child's Behavior through
   Nutrition.* Ledlan Smith, M.D.
*For Your Own Good.* Alice Miller.
*Models of Love.* Joyce & Barry Vissell.

## BOOKS FOR VBAC COUPLES
*Birthing Normally.* Gayle Peterson.
*Silent Knife.* Nancy Wainer Cohen and Lois J. Estner.
*VBAC Stories and Information.* Nan Koehler.
*Transformation Through Birth, A Woman's Guide.* Claudia Panuthos.
*Love Muscle.* Bryce Britton.
*The VBAC Experience.* Lynn Babtiste Richards.

See page 36 for a resource list and get a copy of the *Whole Birth Catalog: A Sourcebook for Choices in Childbirth,* Edited by Janet Isaacs Ashford, The Crossing Press, Trumansburg, N.Y., 14886. $14.95.

Any investment in books or food will pay off in saved hospital bills later!

# Items Required For A Home Birth

*by Kay Mathews*

- Rubber sheet or piece of plastic to cover mattress
- 1 or 2 clean sheets besides the one on the bed
- 6 to 10 large bath towels to soak up liquids
- 2 washcloths — one for wiping brow, 1 extra
- Large disposable diapers or bed pads if you want to avoid soiling towels
- 2 boxes of 4x4 sterile gauze squares
- 4 to 6 large pillows for support

## For the Woman

- Short top for laboring — 1 warm, 1 cool
- 2 or 3 gowns or pj's which open down the front for easy nursing
- Socks for cold feet
- Hospital size sanitary pads, pins or belt
- Disposable diapers to position around Kotex to prevent leakage first two days
- Cornstarch or powder for massage or back rubs
- Heating pad
- Thermometer for post-partum
- Hair clips or bands to keep hair out of face.

## For the Baby

- A supply of diapers. Most diaper services will deliver in advance
- Diaper pins
- Tee shirts
- Gowns and/or terry cloth suits
- Several receiving blankets, plus other heavier blankets
- Plastic underpads
- Alcohol and cotton balls for cleaning umbilical cord
- Bulb syringe for suctioning mucous (small ear syringe)

## Other Supplies

- Large pot for boiling instruments
- Large bowl for catching placenta
- A good portable lamp or strong flashlight
- Wastebasket or box for refuse. Large pillow case for soiled laundry

Have a phone handy. Make arrangements for access to a neighbor's if you don't have one. Have a car gassed up and in dependable running order, should it be necessary to go to the hospital.

Have a supply of juices, herb teas, ice chips, bendable straws, ingredients to make high protein drinks for early labor, soda, crackers, or other easily digestible foods on hand.

# Preparing . . .

### by Donnah Ha

Here are some suggestions of things you can do to prepare yourself and your house for your homebirth:

- Get through prenatal care from a doctor and your midwife
- Attend childbirth education classes
- Get well acquainted with your midwife and assistants
- Practice super nutrition
- Avoid drugs, x-rays and exposure to disease as much as you can
- Exercise adequately

205

# By Two To Three Weeks Before Your Due Date

1. Purchase, collect or borrow the items on the list of needed things. Put them all together in or near the birth room.
2. Make up your bed with plastic to cover the mattress as completely as possible. Use a *heavy* plastic such as a shower curtain. (Ask your midwife if she loans a hand-me-down.) If you want, you can have a sheet on the mattress *under* the plastic too, so that when we strip the bed, it is already made.
3. Wash *all* baby clothes, sheets, diapers, etc. with a mild soap/detergent and rinse extra well. (This includes packaged clothes).
4. Clean your house, with special attention to the birth room and bath room. If you have pets, check them for disease, fleas, etc. Especially if the birth room is small, remove unnecessary objects and clutter. Have a desk or dresser or table top clear for us to use for our equipment.
5. Buy or make a supply of gowns, pjs or shifts which open down the front for easy nursing. Also a couple outfits which are one to three sizes larger than your normal size to wear until your weight declines. It can be depressing to have to wear maternity clothes after the birth, so visit your local thrift store or sew up a couple outfits which can be for the transition period before you return to a smaller size. It's ego boosting to have this taken care of in advance, if you gain a lot.
6. If you wear them, have a couple of nursing or other comfortable bras which are one or two sizes larger than you usually need. When your milk comes in and possibly during the first few months, you will need bigger bras. Do not wear a bra that is too tight. That contributes to breast infections.
7. Stock up on food, perhaps freezing some favorites or arranging with friends or relatives to bring in meals for the

206

first week.

8. Try to keep your laundry caught up.

9. If you are getting diaper service, arrange to have the diapers delivered two weeks before your due date and ask for newborn size (unless you expect a 10 lb. baby!)

10. See a family practitioner or pediatrician *before* the birth and find out when s/he wants to see the baby the first time. Check about the possibility of a home visit. Feel the doctor out about attitudes on homebirth, breastfeeding and perhaps about how s/he feels about your not wanting your baby to have routine eyedrops, vitamin K shots, etc. It will be good to have a pediatrician or other doctor who will not stereotype your home born baby and whom you feel you know and trust in case of any complications.

11. Arrange for someone to help with the running of the house if the mate is not present or must return to work. It's nice to have help the first two weeks, if possible.

12. If you have older children, arrange for help with child-care at least for the first 2 to 4 weeks post-partum. A baby-sitting co-op, friends, relatives, a nursery school or day care center could all be possibilities. Prepare the child(ren) in advance and preferably have them already spending time with the alternative persons. Make pre-arrangements for your older child(ren) to go on special outings with friends and relatives to the zoo, movies, a park, etc. Help them to feel special by asking close friends/relatives to bring small gifts to the older children instead of the baby. You need time for this new baby and yourself. You'll have more positive energy for the older child(ren) if you can have some time alone. Depending on the age of your older child(ren), they will probably enjoy and benefit from the special activities.

13. Lay in a supply of *light* reading matter—library books, magazines, novels—plus some announcements and letter writing materials if you wish, to have on hand to do during the first week or two when you will be resting a lot.

14. If you are going to take pictures, make movies or tape your birth, get all the film, cameras and other equipment ready and check the working order of everything in advance.

15. If you are having guests at your birth, please explain to them in advance that all invitations are conditional — that is it depends completely on the conditions that prevail when you actually go into labor and where your head is at that time. Explain that you or the midwife may ask people to leave if the labor needs privacy to proceed, and that every invited guest should be supportive of that decision.

16. Make alternative arrangements for the care of children at your birth in the event they are not doing well at the birthing or if their presence takes too much energy from the mother.

17. Try to arrange your life and responsibilities in such a way that the last weeks and days of your pregnancy become a time of tranquility and patient, peaceful awaiting. The first priority is to *stay well rested physically* and *keep your head in a positive, happy attitude.*

# Contraindications For Childbirth At Home

*This list should not be taken literally: Very often it is the degree rather than the presence of a certain contraindication which would preclude home birth. Also, in many cases, it would take a combination of these factors to put one in the high risk category. If any of these factors are present they should be discussed with your doctor, but the final decision must rest with the couple.*

## I. Maternal

1. History of problems associated with childbearing such as repeated miscarriages, premature infants, toxemia (eclampsia or pre-eclampsia), diabetes of pregnancy, postpartum hemorrhage or previous Caesaran section.
2. Certain diseases in the mother such as diabetes, thyroid disease, kidney disease, sickle cell disease, heart disease or chronic high blood pressure (hypertension).
3. Viral illness during pregnancy. Any severe infection.
4. Anemia (too few red blood cells): indicated by a hemoglobin below 12 or a hematocrit below 35.
5. Poor nutritional status, heavy smoking, drug addiction.
6. Maternal age less than 16 or more than 40 years.
7. Sixth or more child.
8. Vaginal bleeding in third trimester.
9. Rh sensitization.
10. Inadequate pelvis (too small for baby to pass through).

# II. Fetal

1. Multiple birth (twins, etc.).
2. Hydramnios (too much amniotic fluid).
3. Prematurity (baby's weight under $5\frac{1}{2}$ pounds or born over $2\frac{1}{2}$ weeks before due date).
4. Postmaturity (baby born over $2\frac{1}{2}$ weeks beyond due date).
5. Fetal distress indicated by irregularities in the fetal heart rate or cessation of fetal movement.
6. Suspected stillborn (uterus not enlarging appropriately for gestational age, loss of fetal heart beat, cessation of fetal movement).

# III. In Labor

1. Rupture of bag of waters without commencement of labor within 24 hours.
2. Malpresentation of baby (breech or transverse).
3. Heavy vaginal bleeding.
4. Fetal distress as indicated by great variation in fetal heart rate, meconium stained amniotic fluid, or excessive fetal movement.
5. Failure to progress after 24 hours of labor.
6. Maternal distress (exhaustion, apprehension, abnormal blood pressure and pulse).
7. Fever and other signs of infection.

Reprint 101, c. 2/1976

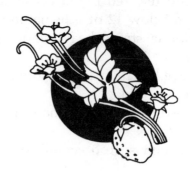

210

# Terminology

Reprinted from Homebirth, Inc.

*Afterbirth:* Placenta and membranes expelled after the birth in the third stage of labor.

*"After-Pains":* Postpartum contractions as the uterus returns to its former size, especially noticeable during nursing. Often more uncomfortable after second or subsequent births.

*Albumin:* A form of protein and tested for in routine urinalysis. Its presence may be related to toxemia of pregnancy.

*Amniotic Fluid:* Water-like fluid contained in the membranous sac surrounding the baby. It supports and permits movement of the baby — acts as a shock absorber and prevents heat loss.

*Amniotomy:* Artificial rupture of the membranes or "bag of waters."

*Analgesics:* Drugs which help raise one's pain threshold, typically narcotics such as Demerol, Nisenthil.

*Anesthesia:* Loss of sensation. May be complete (general); regional (spinal, epidural, paracervical, pudendal, etc.) or local.

*Anterior Presentation:* Most common — the baby lies head down facing the mother's back.

*Anterior Lip:* The front portion of the cervix which sometime persists at the end of first stage of labor.

*Apgar Score:* A 0-10 scale on which the baby is rated at one minute and five minutes after birth. Zero to 2 points are give for five signs: heart rate, respiration, muscle tone, relex response and color.

*Areola:* Pigmented area surrounding nipple-darkens during pregnancy.

*"Bearing-down Urge":* Relex urge to push with the second stage contractions. May take time to establish — occasionally not felt.

211

*Braxton-Hicks Contractions:* Intermittent contractions of the uterus noticed in later pregnancy as uterus prepares for labor. Usually stop with change of position, unlike real labor.

*Breech:* The baby lies so that buttocks, feet or a foot present instead of the head.

*Caput:* Swelling produced on the crown of the baby's head—may be mistaken for the bag of water.

*Centimeters:* Unit of measurement used to describe the progress of dilation of the cervix. Used interchangeably with "fingers" 1 finger = 2 cms.

*Cervix:* The narrow end of the uterus opening into the vagina. This must dilate to five fingers (10 cms) to permit the baby to pass.

*Cesarean Section:* Delivery of the baby by surgical incision of the abdominal wall and uterus. Indications include: unfavorable presentation, fetal distress, fetal head too large for pelvis.

*Coccyx:* The small bone at the end of the vertebral column—"tail-bone."

*Colostrum:* Secretions produced by the breast during pregnancy and after the birth prior to the milk. A high protein substance with some immunity properties and provides a laxative action.

*Contractions:* Tightening and shortening of the uterine muscles during labor which achieve dilation and effacement of the cervix and then the expulsion of the baby and placenta.

*Crowning:* When the baby's head has descended under the pubic arch and no longer recedes between contractions but causes the perineum to bulge.

*Dilation, Dilatation:* Gradual opening of the cervix in the first stage of labor to permit the baby's passage. Measured either by fingers (5 = full dilation) or centimeters (10 = full).

*Effacement:* The thinning and shortening of the cervix measured in percentages. 100% = fully-effaced.

212

*Effleurage:* Lamaze technique — circular stroking of the abdomen during a contractions.

*Engagement:* The stationing of the presenting part of the baby within the pelvic brim.

*Episiotomy:* Incision of the perineum, between the vagina and the rectum, to enlarge the outlet of the birth canal.

*Fetus:* Medical term for baby after third month of pregnancy till birth.

*Fontanels:* Spaces between baby's skull bones which permit molding of the head during birth. Felt as soft spots on top of the head.

*Fundus:* Top of the upper portion of the uterus.

*Gestation:* Period of intra-uterine development: 40 weeks, approximately.

*Hyperventilation:* "Overbreathing" which results in an oxygen surplus for the mother. Symptoms include: dizzyness, tingling or numbness of lips, fingers, toes.

*Induced Labor:* Labor started artifically by rupture of membranes, or by pitocin-like drugs (via mouth or intravenous) or both.

*Inertia:* Of the uterus — sluggish contractions.

*Involution:* Involuntary return of the uterus to normal size after birth — accomplished within six weeks, activated by breastfeeding.

*Labor:* The work done and period of time taken by the uterine muscle to thin (efface) and stretch (dilate) the cervix during Stage I, and to expel the baby down the birth canal in Stage II, followed by the placenta and membranes, Stage III.

*Laceration:* A tear. First degree lacerations of the perineum heal spontaneously — deeper ones require sutures.

*Lamaze:* Method of childbirth preparation named after French physician. Also called psychoprophylaxis (mind-prevention). Emphasis on neuromuscular control, mental concentration (disassociation) and progressive breathing patterns.

213

*Lanugo:* Down-like hair on the newborn.

*"Let-down·Reflex":* Sensation of fullness in the breasts as milk sacs tighten to squeeze milk into the collecting sinuses behind the nipples, thus making milk available for nursing.

*Lithotomy Position:* Delivery position where the mother is flat on her back and legs up in stirrups.

*Lochia:* Discharge of blood, mucus and tissue from the uterus during the postpartum period.

*Meconium:* Greenish-black, tar-like first stools of the baby.

*Molding:* The shaping of the baby's head to the size and shape of the birth canal.

*Mucus Plug:* Accumulation of secretions in the cervix to seal off uterus. Forms a blood-tinged "show" prior to and during labor.

*Neonate:* A baby up to 30 days of age.

*Occiput:* The bony prominence at the back of the baby's head.

*Oxytocin:* The hormone which stimulates the uterus to contract and is also involved in the let-down reflex for breastfeeding.

*Parity:* Refers to the number of births: nullipara—none; primipara—one; multipara—many.

*Pelvic Floor:* Muscular base of the pelvic-abdominal cavity supporting the bowel, uterus, bladder and their passages. Voluntary control of these muscles is important during the birth, and especially afterwards to prevent sexual and/or urinary problems and later "dropping of organs."

*Perineum:* The area surrounding the vagina and anus.

*Pitocin:* A synthetic oxytocin drug used to stimulate labor.

*Placenta:* Oval spongy organ attached to the wall of the uterus. It is attached to the fetus by the umbilical cord via which the baby receives nourishment and waste products are removed.

214

*Posterior Presentation:* The baby lies head down but faces its mother's pubic arch with the occiput against her back. This causes a longer labor with more backache than other presentations.

*Relaxin:* One of the hormones which cause softening of the maternal tissues and ligaments. Exercise in early pregnancy and post-partum can offset the resulting looseness of joints by increasing their muscular support.

*Sacrum:* The triangular part of the pelvis between the coccyx and last vertebra of the spinal column. Counterpressure is often helpful over this area during labor.

*Sphincter:* A ring-like muscle closing openings of the body such as the anus, vagina.

*Station:* Term which refers to the relative position of the baby to the mother's bony pelvis.

*"Stripping of Membranes":* Doctor places a finger inside the cervix and moves it around to free any adhesions of the amniotic sac. This removes the mucus plug and is an artifical stimulation of labor.

*Term:* Completed cycle of pregnancy.

*Toxemia:* A disease of pregnancy. Symptoms, in combination, are: high blood pressure, excess fluid retention and protein (albumin) in the urine.

*Transition:* The phase from 8 to 10 cms. dilation at the end of the first stage of labor. Usually the strongest contractions of all.

*Uterus:* Hollow muscular organ which expands as the baby grows and contracts during labor to open the cervix and then expel the baby and afterbirth.

*Vagina:* The birth canal. It is an expandable passage, softened during pregnancy, leading from the vulva to the uterus.

*Vernix:* The white, greasy substance covering the newborn. It protects the baby from the amniotic fluid and eases delivery.

*Vertex:* Top or crown of the head.

*Vulva:* The external lips or folds surrounding the vaginal entrance.

215

*Excerpt's From Handout*

# *Planning Your Baby's Birth*

*by Penny Simkin and Carla Reinke*

## *Choices in Childbirth*

| MEDICAL PATHWAY | PHYSIOLOGIC PATHWAY |
|---|---|

*(Which of these are routines and which are options in your hospital or birth center? Most parents choose some options from each list.)*

*Labor*

- Mother in wheelchair upon arrival at hospital.
- Shave, minishave, or clipping of long hairs on perineum.
- Enema.

- Partner is asked to leave during prep and exams.

- Mother walks to labor and delivery.
- No shave or clipping of hair.
- Bowels emptied spontaneously, or enema self-administered at home.

- Partner present throughout labor and delivery.

216

- Limit to one support person during labor and birth.
- Confinement to bed and/or one position.
- Induction of Labor.
  Methods: Stripping membranes, amniotomy, oxytocin.
- IV fluids for hydration and energy.
- Frequent vaginal exams.
- Electronic Fetal Heart Monitor.
- Pain Relief through medication: analgesics or anesthetics.

- Presence of other friends, relatives, and siblings.
- Freedom to walk and change positions as desired.
- Spontaneous Labor.
  Alternatives: Making love, breast stimulation.
- Drinking fluid or eating as desired.
- Vaginal exams when requested by mother or for medical reasons.
- Listening to fetal heart with fetal stethoscope.
- Relaxation, emotional support, massage, breathing.

*Birth*

- Lithotomy position or semi-sitting in labor bed for pushing.
- Prolonged breathholding and bearing down for expulsion.
- Limit of two hours on second stage—then forceps or cesarean birth.
- Delivery table for birth.
- Lithotomy position with stirrups for birth.
- Mother not allowed to touch sterile field.
- Catheterization in second stage.
- Episiotomy.

- Forceps or vacuum extraction.

- Choice of position and freedom to move.
- Mother follows her urge to push.
- Allow for longer second stage and position variations to help progress.
- Birth in labor bed, birth chair, or bean bag.
- Sidelying, all fours, squatting, standing with leg up, semi-reclining with back support, no stirrups.
- Mother allowed to touch baby's head as it crowns.
- No catheterization and frequent voiding in first stage.
- No episiotomy: massage, warm compresses, slower delivery, coaching to pant out baby, support to perineum.
  Late episiotomy with no enesthesia.
- Spontaneous delivery.

217

## After Birth

- Intubation I Suctioning.
- Immediate care of baby done out of sight of mother: e.g., identification, Apgar, heat lamp, replace hemostate with cord clamp.
- Limit of 15-20 minutes on third stage followed by manual extraction of the placenta.
- Pitocin drip or injection for contraction of uterus after placenta is born.

- Waiting to see if baby can handle own mucus.
- Care done on mother's abdomen. Baby skin to skin with mother with heat lamp or blanket over them. Delay in non-essential routines.
- Allow for longer time for placenta. Allow mother to move around, nurse baby. Let cord drain.
- Evaluation of uterus before using uterine stimulant routinely.
  Breastfeeding.

## Baby

- Baby to isolette or nursery for 4-24 hours. Mother to recovery room for observation.
- Eye drops – silver nitrate applied shortly after birth.
- Baby's first feeding – glucose water by nurse.
- Baby in Nursery except for scheduled 4 hour feedings.
- Circumcision.
- Home in three or more days after delivery.

- Baby held by mother or father on delivery table and/ or in recovery.
- Omit eye drops or delay administration up to 2 hours. Use of other agent as alternative.
- Colostrum by mother who plans to breastfeed or plain water given by mother.
- Demand feeding, baby to mother when crying. Twenty-four hour rooming in.
- No circumcision.
  Parents present to comfort baby after operation.
- Early discharge from hospital.

## The Unexpected

## COMMON MEDICAL PROCEDURES

## POSSIBLE OPTIONS

### Cesarean Birth

- Scheduled surgery.
- Mother without her support person in surgery.
- General anesthesia.
- Screen to prevent viewing surgery.

- Mother not allowed to wear contacts or glasses.
- Baby sent to Intensive Care Nursery.

- Surgery after labor begins.
- Father present to support mother.
- Spinal or epidural.
- Screen lowered at time of birth or baby held up for mother and father to see.
- Mother to wear contacts or glasses.
- Father to hold baby and mother to see baby, if baby is not in distress.

Mother allowed to breastfeed in recovery if her and her baby's condition permit.

### Premature/Sick Infant

- Baby cared for by professionals.

- Baby rushed to intensive care.
- Baby sent to another hospital or another part of hospital.
- Baby transported to hospital with intensive care unit.

- Limited visits to baby from mother only.
- IV and bottle feeding.

- Parents involved in care of baby, diapering, touching, talking to baby in incubator, feeding baby.
- Mother allowed to hold and see baby, if not distressed.
- Baby close to mother; in same part of hospital.

- Father goes with the transport team, mother goes if she is able.
- Father and/or extended family allowed to see baby.
- Mother allowed to express her colostrum for the baby and encouraged and helped to get started at breastfeeding.

Copyright © 1980, by *The Pennypress*

219

# A Patient's Bill Of Rights*

1. The patient has the right to considerate and respectful care.
2. The patient has the right to obtain from his physician complete current information concerning his diagnosis, treatment, and prognosis in terms the patient can be reasonably expected to understand. When it is not medically advisable to give such information to the patient, the information should be made available to an appropriate person in his behalf. He has the right to know by name, the physician responsible for co-ordinating his care.
3. The patient has the right to receive from his physician information necessary to give informed consent prior to the start of any procedure and/or treatment. Except in emergencies, such information for informed consent should include but not necessarily be limited to the specific procedure and/or treatment, the medically significant risks involved, and the probable duration of incapacitation. Where medically significant alternatives for care or treatment exist, or when the patient requests information concerning medical alternatives, the patient has a right to such information. The patient also has the right to know the name of the person responsible for the procedures and/or treatment.
4. The patient has the right to refuse treatment to the extent permitted by law, and to be informed of the medical consequences of his action.
5. The patient has the right to every consideration of his privacy concerning his own medical care program. Case discussion, consultation, examination, and treatment are confidential and should be conducted discreetly. Those not directly involved in his care must have the permission of the patient to be present.

220

6. The patient has the right to expect that all communications and records pertaining to his care should be treated as confidential.
7. The patient has the right to expect that within its capacity a hospital must make reasonable response to the request of a patient for services. The hospital must provide evaluation, service, and/or referral as indicated by the urgency of the case. When medically permissible, a patient may be transferred to another facility only after he has received complete information and explanation concerning the needs for and alternatives to such a transfer. The institution to which the patient is to be transferred must first have accepted the patient for transfer.
8. The patient has the right to obtain information as to any relationship of his hospital to other health care and educational institutions insofar as his care is concerned. The patient has the right to obtain information as to the existence of any professional relationships among individuals, by name, who are treating him.
9. The patient has the right to be advised if the hospital proposes to engage in or perform human experimentation affecting his care or treatment. The patient has the right to refuse to participate in such research projects.
10. The patient has the right to expect reasonable continuity of care. He has the right to know in advance what appointment times and physicians are available and where. The patient has the right to expect that the hospital will provide a mechanism whereby he is informed by his physician or a delegate of the physician of the patient's continuing health-care requirements following discharge.
11. The patient has the right to examine and receive an explanation of his bill regardless of source of payment.
12. The patient has the right to know what hospital rules and regulations apply to his conduct as a patient.

*Approved by the House of Delegates of the American Hospital Association, February 6, 1973. Reprinted with the permission of the American Hospital Association.

# What It Feels Like To Be Pregnant: One Point Of View

*by Nan Koehler, 1974*

How do you know when you are pregnant? First, if you know when you are ovulating, you'll know whether it's possible to be pregnant or not. Second, if you're in touch with your body, you'll feel different, elated or depressed. The first weeks vary. Toward the end of the first month, your breasts begin to get sensitive. You'll miss your period or have a light one. The second and third month most women (I did anyway, and those I know) definitely feel badly. A friend of mine says hysterical is a better word. Your body is adjusting to very high levels of progesterone and estrogen. The uterus is growing and pressing on your bladder in such a way that you have to urinate all the time — or at least that's how it feels. This symptom is relieved somewhat when the uterus begins to grow up and out of the pelvis. The growing uterus also presses upward on the intestines and stomach so that the stomach is horizontal instead of slanted. This gives you heartburn, etc. Not everyone has these symptoms — it depends on how you eat (snacks or big meals) among other things. Also, the peristaltic action of the digestive track slows down so that food isn't moving through as fast as it was before. Some doctors think that's what causes morning sickness. Actually, when you are hungry and/or tired, nausea is more likely to be a problem. Sometimes the pigmentation of your skin changes. I've read that it is due to a folic acid deficiency what manifests during pregnancy. By the time you have your act together — more sleep, altering your diet to get more protein, vitamin C, calcium, magnesium, iron, and whatever else you need to feel "normal" again — the first trimester or the first three months of

222

pregnancy will be over. The psychologists have another view of this period of pregnancy. Many feel the physical symptoms manifest the mind getting used to being pregnant, but I think focusing on the nutritional aspects of pregnancy is easier to do something positive about, and feel better right away.

The second trimester is the proverbial best time of pregnancy. You know for sure that you are pregnant, having missed three periods; although, technically speaking, you aren't officially pregnant until someone can hear the heartbeat of the baby. All the other signs of pregnancy can be caused by something else! You can now rearrange your life accordingly. Many women find this a very horny time with their sexual interest elevated to new and unusual heights!

The last trimester is difficult again because the baby is getting so big that it's hard to get around, especially in and out of bed. Toward the end, women tend to get spacey and manifest a fantastic nesting urge. I did and everyone else I know did also. If you are lucky, you start laboring in the eighth month, slowly. My first baby came more or less abruptly. Although I had lightened or let down two weeks before (so I knew he was due), I had no Braxton-Hicks contractions (contractions of the uterus before labor) or effacement of the cervix (stretching and thinning). Lightening is when the baby drops (usually head down) into the pelvis shortly before birth. The longer the baby is in that position the more pointed his head will be at birth. Not all babies drop down two weeks before. Joshua, my second, didn't and his head was round at birth.

The first thing that happens in labor, aside from what I just wrote, is a crampy feeling at the base of the abdomen, like menstrual cramps. You also lose the mucus plug in the cervical opening. That's called "show." If you've been laboring awhile, the actual birth will go right into second stage (pushing) labor. Otherwise the uterus has a lot of work to do in a shorter amount of time. As far as I know, no one knows exactly what triggers a birth. It's thought that the placenta matures and initiates the labor. Also, your body has a dif-

223

ferent hormonal balance at the time of birth. Leboyer thinks this is triggered by the child who secretes adrenal hormones when it's ready to be birthed. The size of the baby stretches the uterine muscles to maximum capacity which may be what triggers the uterine contractions. Some women find the first sign that they are laboring is the rupturing of the amniotic sac. But those women I know to whom that's happened all experienced some symptoms of labor, but didn't recognize them as such.

The most important thing a woman can do when in labor is to stay loose or relaxed. The natural childbirth breathing exercises help fantastically. Among some people who have their babies at home, it's the practice to get very high or stoned or whatever and/or make love in early labor. If you remain sexually active as long as you can, you'll probably be looser. Birthing is in some ways like making love. Many of the responses are the same. All the muscles and organs involved are the same. A strong, well controlled Kegel muscle has beneficial results on both activities. Some women experience what's called "birth orgasm" when the baby presses on the clitoris on the way out. You'll never read this in the birth literature, but ask around and you'll hear that I'm not making this up! We all know about the horrors some women experience, but it doesn't help to focus on them. Statistically, they are very rare. Another aspect of birthing that connects it with lovemaking is the experience of those women who have pushed their babies into their husband's or friend's hands instead of a stranger's. It's much easier to spread your legs to someone you love!

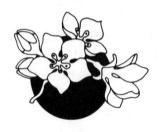

224

# General Instructions For Expectant Mothers

*by Bill Fischer*

## Things to do:

1. Eat a well-balanced diet, moderate protein, iron, vitamins and minerals. Read up on good nutrition and vitamin/ mineral supplements. Eat plenty of fresh fruit, vegetables, whole grains and protein foods.
2. Drink 8 to 10 glasses of water daily. Fruit juices diluted by ½ are good, as are herb teas. Liquids help keep you regular and unconstipated.
3. Get plenty of sleep—eight or more hours at night if you can, plus one or two short naps during the day. Never allow yourself to become totally fatigued during pregnancy. Prop feet up.
4. Exercise in the open air and sun. Walking a mile or so a day is great preparation for labor. Always stop short of fatigue.
5. Dress in loose clothing which does not constrict any part of your body's circulation.
6. Prepare your nipples for nursing. Attending La Leche League meetings and reading about breastfeeding are helpful.
7. Prepare your perineum (the area between your anal opening and your vaginal opening) for stretching by doing perineal massage and kegel exercises. Use no harsh soaps on your perineum and oil it once or twice daily with a pure oil, such as wheat germ oil or vegetable oil from a health food store. Use cotton instead of nylon underwear.

225

# Things to avoid:

1. Avoid white sugar and white flour—all refined food.
2. Avoid heavy use of caffein drinks such as coffee, tea, cola.
3. Avoid smoking cigarettes and being in enclosed areas where heavy smoke is accumulating. Speak up to smokers!
4. Avoid as much as you can the use of foods and beverages which are prepared with artificial colorings, flavor, preservatives and other additives of unknown potential. Read labels carefully.
5. Avoid douching and enemas unless definitely prescribed.
6. Avoid injections of live vaccine. Check carefully the danger potential before having any vaccinations/injections in pregnancy.
7. Avoid use of and contact with pesticides, poisons, volatile paints and varnishes, paint removers, certain glues and adhesives, smoke, soil known to be contaminated with weed killer or other contaminants, and all other chemicals or questionable products. Be alert to such hazards without becoming paranoid!
8. *Avoid rare or raw meat* when pregnant. *Be careful handling cat feces* such as in litter boxes. These are two routes of infections.
9. If you eat meat, especially liver, you may want to purchase the liver from a health food store to decrease the risks of DES concentrations in the liver. If you are concerned about this, do some reading to help you decide what to do.
10. *Avoid protein deficiency.* Use guides to monitor your protein intake. Most professionals recommend about 80 grams of protein daily for pregnant women. The added needs of the growing baby demand conscientious attention to diet.
11. *Avoid all x-rays during pregnancy* unless they are a matter of extreme, undelayable urgency. Always ask for a lead apron to cover your pelvic region *any time* you are x-rayed. During your childbearing years, the safest pro-

226

cedure is to be x-rayed only during your menstrual period (some say only during the first two weeks following a period, but even this is not safe for women who ovulate early or for an egg that has begun to ripen before ovulation). Refuse to be intimidated; do some research and reading. Try to avoid routine x-rays all your life and ask for a skin test instead. Always tell any doctor or medical technician you see that you are pregnant.

12. *Do not take any medication or drugs* when pregnant or nursing *unless it is absolutely unavoidable.* Remember that virtually no over the counter medicine or prescribed drug can be said to be completely safe for the fetus under all circumstances. The earlier it is in your pregnancy, the more vital this advice is. Remember that all of the following are *drugs:* aspirin, cough medicines, throat lozenges, indigestion tablets, sleeping preparations, diet pills, 'water' pills (diuretics), muscle relaxants, tranquilizers, allergy pills, laxatives, headache remedies, etc. etc. Do not use your baby as a guinea pig. Remember that doctors sometimes prescribe drugs for women without asking if you could be pregnant or are pregnant, so it is up to you to be sure that you don't take unnecessary drugs during pregnancy. If you have some illness or condition during pregnancy which seems to indicate drug treatment is necessary, take the time to research carefully before taking treatment. Ask the doctor to check, ask the pharmacist, check in journals, etc. Read *Life Before Birth* by Ashley Montague, and *Your Baby's Brain Before Birth* by Rosen. Especially no aspirin; it interferes with the chemistry of labor and can cause bleeding in the baby.

If you are pregnant and have done some of the 'avoid' things mentioned here, do not become alarmed, but put it in perspective of the whole pregnancy. These are important guides to follow, but not following any of them does not automatically point to problems. For instance, many women who smoke have given birth to perfectly healthy babies — but you still should be made aware that smoking does increase the hazards to the baby. Choices should always be "informed" choices.

These instructions are good for all potentially pregnant *(any woman having intercourse without continual, careful use of reliable contraception)*, as well as pregnant women. The first three months of your pregnancy are the most crucial to fetal development.

# Maintaining Health During Pregnancy

*by Nan Koehler, 1975*

There are many minor discomforts accompanying pregnancy which I always thought were "normal." Recently (during and after my third pregnancy), I've come to hold a different opinion regarding almost all of them. For example, I would read that the discoloration of the skin, especially the facial skin (the mask of pregnancy) was a normal symptom of pregnancy. It is not normal; it is a lack of folic acid.

Pregnancy is a time of stress for the body and any inherent metabolic weakness will show up at that time. Everyone has unique nutritional needs which depend on their personal body chemistry and their life-long eating and living habits. Pregnancy will make them manifest! It does not always help to follow a minimum daily requirement chart, because everyone's needs are different. Each woman has to figure it out for herself. I would recommend reading *Nutrition in a Nutshell* by Roger Williams or *Nutrition Against Disease* also by Roger Williams. A very handy tool for figuring out dietary imbalances is the *Vita-Wheel* sold at the Evelyn Porter Health Food Chain. They are made by Health Wheels, Inc., P.O. Box 4942, Irvine, CA 92664.

228

Maintaining Health During Pregnancy

Here are some of the minor disorders listed in Margaret F. Myles, *Textbook for Midwives*, 7th edition, Churchill Livingstone, London, 1971, p. 131: 1) Morning sickness, 2) heartburn, 3) constipation, 4) backache, 5) varicose veins, 6) hemorrhoids, 7) itching skin, 8) fainting (which I won't mention since it is rare!) and I would add three more: 9) skin discoloration, 10) fatigue, and 11) depressions.

1) Morning sickness. Myles says it may be endocrine in origin or it may be due to "disturbance in metabolism of glucose" with an increased production of ketone bodies and ketosis cause vomiting especially when glucose intake is low. Her remedy is to eat a snach before bed and then tea and biscuits before rising (preferably served by the husband!) that is the standard remedy and usually it works. I have had morning sickness when I was nervous, tired, or hungry. All three together and I would be nauseated for sure. The best remedy for me has been more sleep and the addition to my diet of vitamin B complex, more protein, and calcium magnesium. Another remedy for nausea is to drink the juice of a lemon or peach-leaf tea. 2) Heartburn. This condition is caused by the enlarging uterus displacing the stomach upwards through a diaphram weakened by fatigue. The recommended remedy is to eat smaller meals, drink milk as the last thing before retiring *and sleep more.* Eating raw apple peels is what my mother recommends for heartburn. 3) Constipation. Myles says this is due to the relaxing effect of progesterone on the peristalic action of the intestinal muscles. For me, the best remedy is exercise and rest. Constipation can be due to fatigue. Eat popcorn every night! Add B vitamins, vitamin E, potassium, and especially pantothenic acid to your diet. Also, drink more water. 4) Backache and 5) Varicose veins. No matter how active we think we are, compared to what our bodies are built for, we are terribly sedentary. Both these last two symptoms are the result of not getting enough strenuous exercise. For lower backache from pelvic engorgement, orgasmic release is often the answer. For backaches, also make sure you have

229

enough vitamin C, D, calcium magnesium, and protein in your diet. Drink red raspberry tea as a muscle toner. For varicose veins, take vitamins B, C, and E, plus rutin, lecithin, and spend some time with your legs up. 6) Hemorrhoids. These result from hard feces and lack of muscle tone. Do Kegel exercises and drink more fluids. Make sure you are getting enough vitamins A, $B^6$ and E. Never put off going to the toilet. 7) Itching skin and 8) Itching vulva. It could be that the body is getting rid of wastes. Drink more liquids (two-three quarts of water per day), especially cleansing teas such as alfalfa or dandelion. Be sure the skin and clothes are clean. Sometimes an itchy vulva means one is horny and the best remedy is seminal fluid. Make sure you are taking enough B vitamins. Also smear the vaginal lips with yoghurt as a remedy for itching. 9) Skin discoloration. This condition can result from a lack of folic acid or para-aminobenzioic acid. 10) Fatigue. Take an organic iron, not iron sulfate! Eat organ meats like liver if you are eating meat. 11) Depression. This could be due to many factors. The first thing to consider is whether you have a lack of protein, or second, B vitamins, especially $B^6$ and $B^1$.

Some people may argue that many of these pregnancy discomforts are normal. For me, it has been better to focus on my diet for quick results rather than to accept these symptoms as normal. The body and mind are one and I have discovered that when my body is functioning well, my mind and spirit follow along!

In closing, I would recommend a small book by Jane Kinderlehrer, *Confession of a Sneaky Organic Cook.* Happy pregnancy!

# Common Discomforts Of Pregnancy

by Mary Weiner

There are some common discomforts which may occur at one time or another during pregnancy. Of course, prevention is always preferrable to cure, so ways of possible avoidance are mentioned as well as remedies. The effectiveness of the following remedies varies greatly. If one doesn't work, try another.

## BLEEDING GUMS

Causes—increased blood volume, hormonal changes, inadequate diet

Prevention/remedies—massage gums, floss, use soft tooth brush; increase foods rich in vitamin C, D, $B^6$, calcium vitamin C supplement

## CONSTIPATION

Causes—poor diet; not enough exercise; inadequate calcium absorption; hormonal changes; pressure of uterus on lower intestinal tract

Prevention/remedies—chew food thoroughly; leafy green salad daily; lots of fresh fruits; whole grains, bran; yogurt or kefir daily; increase fluid intake; daily exercise; one cup prune juice daily, at room temperature; limit muscle meats to 2-3 times weekly; calcium/magnesium supplement; tea of senna leaf, alfalfa, dandelion and cascara

CRAMPS are painful spasmodic muscular contractions in the legs (usually the calves, but occasionally the outer thighs).

Causes—pressure of enlarged uterus on nerves supplying the legs; change in calcium and phosphorous balance in muscles; slowed circulation; may be aggravated by poor posture and chilling

231

Prevention—elevate legs and keep them warm; don't point toes; warm milk at bedtime; calcium/magnesium tablets taken with vitamin C before meals; adequate vitamin D (sunshine); exercises to improve circulation (squat, pelvic rock, tailor sit, elevate legs)

Remedies—force toes upward and make pressure on knee to straighten leg; just below site of cramp, stroke evenly and firmly with your knuckles toward the heart

*FATIGUE, SLEEPINESS*

Causes—stress of change; great increase in progesterone, a hormone which relaxes smooth muscles

Prevention/remedies—regular rest periods during day; use relaxation techniques at intervals; proper diet; Brewer's yeast and/or liver

*GAS*

Cause—usually undesirable intestinal bacteria

Prevention/remedies—small frequent meals; chew food thoroughly; avoid constipation; avoid gas-forming foods; yogurt or kefir daily to build "friendly" bacteria in intestines

*HEADACHE*

Causes—tension, fatigue

Prevention/remedies—regular, adequate rest; relaxation techniques; fresh air and deep breathing; tea made with 2 parts camomile and 1 part rose hips; camomile compress to forehead and back of neck

*HEARTBURN* is a burning sensation beginning behind the breast bone and going upward to the throat. Contrary to the implication, it has nothing to do with the heart. Burping, nausea, acid regurgitation and pressure in the stomach area may be present as well.

Causes—pregnant uterus displaces stomach upward; gastric juice backs up into esophagus (food tube); worry, fatigue, improper diet may contribute to its intensity

Prevention/remedies—small frequent meals; avoid greasy, fried and highly-seasoned food; raw apple; peppermint tea with honey or licorice tea; sips of hot water or milk; at night use 2-3 pillows under your head and shoulders or side-lying position; charcoal tabs. ***DO NOT take antacids or baking soda as the sodium content tends to inhibit digestion and absorption of B vitamins and cause gas and water retention.

*HEMORRHOIDS* are veins at the anal opening which are engorged with old blood. They usually disappear after the birth.

Causes — pressure interfering with proper return circulation from the pelvic area; weak perineal muscle; improper diet; constipation

Prevention/remedies — increase Kegel and pelvic rocks; proper toilet position and avoid straining; diet high in roughage and B vitamins (fresh fruit, bran, whole grains, yogurt, blackstrap molasses); drink plenty of fluids; vitamin E and C supplements; three cups corn silk tea and 200 mg. niacinamide daily for 2-3 days; mix crushed garlic with cocoa butter or coconut oil, place in jar with loose lid, put in pan of cold water, simmer 10 minutes, then apply while still warm.

*ITCHING*

Cause — stretching of skin on abdomen and breasts

Prevention/remedies — wear soft clothing next to skin; rub in lanolin, cocoa butter or natural oil; often aggravated by laundry detergent, fabric softeners, etc.; bathe in parsley, rosemary flowers, sage, plantain, comfrey, sarsaparilla, dandelion, lavendar, lobelia

*NAUSEA* or "morning sickness" is usually confined to between the fourth and fourteenth weeks and occurs in about half of pregnant Western women. It usually occurs only in the morning but sometimes lasts throughout the day, especially at mealtime. ***If vomiting occurs, be sure to drink plenty of fluids to avoid dehydration. If it persists, call your health care person.

Causes — anxiety; mere anticipation of nausea; low blood sugar; inadequate B vitamins

Prevention/remedies—try to keep your life peaceful; small frequent meals and snacks high in protein and B vitamins; limit sweets; animal fats, heavy and fried foods; vitamin $B^1$ and B6 5 mg. each daily taken with Brewers yeast or B complex; vitamin $B^6$ 10 mg. with magnesium 50 mg. three times daily; peppermint, spearmint or peach leaf tea (small amount lobelia may be added); cup of water with 1 tsp. apple cider vinegar and honey on awakening, then rest before getting up; hot water; warm milk; juice; Tongue Pull (This may seem very strange, but it sometimes works when nothing else does. Using a handkerchief or any dry cloth, grasp your tongue and pull it straight out until it feels quite uncomfortable. Hold it for 30 seconds.)

*SHARP SENSATION IN GROIN* is usally a cramping of the round ligament which anchors the uterus.

Prevention/remedy—don't favor one side of body; avoid strain

*SHORTNESS OF BREATH*

Cause—uterus presses on the diaphragm

Prevention/remedies—don't lie flat on your back; pelvic rock position to allow uterus to fall forward; go into relaxation; be calm

*SLEEPLESSNESS* is common in late pregnancy.

Causes—baby's position and size; displaced organs; insufficient calcium: nature's way of preparing us for new motherhood

Prevention/remedies—calcium magnesium supplement before going to bed; warm milk; tea made with equal parts of scullcap, catnip, hops and camomile; soak in hot bath with warm drink and candlelight to make you relaxed and sleepy; OR stay up for awhile and read, sew, cook, write letters, etc. until you're sleepy.

*VAGINAL DISCHARGE* is often increased during pregnancy. \*\*\*If there is intense itching, strong odor, or if it is profuse, you probably have a vaginal infection. There are several kinds, and treatment may be different for each. If you begin the remedies and baths as soon as you notice itching and

234

the symptoms are not relieved in two days, consult your health care person. It is very important to identify an infection early. The longer you delay, the more difficult it is to cure. Your baby could pick it up on the way out, so it is very important to take care of it before labor begins.

Causes — hormonal changes of pregnancy; infection may be present

Prevention — air or sunshine on the perineal area; don't wear panties or wear ones with cotton crotch area; cleanse area with water at least once daily; wipe properly after bowel movement from front to back

Remedies — as above; sit in a warm bath containing 1 cup white vinegar for 20 minutes three times daily

*VARICOSED VEINS*

Causes — pressure interfering with return circulation from legs and pelvis; walls of veins become weakened; improper diet; inadequate exercise; hereditary tendency

Prevention — exercises which increase lower body circulation (pelvic rock, squat, tailor sit, elevate legs); well-balanced diet rich in roughage, vitamin C and E; avoid standing in one place; regular exercise (walking, swimming)

Remedies — as above; support stockings (not ace bandages as they do not give even support); vitamin E and C supplements, also rutin and niacinamide; marigold tea and bath

***If a discomfort persists, consult your health care person.*

# *Signs To Report*

- unusual or severe headache
- burning or painful urination or frequent urination in second trimester
- nausea and vomiting after fourth month
- fever, chills
- discharge of clear fluid or blood from vagina
- extreme swelling of hands, feet, legs, face
- blurred vision

© 1976 Enterpoint Foundation.

235

# Recipes For Minor Complaints During Pregnancy

*by Ginny Woods*

## Morning Sickness

- Consider emotional needs and outlets
- Well balanced diet
- Hormonal changes make the lady a walking hormone
- Eat small, frequent meals. Avoid heavy spices, dairy and meats
- Munch dry toast or crackers before getting out of bed
- Brewers yeast is very helpful
- Miso and seaweed soup, watermelon, yams
- Liquids half hour before or after meals

HERBS:

Tea #1
| | |
|---|---|
| 1 tsp. Catnip | Steep 20 minutes, covered, in |
| 1 tsp. Peppermint | 1 cup water. Add lemon or honey to taste. Drink hot. |

Tea #2
| | |
|---|---|
| 1 tsp. Basil | Steep 20 min. in 1 cup water, |
| 1 tsp. Tansy | covered. Take 1 Tbsp. half |
| 1/4-1/2 tsp. Ginger (to taste) | hour before meals. |

Tea #3
| | |
|---|---|
| 1 tsp. Wormwood | Steep 20 min. in 1 cup water, |
| 1 Tbsp. Red Raspberry Leaves | covered. Take 1-3 Tbsp. before meals. |

236

Tea #4
   2 tsp. each Peppermint, Hops, Lemon Balm, Camomile

Steep 20 min. in 1 quart water, covered. Drink as desired for nausea.

Tea #5
   1 tsp. Goldenseal powder

Steep 20 min. in 1 cup water, covered. Stir and strain. Take 1 tsp. tea for nausea. DO NOT take more than 6 tsp. in a 24 hour period or use more than 3 days in a row as goldenseal is cumulative in the body and larger amounts cause abortion.

## Constipation

- Avoid strong cathartics
- Take 1-2 Tbsp. olive oil daily
- Prune, fig, apple, rhubarb juice daily
- 2 quarts liquid daily
- Consider emotional blockages and needs. The emotions rule the intestines.

HERBS:

Tea #1
   For daily use for constipation
   2 Tbsp. Fennel seeds, crushed

Steep in 1 pint water for 20 min.

Tea #2
   4 tsp. Cascara Sagrada

Steep 20 min. in 1 quart water. Drink 1-2 cups before the first meal of the day.

Tea #3
   1 Tbsp. White Oak Bark     Simmer, covered, for 10
                              min. in 1 pint water. Drink
                              1-2 cups daily, before meals.

Tea #4
   1-2 tsp. Uva Ursi          Steep in 1 pint water for 30
                              minutes. Drink 1/2 cupful
                              every 4-6 hours as needed.
                              This herb is oxytoxic in large
                              amounts.

Tea #5
   1 tsp. Buckthorn           Steep 30 min. in 1 pint water.
   1 tsp. Red Raspberry       Drink 1-2 cups daily.
      Leaves
   1/8 tsp. Lobelia

# Mask Of Pregnancy

- Caused by excessive stress on the adrenals.
- Include Brewers yeast, panothenic acid, and whole wheat products in the diet.

HERBS:

Tea
   1 tsp. Scullcap            Steep for 20 min. in 1 pint
   1 tsp. Hops                water. Drink 1/2 cup 4 times
   1 tsp. Valerian            a day.

# Dental Decay

- Due to hormonal changes and fetal demands
- Avoid sugar, molasses, honey, and excessive use of dry fruits.
- Floss teeth daily, brush 2-3 times a day, massage gums and brush tongue and cheeks.

238

- Green Clay water mouthwash. Place 1 tsp. green French clay in 1/2 glassful water. Set in the sun for at least 1-2 hours before use.

HERBS HIGH IN MINERALS FOR TEETH:
- Fresh Comfrey leaves and Nettles
- Teas daily of any of these herbs—Comfrey, Nettles, Oak Straw, Horsetail Fern, Camomile, Borage. Steep 1 ounce herb in 1 pint water for 3/4 hour. Drink daily.

## Tissue Edema

- Rest off feet for 20 minutes doing this 3-4 times a day.
- Salt food to taste, avoiding excessive use
- Exercise, yoga, pelvic rocks and walking daily.
- Eliminate sugars
- Include Yucca tablets, complex supplement or foods, such as brewers yeast in diet

HERBS:
- High potassium herbs such as Alfalfa (sprouts are best), fresh Parsley, and Comfrey
- Teas of Comfrey, Parsley, and Uva Ursi
  For Uva Ursi tea use 1-2 tsp. in 1 pint water and drink 1/2 cup 4 times daily. For other herbs use 1 ounce to 1 pint.

## Hemmorhoids

- Caused by constipation, emotional blockages, poor muscle tone, fetal pressures, vitamin E deficiency
- Maintain soft stools and regularity
- Increase bulk foods
- 200-400IU vitamin E daily
- Increase foods rich in vitamins A, B, E
- 100 kegal exercises daily
- For itching, use compresses of fresh raw Ginger. Mash and place directly on area. Witch Hazel herb works well too.

239

# Heartburn

- Eat small, frequent meals and take liquids between meals
- Avoid sugars, white flour products, fried foods, sodium bicarbonate, and heavy spices
- Papaya and papaya tablets (1-2 per meal) are beneficial

HERBS:

Tea

| | |
|---|---|
| 1 tsp. Peppermint | Steep in 1 cup water for 20 min. |
| Tincture of Peppermint | 5 drops in 1/4 cup water, taken all at once. Repeat as necessary. |

# Backache

- Pelvic rocks, hands and knees position, yoga, massage and sleep on firm surface.
- Include brewers yeast, vitamins C, D, and minerals in daily diet
- Orgasms are good for relieving pelvic congestion

HERBS:

Use high mineral herbs like Borage, Nettles, Oak Straw, Comfrey, Camomile, Parsley, Watercress. These teas can be used 1 oz. to 1 pint water, steep for 3/4 hour, covered. Many of these herbs are best eaten fresh.

# Varicose Veins

- Increase vitamins C and E, and include lecithin and rutin in daily foods.
- Green peppers eaten raw
- Elevate legs above hips three times daily for 20 minutes.

240

## Skin Itching

- Due to stretching of skin and possibly an internal cleansing
- Massage olive, apricot, avocado or almond oil into the skin daily.
- Include more vitamin E foods in diet. E can also be massaged into the skin.

HERBS:
- Use herbs which will further the cleansing process
- Eat fresh or drink as teas daily: Parsley, Alfalfa, Wheatgrass, Comfrey, Watercress. Use 1 oz. herb to 1 pint water.

## Irritability

- Consider emotional and sleep needs
- Vitamin B foods: wheat germ, brewers yeast, whole grains, dairy foods.
- Perhaps a good cry

HERBS:
- Calming herbs are helpful: Catnip, Lemon Balm, Camomile, Hops, Valerian, Scullcap, Comfrey, Peach Leaves and Red Raspberry Leaves.

## Vaginal Itch

- Much more common during pregnancy
- 1 tsp. pure plain yogurt swabbed about the vagina 2-3 times a day.
- Acidophilus tablets or drink, yogurt, miso, sauerkraut
- No douching

Reprinted with permission of Ginny Woods. She is married (18 years) with four children, boy 14, girl 11, boy 4, girl 3. She's been an RN for 16 years, midwife for 14 years, attended over 1500 births. She also studies and practices herbology, homeopathy, acupressure. Ginny is currently practicing midwifery. Her mailing address is 20278 Pleasant Valley Road, Smartville, CA 95977.

# Source of Headaches

*Taken from an old herbal, author unknown*

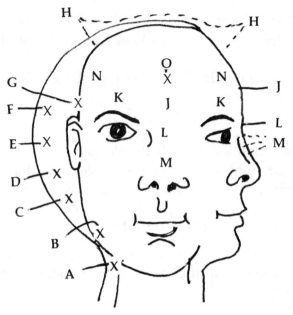

A — Pain and aches at upper side of neck/lower jaw may indicate pharyngitis, laryngitis, diptheria, or trigomonial neuralgia.

B — Aches below lateral of C may indicate nervous disorders, stomach troubles, spinal irritation, impending rheumatism or disease of cervical vertebra.

C — Ache at back of neck, near base of brain may indicate nervous disorders, nephritis, diseases of spinal cord or middle ear disease.

D — Ache at mastoid processes may indicate mastoid troubles, pus etc.

E — Ache near and below F may indicate constipation causativeness.

F — Ache at center back of head may indicate eye trouble-refraction myopia.

G — Ache at back side of head over ears may indicate poor blood or uterine trouble.

242

H—Ache over entire top of head may indicate female disorders, bladder trouble, hysteria, neurasthenia, anemia, chlorosis, epilepsy, or ovarian trouble.

J—Ache in center of forehead just above L may indicate trouble with nose, eyes, or intestines.

K—Aches over or around each eye may indicate dyspepsia, stomach trouble or occular disturbance.

L—Ache above bridge, between eyebrows may indicate constipation, stomach trouble, faulty refraction or decayed teeth.

M—Ache around eye and bridge of nose may indicate stomach, eye, or nose trouble.

N—Ache of bandlike character around forehead may indicate anemia.

O—Ache in upper center of forehead may indicate cattarre of nose or throat.

To help with all of the above conditions, drink more water!

# Pregnancy and Childbirth, Nature's Way

*by Rosemary Sutton*

"Nothing is so beautiful as a ship at full sail, or a woman great with child."

When a woman is pregnant and "great with child," she feels, with deep heart's instinct, her oneness with the flow of creation, the birth/death cycle. Divine Mother sends her gifts of guidance to her daughters: the strengthening and healing herbs, grasses, and flowers. Almost half-remembered in their use.

243

Tonic teas should be drunk throughout pregnancy, to insure an easy birthing. Raspberry leaf tea is the tried and true tonic to the uterus, as are squaw vine and wild yam root. For the unsettled stomach, which is sometimes felt in the early months, teas of fennel leaf or seed, wild yam root, mint, or a pinch of golden seal are in order.

Nutritional requirements are high during pregnancy. Calcium is essential for bone and tooth formation: good sources are salads of amaranth, borage, comfrey, coriander, dandelion, mustard greens, and watercress. Iron is found in these too, and in chives and burdock root. Folic acid is abundant in all leafy greens.

Begin early to condition the skin, preparing for smooth stretching. Add a strong tea of comfrey leaf or root to the bath, or take as a sitz bath. After bathing, body oil is helpful to lubricate the skin and maintain its elasticity. An oil I like is made by *gently* heating together 2 cups of oil (olive, sesame, almond, or the like) with a handful each of elder blossoms and comfrey. Part of the oil could be wheat germ oil or capsules of Vitamin E could be opened and added. The heat of a summer's day, or perhaps two, is enough to steep the oil. After cooling, add finely crushed pollen, an incredible skin builder, and a few drops of a pure essential oil, for the senses.

The perineum, the skin below the vagina, should be conditioned throughout pregnancy with sunlight, fresh air, and massage with the body oil. If it should tear, a poultice of good ole comfrey (fresh, preferably) will be healing.

As your time approaches, have your medicine chest well stocked. Have on hand pennyroyal leaf and oil, tansy, and blue cohosh. These herbs, valued as they are for bringing on a delayed menstrual flow, are not normally called upon in pregnancy. But if you wish to hasten a long labor, or bring on labor when the water has broken, but contractions not yet begun, then use these herbs. The scent of the pennyroyal oil would be inhaled, or the oil could be poured in simmering water to vaporize the room. The pennyroyal leaf, tansy, and blue cohosh would be taken as teas.

For normal labor, a gentle relaxant tea of chamomile and catnip, flavored with hibiscus flowers, is useful to moisten dry lips and face, and is a delicious celebration drink later.

The little stem of the umbilical cord will usually not need any special care. Comfrey leaves, crushed and wrapped inside a cabbage leaf could be laid across the navel (the origin maybe of the legend of finding the baby under a cabbage?). Indians of this area used mugwort leaves to hasten healing.

Milk will flow in abundance to the mother getting enough rest and good liquids. Fennel tea is a galactgogue: it increases the milk. An old legend says that placing pimpernel roots next to the breats will cause a copious flow. Sage and parsley tend to dry up the milk.

Remember that the essential oils of herbs, along with garlic and onions, are not, unlike other foods, filtered by the mother's body, but instead pass directly into her milk. The babe then receive the benefits and effects of all herbs the mother ingests. So if your colicky child refuses chamomile tea (though few will!), drink large amounts yourself and rest assured.

For sore nipples, mix the body oil with pure lanolin and rub in. If a breast infection develops, drink echinacea tea and take golden seal and myrrh gum capsules, as natural antibiotics. Hot poultices of potato, or alternate hot and cold applications of cloths wrung out in tea will give relief.

Bathing is a wonderfully relaxing experience after a full day of child care. Add a bit of pine needle essence to your bath to really unwind. To soothe the babe's skin, a gentle infusion of chamomile and bran can be strained and added to the water. Soap can irritate tender skin. If really dirty, the little one can be scrubbed with oatmeal tied in a kerchief. It forms a creamy liquid in water. Be sure to rinse well. Oiling the diaper area with good quality olive oil is a rash preventative.

Ideally, of course, each and everyone should have an herb garden: perhaps tucked amongst the vegatables and flowers, or a separate space, to wander in and dream of a babe's sweet face.

# Herbs and Pregnancy

## By Sherry Madrone

Pregnancy is a time of being close to the Earth. The nearness to seeds, flowers blossoming, nesting, harvest, and the flow of the seasons is obvious. Turn to the lessons of Nature and you will find a true friend. The natural leaf, flower, bark or root has none of the harmful side effects found in pharmaceuticals, which discard most of the plant and usually synthesize the remaining part which they think will give the same effect. The plant was created in its whole to provide the healing we seek.

Here are a few remedies and tonics which I've tried and found useful. They must always be accompanied by thankfulness and respect for their assistance.

*Morning Sickness:* Your body may be purifying and preparing for a healthy pregnancy. Avoid overeating. Omit white flour, sugar and salt if they are in your diet. Brew peach tree leaves, or peppermint or ginger and cinnamon, or raspberry leaves. Increase intake of Vitamin B.

*Prevent miscarriage:* Alfalfa, peppermint, rose hip tea.

*Water retention:* Burdock root tea, and *lots* of water! Drink 12 cups a day. Your kidneys will work better, and eliminate toxins.

*Calcium and Iron:* Amaranth, borage, comfrey, coriander, dandelion, mustard greens, watercress, nettles, burdock root, dock, kelp, parsley.

*Tonic:* Raspberry leaf: very important to drink throughout pregnancy. Flaxseed: enrich blood, strong nerves, laxative. Crush one tsp. and add a cup of boiling water.

*Prevent bleeding at birth:* eat alfalfa sprouts daily through pregnancy.

*Yeast infections:* Slippery elm, white oak bark, oatstraw. Equal parts. Douche and tea.*

*Trichimonas:* Yellow dock root, or chaparral and slippery elm douche.*

246

*Avoid:* blue cohosh, LSD, goldenseal, mistletoe, pennyroyal, tansy, osha, rue, and yarrow.

Make your labor a labor of love. Relax and totally surrender to the experience of a new being who has chosen you to come into this world through. Remember that Nature will take care of everything if you just relax and let it happen. Prepare your environment for this holy day. Hang live herbs about the room. Make wildflower and herb arrangements to soothe and protect you. Consider combinations of:

Sweet Woodruff: tonic and calm
Mint: strength
Rosemary: protection
Lavendar: ease birth
Marjoram: nerves
Bay Laurel: ease birth
Basil: nerves and nausea
Balm: calming
Borage: courage
Calendula
Clary Sage
Costmary

These herbs and others have been used around the world by women in labor.

Herbs were often crushed in the laboring woman's hand during contractions and the aroma would aid their birth. Perhaps a pillow made from herbs would be a welcome aid. Try a combination of:

Borage, for courage
Rosemary, to protect
Mint, to lift the spirit
Lavender or Camomile, to soothe

Some herbs can be burned to release their aroma, especially: rosemary, orris root, scotch pine, juniper, elecampane, mullein, lavender. This is especially nice to freshen the room during a long labor or after the birth.

*Prolonged labor:* Bathe with any of the forementioned herbs. Drink camomile and catnip tea if rest is in order. If you feel your strength is up and you wish to get your labor going stronger, drink blue cohosh tea and/or chew osha root. Do not use teas to hurry a labor due to your own impatience. This is an abuse of our natural friends, and a denial of the process of natural childbirth.

*Minimize bleeding:* alfalfa and sheperds purse tea.

*Expel Placenta:* angelica root, basil, feverfew, lavender.

*Stabilize blood pressure:* black cohosh, linden flowers, sheperds purse tea with honey. Low blood pressure is often due to dehydration and/or low blood sugar as well as loss of blood. Make sure you drink plenty of fluids during labor. Include juices. Keep your bladder empty.

*Heal tears or stitches:* Comfrey sitz baths four times a day for at least five days. Drink at least four cups of comfrey tea a day. You will find this such a soothing pleasure that you will look forward to it! Squirt comfrey tea over the area when you pee to avoid the stings too.

*Milk:* increase with blessed thistle, fenugreek seed, camomile, fennel, sassafrass, or hops. Decrease with parsley or sage.

*Mastitis:* Comfrey leaf poultice, or elderblossoms.

*Tea after birth:*
    angelica root: expel placenta
    comfrey or raspberry leaf: strength
    yarrow or sheperds purse: bleeding
    Mu Tea: balance

*Sore nipples:* rub with almond oil and honey, or hydrous lanolin. Start rubbing your nipples early in pregnancy and this should never be a problem. Rub vegetable oil with vitamin E or wheat germ oil into your abdomen daily during pregnancy too and stretch marks should be minimal.

*Renew Body:* with this combination brew: black cohosh for a uterine tonic; sarsparilla to strengthen the blood; licorice root as a laxative and for adrenal hormones; American

248

ginseng for hormones; false unicorn as a uterine tonic and squaw vine as a uterine tonic. Drink as a tea or cap or mix with honey or wrap in rice paper.

HAPPY BIRTHDAY!!

*If your doctor advises against douching, just sit in a pan of tea.

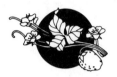

# Treating the Common Cold

*by Nan Koehler*

The genesis of most potentially serious ailments (ear infections, tonsillitis, mastitis, pneumonia, and fevers of all sorts) is the good old common cold. It can spiral into the "flu" and from that into any number of other ailments elaborately described in the medical texts. Good health doesn't just mean lack of a chronic condition, it means lack of that nagging recurring cold; it means feeling good all the time. I hope these suggestions will help you achieve that goal.

When using home remedies, it's important to CATCH IT EARLY! At the first sign of a cold, that vague uneasy feeling, usually centered in the stomach, often preceded by subtle intestinal upset of gas, *stop eating.* Headache, sore throat, weak limbs, crabbiness, free flowing mucus, or stomach ache mean you've already come down with a cold. To cure the cold by fasting is definitely the secret. Usually it takes only one meal; but, depending on how quickly you perceive what's happening to your body, it might mean fasting 24 hours. Along with the short fast, go to bed early and/or nap, drink lots of liquids — blood purifying teas are best (dandelion, alfalfa, peppermint, clover, comfrey, echinachea root (more potent), or mugwort which is heavy but very effective, and 2-3 quarts of water a day. Take extra vitamins: A (up to 100,000 IU/day), B complex (100 mg/day), C (1000 mg/hr.). Whenever taking vitamins, it's wise to take minerals as well: at least 1000 mg/day of calcium and 500 mg/day of magnesium. To restore intestinal balance take 1-2 tsp. of liquid acidophilus 3 times daily.

For really fast results, drink apple cider vinegar tea. In a quart of warm water put 2 tsp. of apple cider vinegar and sip continually, refilling as needed throughout the day. If you don't want to fast on the second day, do the alkaline diet (see attached sheet) until you feel perfectly normal.

Once you have a cold you have no choice but to do the complete 24 hour fast or your condition will take many days to resolve. For earache and swollen glands smear your throat with some kind of aromatic rub, put garlic in your ears either directly or as an oil. Nature's Herb Co. has a wonderful ear oil which you can drop in your ears to fumigate the sinuses. Then place cotton in your ears or a scarf over your head to keep the head warm and the garlic in place. Caution: whole garlic cloves must be sliced in their largest dimension then stabilized in the lower part of the outer ear with fumigant ointment so that it doesn't get stuck down in the ear canal or burn the ear tissue.

For headache, do a facial steam. Put an aromatic herb (Bay, Rosemary, or Camomile) in an enamel pot with a lid, bring to a boil and when you can smell the herb take the pot off the flame with the lid on. Put a towel over the pot, your head under the towel then take the lid off. Stay under that canopy as long as you can.

When you have a cold, your sensory input is dampened, your mind seems to work differently. Mother Nature intends that you "shut down," retreat within, and rest. A friend, Nancy Cohen, suggests colds "can be blocked sadness — a good cry can help a lot."

# Treating Hayfever and Allergies in General

*by Nan Koehler*

It will be much easier for you to "control" your body's reaction to "summer-coming" if you look inside yourself rather than outside for help. I mean inside your own body-system, your body-mind-spirit system. This is especially important for women who are pregnant, about to be pregnant, nursing or going through changes because the commercially available aids for hayfever are potential hazards to your health.

1. If you know that this is going to be a hard time of year for you, i.e. you are congested, have irritated eyes and a runny nose, headache, etc., then before it's all out-of-hand *get more rest.* Go to bed systematically an hour earlier than usual and try to rest some in the early afternoon. Your body can deal with everything better when it is well rested. (People with allergic tendencies have weak adrenal glands.)

2. Drink more water. Drink 4-6 quarts of water each day. Many of us are marginally dehydrated and especially anyone with breathing difficulties is bound to have this problem. Your mucus will be runnier and flow out more easily when you are well hydrated. Your kidneys and liver also work better to rid your body of toxic chemicals. Flush and sweat it out! You should be urinating every 2-3 hours, except at night.

3. Don't eat any starches, sugar, *or* honey. Just concentrate on fruits, vegetables and proteins. Begin doing this before your body is "over-the-hill." Anticipate the spring grass season and begin the rest, water, no starch regime before your symptoms are extreme. Nip it in the bud, in other

words.

If this regime doesn't work, then you might want to restrict your diet even more. This means doing an alkaline diet until you feel okay and then slowly introducing other foods—except for the starches, sugar, honey. An alkaline diet means no animal proteins (no butter, milk, cheese, eggs, or meat) rather mainly vegetables. (Most fruits are acid, but some aren't. Melons and bananas are alkaline.) I have a list of alkaline foods, or you can get one in any number of health food books.

4. To desensitize your body, you might want to make a tea of the flowering grasses (with yellow dock flowers) each day in a glass jar and sip that throughout the day to keep the level of the herb steady in your body—like you do when taking medicine four times a day. If you can do this, it is very very effective in minimizing hayfever symptoms.

5. Take an extra does of vitamins during this time. Vitamin C—2000 mg/day, Vitamin A—50,000 IU/day, Vitamin E—800 IU/day, B Complex—100 mg/day and some mineral suppliment. Take the vitamins two times a day with breakfast and dinner.

6. Some good books: *Goodbye Allergies*, Judge Tom Blaine; *Are you Confused?*, Paavo Airola; *Food Is Your Best Medicine*, Henry Bieler; *The Yeast Connection*, William G. Cook, M.D.; in *Mothering Magazine*, 29, Fall, 1983.

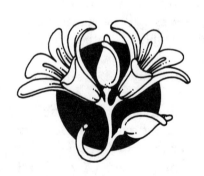

# Woman's Herbs

*Compiled by Nan Koehler, December, 1976*

## Menstruation

- Mugwort (tonic for all woman's disorders)
- Yarrow, Cranesbill (decreases excess flow)
- Wild carrots (increases flow)
- Clover (sooths nerves)
- Pennyroyal, Rue, Tansy, Cohoshes, Skullcap, Spicebush, White Cedar (cause contractions of the uterus)
- Parsley directly in the vagina promotes menstrual flow! It works.
- See "Other" for herbs used to relieve symptoms of menstruation.

## Prenatal

- Alfalfa (for juandice, anemia, constipation and toxemia)
- Clover (reduces acidity and helps iron assimilation)
- Squaw vine (*Mitchella Repens* — take in last two weeks of pregnancy)
- Plantain (for potash)
- Red Rasberry (tones uterine muscles)
- Comfrey (helps protein synthesis and general tonic)
- Mint, Peach leaf, Blackberries, Red Rasberry (used for nausea)
- You can order already capped: Red Rasberry, Pennyroyal, Squaw vine, Black Cohosh root, Lobelia, or Blessed Thistle from: Harmony Products (Prenatal Herbs) #7, South Gate, CA 90280

Take: 2 caps 4 times a day 5 weeks before birth, then 3 caps 4 times a day 2 weeks before birth.

253

# Birth

- My favorite Birth tea is: Basil, Lavender, Nutmeg, and Red Rasberry.
- Angelica root, Pennyroyal, Camomile, or Basil tea is used to expell placenta

# Afterbirth

- Comfrey (to heal the placental site)
- Plantain (same as Comfrey)
- Yarrow, Nettle (stops excess bleeding)
- Alfalfa (restores blood)
- All these are taken to aid nursing: Fennel, Camomile, Bedstraw, Filaree, Bayberry, Hops, Lavender, Milkwort, Blessed Thistle.
- Sage (makes milk taste bad)
- Good tea for increasing milk: Simmer in enamel pot ½ oz. each Marsh Mallow root, Star Anise and/or Anise seeds, Fennel seeds for 15 min. in 1 pt. water. Add Alfalfa and Borage steep for another 15 min. Sip throughout day.

# Other

- Mugwort (benefits all disorders)
- Wild carrot, plantain (use for bladder infections)
- *For constipation:* Rhubarb root, Camonile, Saffron, Catnip, Cascara sagrada, Licorice root, and *lots of water*
- Senna Pods (careful).
- *For vaginitis* (non-specific or yeast). Here are recipes for sitz baths. Choose the one you can do regularly.
  1. 4-5 tbp. acidophilus in qt. warm water 3-4 times a day
  2. or apple cider vinegar — ¼ c. in qt. warm water 3 times a day, then tapper off for two weeks or baking soda — if the vinegar doesn't work — 2 tsp. in qt. warm water
  3. or liquid chlorophyl, 2-3 tsp. in qt. water 3-4 times a day — decrease to two weeks

4. or tea made from Comfrey, Golden Seal, Camomile, and Sage ($\frac{1}{2}$ the amount). Serve 1-3 times a day. Mild every other day.
- *For Trichomonas:* Flagel (if you are pregnant you can't take flagel, but can keep the organisms under control by adding 3 cloves garlic to any of the vaginitis douches above)
- For all vaginitis, rest more, drink more water and take more vitamins. (Vitamins C, A & B's)

# Dr. Jensen's Balanced Daily Eating Regimen

Make a habit of applying the following General Diet Regimen to your everyday living. This is a healthy way to live *because*, when followed, you do not have to think of vitamins, mineral elements or calories. I will give you more specific instruction for your troubles after you have made this daily regimen automatic.

The best diet, over a period day, is two different fruits, at least four to six vegetables, one protein and one starch, with fruit or vegetable juices between meals. Eat at least two green leafy vegetables a day. 50% to 60% of the food you eat daily should be raw. Consider this regimen a dietetic law.

## Rules of Eating

1. Do not fry foods or use heated oils.
2. If not entirely comfortable in mind and body from the previous meal time, you should miss the next meal.
3. Do not eat unless you have a keen desire for the plainest food.
4. Do not eat beyond your needs.
5. Be sure to thoroughly masticate your food.
6. Miss meals if in pain, emotionally upset, not hungry, chilled, overheated, and during acute illness.

## *Impositions for Getting Well*

- Learn to accept whatever decision is made.
- Let the other person make a mistake and learn.
- Learn to forget and forgive.
- Be thankful and bless people.
- Live in harmony — even if it is good for you.
- Do not talk about your sickness.
- Gossip will kill you. Don't let anyone gossip to you either. Gossip that comes through the grape vine is usually sour.
- Be by yourself every day for ten minutes with the thought of how to make yourself a better person. Replace negative thoughts with uplifting, positive thoughts.
- Skin brush daily. Use a slant board daily.
- Have citrus fruit in sections only, never in juice form.
- Have only a limited amount of bread (with a lot of bowel trouble, no bread).
- Exercise daily. Keep your spine limber. Develop abdominal muscles. Do sniff breathing. Have a daily set of exercises.
- Grass walk and sand walk for happy feet.
- No smoking, drinking, spitting or cussing. Keep away from "spitty" people.
- Bed at sundown, 9 p.m. at the latest, if you are at all tired, fatigued and unable to do your work with vim and vigor. If you are sick you must rest more. Sleep out of doors, out of the city, in circulating air. Work out problems in the morning, don't take them to bed with you.

## *Food Healing Laws*

1. *Natural food* — 50% to 60% of the food eaten should be raw.
2. *Your Diet should be 80% alkaline and 20% acid.* Look at the acid — alkaline chart in "Vital Foods for Total Health," page 100.
3. *Proportion* — 6 vegetables daily, 2 fruits daily, 1 starch daily and 1 protein daily.

256

4. *Variety* — vary sugars, proteins, starches, vegetables and fruits from meal to meal and from day to day.
5. *Overeating* — you can kill yourself with the amount of food you eat.
6. *Combinations* — separate starches and proteins. One at lunch and the other at supper. Have fruits for breakfast and at 3:00 p.m.
7. *Cook without water* — Cook without high heat. Cook without air touching hot food.
8. *Bake, broil or roast* — If you eat meat, have it. Have lean meat, no fat, no pork. Use unpared vegetables if possible and eat them as soon after picked as possible.
9. *Use stainless steel, low-heat cooking utensils* — It is the modern health engineered way of preparing your foods.

. . . BEFORE BREAKFAST:

Upon arising, and one-half hour before breakfast, take any natural, unsweetened fruit juice, such as grape, pineapple, prune, fig, apple or black cherry. Liquid chlorophyl can be used — take 1 teaspoonful in a glass of water.

You can have a broth and lecithin drink if you desire it. Take 1 teaspoonful of vegetable broth powder and 1 table-spoonful of lecithin granules and dissolve in a glass of warm water.

On doctor's advice, you may have citrus fruits such as orange, grapefruit, lemon or tomato.

Between fruit juice and breakfast, follow this program:

Skin brushing, exercise, hiking, deep breathing or playing. Shower. Start warm and cool off until your breath quickens. Never shower immediately on arising.

BREAKFAST:

*Stewed fruit, one starch* and *health drink* or *two fruits, one protein* and *health drink*. (Starches and health drinks are listed with the lunch suggestions.) Soaked fruits, such as unsulphured apricots, prunes, figs. Fruit of any kind — melon, grapes, peaches, pears, berries or baked apple, which may be sprinkled with some ground nuts or nut butter. When possible, use fruit in season.

257

# Suggested Breakfast Menus

MONDAY
Reconstituted Dried Apricots
Steel-Cut Oatmeal — Supplements
Oat Straw Tea
Add Eggs, if desired.
*or*
Sliced Peaches
Cottage Cheese — Supplements
Herb Tea

TUESDAY
Fresh Figs
Cornmeal Cereal — Supplements
Shave Grass Tea
Add Eggs or nut butter, if desired.
*or*
Raw Apple Sauce and Blackberries
Coddled Egg — Supplemlents
Herb Tea

WEDNESDAY
Reconstituted Dried Peaches
Millet Cereal — Supplements
Alfamint Tea
Add Eggs, cheese or nut butter, if desired
*or*
Sliced Nectarines and Apple
Yogurt — Supplements
Herb Tea

THURSDAY
Prunes or any reconstituted dried fruit
Whole Wheat Cereal — Supplements
Oat Straw Tea
*or*
Grapefruit and Kumquats
Poached Egg — Supplements
Herb Tea

FRIDAY
Slices of Fresh Pineapple with
Shredded Coconut
Buckwheat Cereal — Supplements
Peppermint Tea
*or*
Baked Apple, Persimmons
Chopped Raw Almonds, Acidophilus Milk
Supplements
Herb Tea.

SATURDAY
Museli with Bananas and Dates
Cream — Supplements
Dandelion Coffee or Herb Tea.

SUNDAY
Cooked Applesauce with Raisins
Rye Grits — Supplements
Shave Grass Tea
*or*
Cantaloupe and Strawberries
Cottage Cheese — Supplements
Herb Tea.

## *Preparation Helps*

*Reconstituted dried fruit* — Cover with cold water, bring to boil and leave to stand overnight. Raisins may just have boiled water poured over them. This kills any insects and eggs.

*Whole grain cereal* — To cook properly with a little heat as possible, use a double boiler or thermos — cook your cereal.

*Supplements* — (Add to cereal or fruit) Sunflower seed meal, rice polishings, wheat germ, flaxseed meal (about a teaspoonful of each.) Even a little dulse may be sprinkled over, with some broth powder.

259

10:30 A.M.:
Vegetable broth, vegetable juice or fruit juice.
LUNCH:
*Raw salad,* or as directed, *one* or *two starches,* as listed and a *health drink.* Get salad suggestions from Dr. Jensen's Cook Book and Food Guide "Vital Foods for Total Health."
*Note:* If following a strict regimen use only one of the first seven starches daily. Vary the starch from day to day.

RAW SALAD VEGETABLES:
Tomatoes (citrus). Lettuce (green leafy type only, such as romaine). Celery, cucumber, bean sprouts, green peppers, avocado, parsley, watercress, endive, onion (s), cabbage (s). (s) are sulphur foods.

STARCHES:
1. Yellow corn meal. 2. Baked potato. 3. Baked banana (or at least dead ripe). 4. Barley—a winter food. 5. Steamed brown rice or wild rice. 6. Millet—have as a cereal. 7. Banana squash or Hubbard squash.
Steel-cut oatmeal, whole wheat cereal, Dr. Jackson's meal, whole grain, Roman meal, shredded wheat bread (whole wheat, rye, soy bean, corn bread, bran muffins, rye krisp preferred.)

DRINKS:
Vegetable broth, soup, coffee substitute, buttermilk, raw milk, oat straw tea, alfamint tea, huckleberry tea, papaya tea, or any health drink.

## *Suggested Lunch Menus*
MONDAY
Vegetable Salad
Baby Lima Beans, Baked Potato
Spearmint Tea

### TUESDAY
Vegetable Salad — with health
mayonnaise if desired.
Steamed Asparagus
Very ripe bananas or Steamed,
Unpolished Rice
Vegetable Broth or Herb Tea.

### WEDNESDAY
Raw Salad Plate — Sour Cream Dressing
Cooked Green Beans, Corn Bread
and/or Baked Hubbard Squash
Sassafras Tea

### THURSDAY
Salad — French Dressing
Baked Zucchini and Okra
Corn-on-cob, Rye Krisp
Buttermild or Herb Tea.

### FRIDAY
Salad
Baked Green Pepper stuffed with
eggplant and tomatoes
Baked Potato and/or Bran Muffin
Carrot Soup or Herb Tea.

### SATURDAY
Salad
Steamed Turnips and Turnip Greens
Baked Yams, Catnip Tea.

### SUNDAY
Salad
Lemon and Olive Oil Dressing
Steamed Whole Barley
Cream of Celery Soup, Steamed Chard
Herb Tea.

*Salad Vegetables:* Use plenty of greens. Choose four or five vegetables from the following: Leaf lettuce, watercress, spinach, beet leaves, parsley, alfalfa sprouts, cabbage, young chard, herbs, any green leaves, cucumbers, bean sprouts, onions, green peppers, piminentos, carrots, turnips, zucchini, asparagus, celery, okra, radishes, etc.

*"Vital Foods For Total Health," Nature's Own Cook Book, by Bernard Jensen, D.C. is a complete food guide.* Tables for vitamin and mineral guidance, acid and alkaline tables — with complete instructions for perfect combinations to assure you a correct daily balance . . . designed to get you well and keep you well.

Shows how to cook, prepare and serve foods healthfully the natural food way. Illustrated with charts and recipes. Have your own copy.

3:00 P.M.:
Health Cocktail, juice or fruit.

DINNER:
*Raw salad, two cooked vegetables, one protein* and a *broth* or *health drink* if desired.

*Cooked Vegetables:* Peas, artichokes, carrots, beets, turnips, spinach, beet tops, string beans, swiss chard, eggplant, zucchini, summer squash, broccoli (s) cauliflower (s), cabbage (s), sprouts (s), onion (s), or any vegetable other than potatoes.

*Drinks:* Vegetable broth, soup, or health beverage.

PROTEINS:
*Once a Week:* Fish — use white fish, such as sole, halibut, trout or sea trout.

*Vegetarians* — use soy beans, lima beans, cottage cheese, sunflower seeds and other seeds, also seed butters, nut butters, nut milk drinks, eggs.

*Three Times a Week:* Meat — use only lean meat. Never pork, fats or cured meats.

*Vegetarians* — use meat substitutes or vegetarian proteins.
*Twice a Week:* Cottage cheese or any cheese that breaks.
*Once a Week:* Egg Omelet.

If you have a protein at this meal, health dessert is allowed, but not recommended. Never eat protein and starch together. (Notice how they are separated.)

You may exchange your noon meal for the evening meal, but follow the same regimen. It takes exercise to handle raw food, and we generally get more after our noon meal. That is why a raw salad is advised at noon. If one eats sandwiches have vegetables at the same time.

## Suggested Dinner Menus

### MONDAY
Salad
Diced Celery and Carrots
Steamed Spinach, waterless-cooked
Puffy Omelet, Vegetable Broth

### TUESDAY
Salad
Cooked Beet Tops; Steak, broiled
or Ground Beef Patties — Tomato Sauce
Cauliflower, Comfrey Tea

### WEDNESDAY
Cottage Cheese, Cheese Sticks
Apples, Peaches, Grapes, Nuts
Apple Concentrate Cocktail

### THURSDAY
Salad
Steamed Chard, Baked Eggplant
Grilled Liver and Onions
Persimmon Whip (Optional)
Alfa-mint Tea

FRIDAY
Salad
Yogurt and Lemon Dressing
Steamed Mixed Greens, Beets
Steamed Fish with slices of Lemon
Leek soup

SATURDAY
Salad
Cooked String Beans, Baked Summer Squash
Carrot and Cheese Loaf
Cream of Lentil Soup
or Lemongrass Tea
Fresh Peach Jello, Almond-Nut Cream

SUNDAY
Salad
Diced Carrots and Peas, Steamed
Tomato Aspic, Roast Leg of Lamb
Mint Sauce

*Vegetarians* — use vegetarian dishes in place of meat dishes.

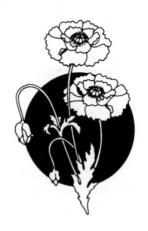

# But Where Will I Get My Calcium?

| Food | Amount | Calcium | Protein | Fat |
|---|---|---|---|---|
| DAIRY | | | | |
| Cheddar cheese | 1 cup (8 oz.) | 2048 mg. | 68.8 g. | 88.0 g. |
| whole milk | 1 cup | 287 mg. | 8.5 g. | 8.8 g. |
| SEEDS AND NUTS | | | | |
| Brazil nuts | 1 cup | 558 mg. | 42.0 g. | 201.0 g. |
| almonds | 1 cup | 328 mg. | 26.0 g. | 76.0 g. |
| sesame seeds | 1 cup | 253 mg. | 42.0 g. | 123.0 g. |
| LEAFY GREEN VEGETABLES | | | | |
| collards, steamed | 1 cup | 376 mg. | 7.2 g. | 1.4 g. |
| turnip greens, steamed | 1 cup | 267 mg. | 3.2 g. | .3 g. |
| dandelion, steamed | 1 cup | 252 mg. | 3.6 g. | 1.1 g. |
| brocolli, cooked | 1 cup | 132 mg. | 4.6 g. | .4 g. |
| SEAWEEDS | | | | |
| Kelp | 1 cup | 2405 mg. | 16.5 g. | 2.4 g. |
| Irish moss | 1 cup | 2022 mg. | – | – |
| dulse | 1 cup | 676 mg. | – | – |
| agar | 1 cup | 567 mg. | – | .3 g. |
| SHELLFISH | | | | |
| shrimp, cooked | 1 cup | 162 mg. | 46.0 g. | 24.0 g. |
| lobster, steamed | 1 med. | 130 mg. | 37.0 g. | 3.0 g. |

*Eastwest Journal*, July, 1978.
Source, *Nutrition Almanac*, by Nutrition Search, Inc. (McGraw Hill, 1973).
Reprinted with permission.

# The Cereal Grains – Some Of Their Special Characteristics

by Dr. Royal Lee, January, 1953

*Wheat:* Possibly the reason wheat has become so popular is because its protein is best for bread making; other cereals

265

refusing to make a light loaf as their protein has not the proper texture to form gas bubbles. Moreover, wheat will not grow on soil low in phosphorus, so all wheat has a fairly high content of this essential mineral. (The calcium that must be combined with phosphorus to calcify bone may be obtained from hard water — cattle cannot be profitably produced except on land underlaid with limestone to supply the hard water.)

This is a characteristic common to all cereals. They supply only one of the two important bone minerals. Unless the other mineral element is available from other sources, cereal foods fail to properly support bone growth. In general, the grasses and leaves of animal feeds help in supplying the calcium and other alkaline elements to complete the nutritional pattern. The ash of cereals, like the ash of the meat foods, is acid and must be balanced by the alkaline ash of leaf and root vegetables. Hogs and chickens are fed alfalfa leaf meal for the purpose of neutralizing the acid ash of the cereal feeds.

Milk is neutral, and cannot correct unbalances.

*Rice:* More people live on rice than on wheat. The protein of rice has the highest biological value of all vegetable source proteins with the possible exception of potato protein. The Oriental rice-eating people are able to maintain a high standard of health on brown rice and a little meat or fish as a protein supplement. Heart disease, arthritis and high blood pressure are almost non-existent in China.

*Rye:* Rye, as distinguished from wheat, will grow on any soil. If a farmer had a sand field that will not grow anything else, he plants it in rye. He will get a good crop if it rains, but the grains will be almost devoid of minerals and vitamins. If rye is grown on the same soil as wheat, it is a better food than the wheat. Animal tests have shown that rye develops muscle, while wheat promotes fat formation. This characteristic of rye is shown up in the feats of rye-eating athletes. Finnish competitors walk away at the Olympic Games with ten times their normal share of trophies where endurance is the test. In Reader's Digest of September, 1952, is the account of a 66 year old bicycle rider who won a 1000 mile race over 50 young contestants, in Sweden. His main item of diet seems to have been rye bread.

The Finns live on rye bread, fish and fruit. Alfred McCann, in his book (1926), "The Science of Keeping Young," had a chapter on the Finns, calling them the "super-man race," the only modern nation getting a rational diet.

*Barley:* Barley, because of its adhering husk that must be "pearled" off to make it acceptable in the culinary arts, has not had the recognition its merits demand. Barley water has been a household remedy for many years for the ills of the teething baby and for many other disorders. It seems to allay any irritation due to a lack of available calcium. This includes not only the troubles of the teething baby, but allergies in general, and low resistance to infection, gastritis, stomach ulcers and colitis, nervous states, even insomnia.

Beer is barley water, plus the barley carbohydrates, rendered soluble by the malt enzymes. These sugars offset the possible benefits of the barley extract, beer drinkers seemingly being almost as susceptible to polio as the soft drink user. Sugar in any form in excess causes the periodic between-meal release of free phosphate radical (from phosphagen turn-over) which destroys vital blood bicarbonate of calcium, our defender against viruses. Potassium bicarbonate and inositol are two factors that combat this calcium bicarbonate deficiency. It is probable that no virus could harm us unless we first prepared a welcome for it by permitting this temporary loss of blood calcium bicarbonate. (Calcium lactate or gluconate can form the bicarbonate after ingestion. Bone calcium, the phosphate, cannot.)

Our normal source of calcium bicarbonate is in hard water. The city of Des Moines, Iowa, had one of the lowest rates of incidence of polio. After the installation of water softening equipment at the city water works, the polio incidence went almost to the opposite extreme. Many physicians have discovered the shortcomings of softened water by noting that soft water drinkers have a reduced state of vitality.

*Oats:* Oats should rank next to rye as a muscle builder—look at the horse. Or the traditionally lean Scotchman. By the way, oats grown in the silt valleys of Scotland sell (in Scotland) for twice the price of English oats, we are informed, because of the superior flavor. No doubt again, the effect of good soil, as in the case of rye.

The protein content of oats is relatively high—oatmeal usually running 15%. (The national average for wheat is 9%, the best Deaf Smith County wheat being 16 to 17%.)

The best oatmeal to buy is steel-cut meal at a health food store. The packaged cereals are all treated with bug poisons, the flavor alone shows their inferiority.

The general practice of fumigating grains to kill bugs is very unfortunate. It is almost impossible to get unfumigated grains today unless you buy direct from the grower and store it yourself. These fumigating gases are poison, and are absorbed in the grain. (Look up the technique of Chromatographic Absorption in analysis if you think there is any doubt of the possiblity of this contamination.) (Starch is one of the best of all chemicals to pick up these poison gases.)

Rolled oats is a poor cereal. Its previous moistening and cooking destroys much of its vitamin value, and damages the protein. If you buy rolled oats in a feed store where they sell animal feeds, you will get a better grade. The grocery store kind could not be used as animal feed—chickens will die if fed precooked grains. Feed stores get a different grade in 100 pound bags, will sell you 5 pound lots at much less than the usual grocery price. You will find its flavor outstanding.

*Corn:* Corn has a poor reputation as food for the human family, is low in protein, and the protein is low in tryptophane, the precursor of niacin, and predisposes to pellagra, like white rice causes beri-beri. However, the use of refined corn seems to be the main cause, as all commercial corn meal today has the germ removed. But where corn is grown on good soil, and is ground in the kitchen as it is prepared (Mexican style), the grain seems to compare favorably with any

268

cereal. Hybrid corn, the only kind now commercially available in this country, is a refined abomination, refined by nature, as it will not reproduce, its ability to produce more per acre is a direct consequence of its lack of the power plant, the germ, in the seed. Vitamin $B_{12}$, an important component of natural corn, is totally missing in the hybrid variety. Its feed value is impaired, molasses being commonly used to supply the missing elements; without the molasses supplement, it is hard to get hogs or cattle to eat it. Popcorn, freshly ground, makes delicious corn cakes or muffins. Poor food is usually characterized by its lack of a normal flavor, in fact it is obvious that our sense of taste is our natural guide to the best food.

Makers of counterfeit foods know this. That is why an essence of cultured milk is used in oleo to make it taste like butter, just as you would have to perfume green-dyed shavings with essence of new mown hay to make it acceptable to a horse. To insult our sense of taste with counterfeit foods is as stupid as to let someone give us "gold bricks" or counterfeit money. We are told that Corn Flakes must be artificially colored and flavored, that otherwise they are as white and tasteless as tissue paper — and as nutritional. Really, they are worse. They add to an already overburdened state of refined carbohydrate excess. If paper, they would be indigestible, simply add useful bulk to the intestinal content. People today are buying as Methyl-Cellulose, a paper by-product, just for that purpose.

*Starch:* Where recipes call for starch, use tapioca flour, arrowroot, or home-ground whole corn flour. Tapioca has been found much superior to rice (used as a 25% blend with 75% rice) in feeding tests on human subjects in that nitrogen retention and calcium and phosphorus assimilation was improved. (A 50% increase in calcium and phosphorus assimilation.) (Reported in Am. Jol. Clincial Nutrition, vol. 2, No. 6, p. 446.)

Arrowroot was once widely used in baby formulas as a superior carbohydrate, experience having shown it agreed with babies better than any other starch or sugar. We now find the reason—it is the only starch product with a calcium ash. Arrowroot only thrives on tidal flats, where the sea minerals are available. Its known health building properties may be due to race minerals from the sea, as well as from the calcium it gets from the sea water.

Used in ice cream formulas in place of cornstarch, arrowroot imparts a vanilla-like flavor, a smooth texture. Arrowroot, as it comes to you, is not a refined product, it is simply the dried and powdered root.

There is much evidence to show that polio and other infectious diseases can only invade our bodies after we become depleted in calcium and trace minerals (maganese, cobalt, copper and iodine). The only successful defense against undulant fever has been the use of these minerals, both for the cow as well as the human. We might call it the automatic punishment for us to have permitted the soil depletion which is now becoming acute.

Pliny the Elder in his Encyclopedia of Roman times (published 77 A.D.) commented that the first six hundred years of the Roman Empire was marked by the fact that there were no doctors in the country, and none needed. (From "The Wheel of Health" by G. T. Wrench, M.D., an abosrbing book on food and health, $2.00 postpaid, Lee Foundation for Nutritional Research, Milwaukee, Wisconsin.)

Note: Lee Foundation for Nutritional Research is a non-profit, public-service institution, chartered to investigate and disseminate nutritional information. The attached publication is not literature or labeling for any product, nor shall it be employed as such by anyone. In accordance with the right of freedom of the press guaranteed to the Foundation by the First Amendment of the U. S. Constitution, the attached publication is issued and distributed for informational purposes.

Copyright Lee Foundation for Nutritional Research, 2023 West Wisconsin Avenue, Milwakee, WI 53201.

Reprint No. 38B, price—$.05.

# Reading List For Home Remedies And Nutrition

Ruth Adams and Frank Murray, *Body, Mind and the B-Vitamins*
Dr. Paavo Airola, *Are You Confused? Everywomen's Book*
Dr. Henry Bieler, *Food Is Your Best Medicine,* Bantum Books
Dr. Richard Burack, *The Handbook Of Prescription Drugs,* Ballantine
Dr. Sheldon C. Deal, *New Life Through Nutrition,* New Life Publication, Tucson, Arizona
*East West magazine,* July, 1978 and others.
Joy Gardner, *Healing Yourself; Healing Pregnancy*
Dr. Joan Gomez, *A Directory Of Symptoms,* Bantam Books
Dr. Jarvis, *New England Folk Medicine*
Jane Kinderlehrer, *Confessions of a Sneaky Organic Cook*
Frederick LeBoyer, *Loving Hands*
Juliette de Bairacli Levy, *Nature's Children*
John Lust, *The Herb Book*
Joseph Meyer, *The Herbalist,* Clarence Meyer, Ind. Botanical Gardens
*Mothering Magazine*
*Prevention Magazine*
Laurel Robertson, et al, *Laurel's Kitchen,* Nilgiri Press, Berkeley, CA
Jeanne Rose, *Herbs and Things; Modern Herbal*
Herbert Shelton, *Fasting Can Save Your Life,* Natural Hygiene Press
Dr. Jean Valnet, *Organic Garden Medicine,* Erbonia Books
Michael Weiner, *Earth Food, Earth Medicine,* Macmillan Co.
Emrika Padus, *The Woman's Encyclopedia of Health and Natural Healing,* Rodale Press
Dr. Rober Williams, *Nutrition Against Disease,* Bantum Books
Peter Wingate, *The Penguin Medical Encyclopedia,* Penguin Books
Lendon H. Smith, *Feed Your Kid Right*
Jeannine Parvati, *Hygieia: A Woman's Herbal,* Freestone Press
Robert Conrow and Arlene Hecksel, *Herbal Pathfinders,* Woodbridge Press
Gabriel Cousens, *Spiritual Nutrition and the Rainbow Diet,* Cassandra Press, Boulder, CO 80306
Svevo Brooks, *Common Sense Diet and Health,* Botanica Press, Capitola, CA
Gary Landgrebe, *Tofu Goes West,* Fresh Press, 1978
Frances Moore Lappe, *Diet for a Small Planet*
John Robbins, *Diet for a New America,* Stillpoint Publishing
David Hoffman, *The Holistic Herbal*

271

# Alkaline Foods

### by Dr. Paul Lynn

An alkaline diet is an effective nutritional aid which helps to restore balance in physical and mental functions that are thrown into disharmony by unconcious health and eating habits. This simply means to eat predominately of the foods which give to the body alkaline elements in abundance when broken down by digestion. The entire eliminative system of the body is strengthened and the nervous system is able to return to a more relaxed tone. The body seems to function best when 70%-80% of the diet is composed of alkaline foods.

| PROTEIN | | SUGARS, FATS & OILS | |
|---|---|---|---|
| buttermilk | ac | brown sugar | ac |
| cottage cheese | ac | white sugar | ac |
| yogurt | ac | milk sugar | ac |
| eggs | ac | maple syrup | ac |
| cheeses | ac | cane syrup | ac |
| *soybeans* | *al* | malt syrup | ac |
| yeast | ac | *honey* | *al* |
| *raw mild (nonfat)* | *al* | blackstrap molasses | ac |
| raw milk (whole) | ac | *olive oil* | *al* |
| fish | ac | *soy oil* | *al* |
| fowl | ac | *sunflower seeds* | *al* |
| meat | ac | *sesame oil* | *al* |
| VEGETABLES | | *corn oil* | *al* |
| *All vegetables are alkaline.* | | butter | ac |
| MELONS | | cream | ac |
| *All melons are alkaline.* | | nut oils | ac |
| SEEDS & NUTS | | *margarine* | *al* |
| sesame | ac | *avocado oil* | *al* |
| pumpkin | ac | *cottonseed oil* | *al* |
| flax | ac | CARBOHYDRATES | |
| chia | ac | dried split pea | ac |
| sunflower | ac | *lima beans* | *al* |
| walnuts | ac | *parsnips* | *al* |
| *almonds* | *al* | beans (baked) | ac |
| filberts | ac | bread | ac |
| macadamia | ac | rice (brown) | ac |
| pecans | ac | *corn* | *al* |

# Alkaline Foods

| | | | |
|---|---|---|---|
| *potatoes (white)* | al | *gooseberry* | al |
| lentils | ac | *grapes* | al |
| *potatoes (sweet)* | al | *guava* | al |
| beans (navy) | ac | *huckleberry* | al |
| cereals | ac | *mango* | al |
| chestnuts | ac | *nectarine* | al |
| peanuts | ac | *olive* | al |
| oats | ac | *papaya* | al |
| wheat | ac | *peach* | al |
| rye | ac | *pear* | al |
| barley | ac | *persimmon* | al |
| dhal | ac | *plum* | al |
| aduki | ac | *quince* | al |
| cashews | ac | *raspberry* | al |
| millet | ac | *rhubarb* | al |
| buckwheat | ac | *sapodilla* | al |
| ACID FRUITS | | *dried fruit* | al |
| cranberry | ac | *citrus fruits* | al |
| current | ac | (except oranges) | |
| kumquat | ac | | |
| loganberry | ac | | |
| loquat | ac | | |
| pineapple | ac | | |
| pomegranate | ac | | |
| strawberry | ac | | |
| sour apple | ac | | |
| sour grape | ac | | |
| sour plum | ac | | |
| tangelo | ac | | |
| tomato | ac | | |
| ALKALINE FRUITS | | | |
| *apples* | al | | |
| *apricots* | al | | |
| *bananas* | al | | |
| *blackberry* | al | | |
| *breadfruit* | al | | |
| *cactus fruit* | al | | |
| *cherry* | al | | |
| *coconut oil* | al | | |
| *date* | al | | |
| *elderberry* | al | | |
| *fig* | al | | |

# Vitamins and Minerals

Reprinted with permission
*Alice Feinberg, *Macrobiotic Pregnancy*, pp 56-62, George Ohsawa Macrobiotic Foundation, 902 14th Street, Oroville, CA 95965.

| NAME | NATURAL SOURCES | FUNCTION | SIGNS OF DEFICIENCY | MDR* |
|---|---|---|---|---|
| Vitamin A | Parsley, carrot, spinach, kale, dandelion greens, watercress, cabbage leaves, cauliflower, turnip greens, cantalope, crab, liver, peaches, rosehips, green and red pepper, sweet potato, banana, corn, butter, tomato, string bean, pumpkin, beet, miso | Builds resistance to infections, especially of the respiratory tract. Helps maintain a healthy condition of the outer layers of many tissues and organs, promotes growth and vitality, permits formation of visual purple in the eye, counteracting night blindness and weak eye-sight, promotes healthy skin, essential for pregnancy and lactation. Note: (1) absorption in digestive tract is aided by sesame oil, (2) does not occur in vitamin form in vegetables or fruits, but as provitamin carotene which is trans- | May result in night-blindness, increased susceptibility to infection, dry and scaly skin, lack of appetite and vigor, defective teeth and gums, retarded growth, kidney disorders, eye disorders, sterility | 5,000 I.U. |

| | | | |
|---|---|---|---|
| Vitamin B Complex | Whole grains, seeds, green leaves, nuts, chestnuts, eggs, animal flesh, milk | A complex of different elements vital to proper digestion – unless present foods are not broken down to use as fuel formed by the body into Vitamin A. | |
| B-1 (Thiamine) | Whole grain rice, soybeans, beans, lentils, almonds, kelp, wheat and rye, dried yeast, wholewheat, oatmeal, peanuts, most vegetables, pork, milk, soy flour, abalone, seeds, spinach, dandelion, miso | Promotes growth, aids growth and digestion, essential for normal functioning of nerve tissues, muscles, heart | Loss of vigor, weight, poor appetite, insomnia, swelling and retention of fluid in body, heart irregularities, lowered resistance, depression, vague aches and pains, impaired growth in children | 1.0-1.3 mg. |
| B-2 (Riboflavin) | Soybeans, wholewheat, whole rye, turnip greens, soy flour, peas, most sources of B-1, liver, kidney, broccoli, eggs, wheat germ, miso, spinach, kale, cabbage | Improves growth, essential for health, eyes, skin, mouth, promotes general health | Nose dermatitis, mouth sores, itching and burning, of eyes, cracking of lip corners, inflammation of mouth and bloodshot eyes, purplish tongue | 15-20 mg. |
| Niacin | Sesame seeds, whole barley, buckwheat, fish, | Important for proper functioning of nervous | Pellegra-symptoms: inflammation of skin, | 15-20 mg. |

275

| | | | MDR N.D. |
|---|---|---|---|
| | soybeans, peanuts, rice, brewers yeast, liver, beans, green vegetables, wholewheat products | system, prevents pellegra, promotes growth, maintains normal function of the gastro-intestinal tract, necessary for metabolism of sugars, maintains normal skin condition | tongue, gastro-intestinal disturbances, nervous system disfunction, headaches, fatigue, mental depression, vague aches, pains, irritability, loss of appetite, weight, insomnia, neuritis, weakness |
| Folic Acid | Deep green leafy vegetables, mushrooms, sprouted grains, soybeans, brewers yeast, wheat germ | Essential to the formation of red blood cells, by its action on the bone marrow, aids in protein metabolism and contributes to normal growth | Nutritional anemia |
| B-12 | Seaweeds (esp. high in dulse) fertile eggs, whole grains, yogurt, miso, liver, beef, pork, milk, cheese | Helps in the formation and regeneration of red blood cells, helps prevent anemia, promotes growth and increases appetite in children | May lead to pernicious anemia, poor appetite, growth failure in children, tiredness — 5-8 mcg. |
| Vitamin C | All vegetable greens, broccoli, sweet potato, green pepper, chives, watercress, parsnips, | Necessary for healthy teeth, gums and bones, strengthens all connective tissue, promotes | May lead to soft gums, tooth decay, loss of appetite, muscular weakness, skin hemorrhages, — 70-75 mg. |

276

| | | | |
|---|---|---|---|
| | parsley, kale, carrot, cabbage, berries, citrus fruit, tomato, cantalope, dandelion, bean sprouts, endive | wound healing, helps promote capillary strength and permeability, important in maintaining sound health and vigor | capillary weakness, anemia | |
| Vitamin D | Cod-liver oil, dried fish, swiss chard, spinach, dandelion, all bran cereal, whole wheat and whole wheat flour, liver, milk, eggs, cod, salmon, fish-liver oils, fats and oils, butter, "sunshine" | Regulates the use of calcium and phosphorous in the body and is necessary for proper formation of teeth and bones, very important in infancy and childhood | Lowered resistance, bone weakness and muscle weakness, retarded growth, dental caries, rickets, lack of vigor | 400 I.U. |
| Vitamin E | Green leafy vegetables, brown rice and all whole grains, nuts, bran, whole wheat and whole wheat products, butter, liver, milk | Exact function not known, used in prevention of sterility in the treatment of threatened abortion, in muscular dystrophy, in treating heart conditions | Aging symptoms, retarded growth, mentally slow, wasting muscles, anemia in children, possibly associated with loss of reproductive powers and muscular disorder | 25-30 I.U. |
| Vitamin K | Unrefined oil, brown rice, alfalfa and all green leafy vegetables, soybean, egg-yolk, cauliflower, cabbage, lettuce, | Essential in production of prothrombin (a substance which aids blood clotting), important to liver function | Slow blood coagulation, hemorrhagic diseases, circulatory failure, weakness | 0.5 mg. |

277

| | | | MDR |
|---|---|---|---|
| Vitamin P | spinach, broccoli, kale, nettles, produced by the intestinal flora | | N.D. |
| | Kale, broccoli, buckwheat, lemon juice, turnip greens, green pepper | Maintains walls of small blood vessels, helps combat disease of joints, diabetes, tuberculosis | Low blood pressure, pink toothbrush, migraine headaches, varicose veins, nose bleed, scurvy |
| Calcium | All seaweeds, green vegetables, sesame seeds, kale, nuts, seeds (esp. sunflower) whole grains, cabbage, broccoli, eggs, milk, cheese, nuts, dried fruit | Builds and maintains bones and teeth, helps blood to clot, aids vitality and endurance, regulates heart rhythm, normalizes some enzymes | Retarded bone and tooth development, fragile bones, stunted growth, rickets, nervousness, muscular sensitivity | 0.8 Gm. |
| Copper | Currants, kale, potato, asparagus | Necessary for absorption and utilization of iron, formation of red blood cells | Retards hemoglobin production, defective respiration, general debility, limited growth | 2 mg. |
| Fluorine | Carrot, cabbage, cauliflower, cucumbers, parsley, watercress, almonds, egg yolk, dandelion, beet green | Organic variety combines with oxygen and potassium and sulphur to form blood, skin, nails and hair | Decay of teeth, spinal curvature, weakened eyesight | MDR N.D. |
| Iodine | All seaweeds (esp. kelp | Necessary for proper | Goiter, cretinism, sensi- | 15-30 mg. |

278

| Mineral | Food Sources | Function | Deficiency Symptoms | Daily Requirement |
|---|---|---|---|---|
| | and dulse), swiss chard, all green vegetables, watermelon, carrot | function of thyroid gland, essential for proper growth, energy and metabolism, stimulates circulation, aids oxidation of fats and proteins | tivity to infections, slow body metabolism and mental activity, nervous disorders | |
| Iron | Pumpkin seeds, lima beans, beets, broccoli, brussel sprouts, chard, kale, mixed greens, green peas, pumpkin, spinach, cabbage, carrot, cauliflower, nuts, berries, parsley, nettles | Required in manufacture of hemoglobin, helps carry oxygen in the blood, vital to cell oxygenation, essential in bone, brain and muscle tissue formation | Anemia, paleness, limited growth, poor vitality | 10-12 mg. |
| Magnesium | Dulse, beans (esp. soybeans), lentils, leafy green vegetables, dried fruit, most nuts, nettles, endive | Necessary for calcium and Vitamin C metabolism, essential for normal functioning of nervous and muscular system, activates enzymes in carbohydrate metabolism, helps build blood, nerves and muscles | Soft bones, digestive disorders, exhaustion, irritibility, nervousness, heart acceleraton, convulsions | 300 mg. |

279

| | | | |
|---|---|---|---|
| Manganese | Whole grains, almonds, walnuts, beets, carrot, chives, watercress, kale, apples, apricots | Activates various enzymes and other minerals, related to proper utilization of Vitamins B-1 and E, involved in reproductive process, combines with oxygen, hydrogen and iron to form lymph and hemoglobin | Weak tissue response, restricted growth, glandular disorders, defective reproductive functions | 15-25 mg. |
| Phosphorous | Green peas, sunflower seeds, nuts, beans, lentils, whole grains and cereals, seaweed, dried fruit, watercress, leeks, turnips | Needed for normal bone and tooth formation, interrelated with action of Calcium and Vitamin D, normalizes metabolism, blood coagulation, transports fatty acids, important to brain growth and function | Poor mineralization of bones, poor growth, rickets, decrease in weight, general weakness | 1.2 Gm. |
| Potassium | Dulse and all seaweeds, soybeans, dried fruits, nuts, vegetables | Necessary for normal muscle tone, nerves, heart action and enzyme reaction, aids in elimination, regulates heartbeat, formation of glycogen from glucose, | Affected growth and elimination, weak muscle control, incomplete digestion | 3 Gm. |

280

| | | fats from glucose | | |
|---|---|---|---|---|
| Sodium | Dulse and all seaweeds, green leafy vegetables, dried fruit | Maintain water content of cells, helps to build skin, nerves, mucous membranes, aids in formation of digestive juices, aids elimination of sulphur dioxide | Defective intestinal absorption, restricted growth | 0.5 Gm. |
| Sulphur | Most nuts, brussel sprouts, cabbage, cauliflower, apples, cranberries, most beans, watercress, kale, currants | Vital to good skin, hair and nails, combines with carbon, oxygen and potassium to make up blood, important in liver and skin-cell metabolism | Eczema, restricted growth, dermatitis, poor growth of nails and hair | 0.3 Gm. |
| Zinc | Whole wheat and whole wheat products | Helps normal tissue function, protein and carbohydrate metabolism | Defective intestinal absorption, restricted growth | 10-15 mg. |

I.U. – International Unit
M.D.R. – Minimum Daily Requirement
N.D. – Not Determined
Gm. – Gram
mg. – Milligram
mcg. – Microgram

281

# The New American Diet Contains Major Changes

by Letitia Brewster and Michael Jacobson

(The authors are affiliated with the Center for Science in the Public Interest. The following is excerpted from the opening chapter of "The Changing American Diet," an 80-page booklet issued last week by CSPI. Copies are available at $2.50 each from CSPI, 1755 "S" Street, N. W., Washington, D. C. 20009.)

"People's food habits change very slowly," say most anthropologists. Yet, if our great-grandparents spent a day eating with us, they would be wide-eyed and shocked. And if they were plopped down in a modern supermarket, they would probably not know for sure whether they were in a toy, hardware, or grocery store.

The New American Diet, for example, includes such traditional foods as milk, honey, and broccoli. But it also includes enormous quantities of soft drinks, frozen French fries, and other food products of the industrial age.

Many factors have contributed to our nation's dramatic, almost unprecedented dietary changes. They include:

- New technologies. Technological "advances" such as freezing, dehydration, and food additives have made it possible to produce frozen orange juice, dried soup mixes, and imitation eggs at prices consumers can afford.
- Affluence. As our nation became more affluent, people switched from bread and potatoes to eat meat, chicken and sweets.
- Government programs. Federal food programs made more food available to more people. Over $7 billion dollars a

282

year worth of food stamps, subsidized school lunches and breakfasts, and other programs are enabling low-income families to eat more food than they were able to 30 years ago.

- Working parents. In more and more families, both husband and wife have jobs. Parents who work are less likely to prepare a bacon and egg breakfast and more likely to serve a dinner made from packaged convenience foods than their non-working counterparts.
- The end of the baby boom. Foods that are more popular among children than adults (such as baby foods, candy, and milk) are beginning to show declines in consumption or slower increases now that the average age of Americans is increasing. On the other hand, the consumption of "adult" foods (such as alcoholic beverages, shellfish, and broccoli) is picking up.
- Health concerns. About one-fourth of the 1400 respondents to a 1976 USDA survey said that someone in their household had changed his or her diet as a result of a health problem (overweight, high blood pressure, etc.). Another quarter of the respondents said that someone in their household was now choosing different foods and beverages to prevent such health problems.

This nation's mammoth food industry plays a major role in influencing food habits. Manufacturers cater to (some would say "take advantage of") the public's desire for a particular taste or for convenience. After all, there's a lot at stake: the American appetite is worth over $200 billion a year.

Not surprisingly, the industry chooses to market most aggressively those foods that are most profitable. The food industry spends about $6 billion a year, or three percent of our food bill, on advertising and other forms of promotion to encourage us to buy certain products. In addition, we pay about $26 billion, or 13 percent of our total food bill, on packaging — often just another form of advertising.

Not all foods are promoted equally. Nobody sponsors full-page magazine ads for breast milk or homemade soup, but there are plenty of such ads for infant formula and canned soups. Sugary breakfast cereals ("breakfast candies"), candy bars, and snack cakes comprise the great bulk of advertising on children's TV shows. But you'll find few ads for potatoes or whole wheat bread on those same shows.

## CHANGES IN FOOD CONSUMPTION

| Food | | Change in Consumption (per person) |
|---|---|---|
| Apples, fresh | 1910-76 | -70% |
| Beef | 1910-76 | +72% |
| | 1950-76 | +90% |
| Butter | 1910-76 | -76% |
| Cabbage, fresh | 1920-76 | -65% |
| Candy | 1968-76 | -18% |
| Chicken | 1910-76 | +179% |
| Coffee | 1910-76 | +22% |
| | 1946-76 | -44% |
| Corn Syrup | 1960-76 | +224% |
| Fish, fresh and frozen | 1960-76 | +42% |
| Food Colors (certified dyes) | 1940-77 | +995% |
| Fruit, fresh | 1910-76 | -33% |
| Grapefruit, fresh | 1910-76 | +800% |
| Margarine | 1910-76 | +681% |
| Potatoes, fresh | 1910-76 | -74% |
| Potatoes, frozen | 1960-76 | +465% |
| Soft Drinks | 1960-76 | +157% |
| Sugar and other calorie sweeteners | 1909-76 | +33% |
| Tuna, canned | 1926-76 | +1,300% |
| Turkey | 1910-76 | +820% |
| Vegetables, frozen | 1960-76 | +44% |
| Wheat flour (including flour used in bread, spaghetti, etc.) | 1910-76 | -48% |

In general, "differentiated" foods—those that are unique and can be sold by brand name—bring higher returns to manufacturers than do basic commodities, which are highly competitive. The higher profits permit more extensive ad budgets . . . and the ads certainly influence buying decisions.

Retailers also guide our food choices. The placement of food in supermarkets exercises a subtle influence on our buying decisions. The "end of aisle" displays are prime sales areas, and candy and other "children's" foods are often placed at the child's eye level.

The places where we purchase our food have also been changing. One hundred years ago, many people lived on farms and had gardens. Most food was fresh and locally grown. Now, only a few million people live on farms and only a fraction of the population has extensive gardens.

Of course, vending machines were rare a hundred years ago. Now, about five percent of our food dollar—$10 billion a year—is spent at these machines, where a few coins will bring us a candy bar, cup of coffee, or can of soup.

## Fast Food Spending

But the big growth industry as far as food is concerned has been restaurants. Greater affluence, more vacations, and more people holding down jobs has resulted in our spending one out of three food dollars away from home, mostly in restaurants. This figure is expected to rise to one-half of our food dollar by 1990.

Fast food restaurants gobble up much of that money. They have been a major influence on our changing food habits. The limited choices that are available in a typical fast food restaurant have encouraged a trend toward a diet composed of relatively few different foods. The rise in potato consumption during the last 15 years has been due almost entirely to the purchase of French fries at franchised restaurants. Catsup, pickles, beef, chicken, fish, and ice milk (used in fast food shakes and cones) have also shown dramatic increases.

This narrowing of our eating habits has brought some companies big profits. The largest fast food chain, McDonald's,

285

grew twenty fold from sales of $129 million in 1964 to sales of $2.7 billion in 1976. During 1976 alone, McDonald's spent over $100 million in advertising.

In most cases, food marketers seek to influence our decision, but some, at least, give us a choice. You can still get fresh vegetables, fresh fruit, and fresh eggs in supermarkets. Sometimes, however, we are deprived of that freedom of choice: try to get your hamburger on a whole wheat bun at a fast food restaurant . . . try to talk that vending machine into giving you a can of tomato juice instead of a can of soda pop . . . ask for an apple at a refreshment stand in a national park or football stadium.

Some of the changes in food consumption have been remarkably great. Other changes are surprisingly slight. From a nutritional point of view, the most significant changes in the American diet in the last 65 years have been:

- the increase in fat consumption. Fat provided 42 percent of our calories in 1976, 31 percent more than the 32 percent of our calories that fat supplied in 1910.
- the decrease in complex carbohydrates (basically starch) consumption. Complex carbohydrates accounted for only 21 percent of our calories in 1976, 43 percent less than the 37 percent of calories that complex carbohydrates provided in 1909-13.
- the increase in sweetener consumption. Refined sugar, corn syrup and other caloric sweeteners supplied 18 percent of our calories in 1976, a full 50 percent more than the 12 percent of calories that sweeteners furnished our grandparents in 1910.

These changes would be of only academic interest if they were not linked to important changes in the public's health. But our "new" diet, in combination with our sedentary lifestyle, has contributed to what must be considered a national epidemic of obesity, diabetes, heart disease, stroke, and tooth decay. (Smoking, of course, has also contributed enormously to heart disease, as well as lung cancer.) These health problems cost American tens of billions of dollars a year in direct medical expenses and indirect losses to the economy.

The massive power of the food industry to direct eating habits, the relative powerlessness of the consumer, and the catastrophic health consequences of the New American Diet indicate the need for a comprehensive federal program to change the American diet. In most cases, federal actions should aim to provide people with more choices and more information than they now have. Measures that the federal and local governments should consider include:

### CHANGES IN NUTRIENT CONSUMPTION

| Nutrients | | Change in Consumption Per Person |
|---|---|---|
| Calories | 1910-76 | - 3% |
| Fat | 1910-76 | +28% |
| Carbohydrates | 1910-76 | -21% |
| Protein | 1910-76 | + 1% |
| Dietary fat from separated fats and oils (butter, margaine, oil, etc.) | 1921-76 | +56% |
| Grams of carbohydrates from sugars | 1909-13 – 1976 | +31% |
| Grams of carbohydrates from starches | 1909-13 – 1976 | -45% |

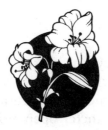

Reprinted from "The Changing American Diet," which is available from the Center for Science in the Public Interest, 1755 S Street, N. W., Washington, D. C. 20009, for $4.00, copyright 1982.

287

# The Kegel Muscle — Keep It Toned For Easy Birthing And Good Sex

*by Nan Koehler*

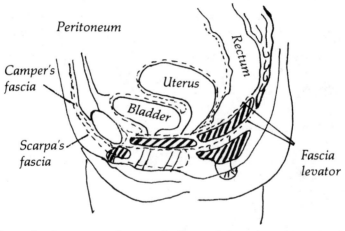

The *striped areas* are the muscle floor of the pelvis through which pass the three openings; the urethra, the vagina and the anus.

The kegel or pubococcygeus muscle holds your insides in the proper place from your tail bone to your pubic bone. It is a complicated muscle which has several parts. Part of the muscle consists of the sphincter openings of the bladder, the vagina and the rectum. In the man, the sphincter openings are analogus with the urethra running up the center of the penis.

## Kegel Muscle

These drawings are a good example of what can happen when the kegel muscle is weak.

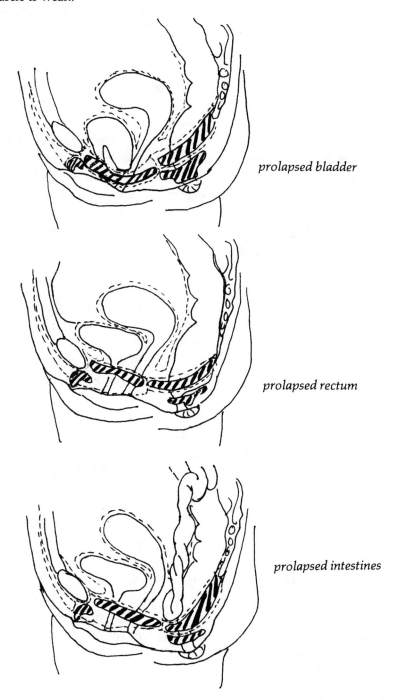

*prolapsed bladder*

*prolapsed rectum*

*prolapsed intestines*

289

A tight kegel muscle assures:

1. Control at the moment of birth. The vagina can be relaxed when pushing the baby out and the likelihood of tearing is greatly reduced.
2. Speedy recovery from birthing and reducing the need for episiotomies. Bladder and rectal control can be regained right away. Prevention of and relief from hemorrhoid symptoms.
3. Better orgasms for men as well as women. (Sexual problems are sometimes related to a loose kegel muscle.) The stronger the kegel muscle, the stronger will be the spasms of orgasm and the stronger the pleasurable sensations.

Exercises:

1. When peeing, stop and start the flow of urine in small amounts by contracting the muscle.
2. Several times during the course of the day, practice a series of five very slowly: hold-release, hold-release.
3. Several times a day practice slowly, five times, contracting the muscle to the count of five, then release the muscle to the count of one.
4. Reverse exercise #3 by contracting to the count of one, then slowly releasing the muscle to the count of five.

# *The Rhythmic Second Stage*

*by Shelia Kitzinger*

Far too often the second stage of labor constitutes an assault course on delivery. Physiological rhythms are ignored and with urgent, repetitive, often shouted, commands to 'try harder' and 'go on pushing,' a ritual contest is created between the woman and her own body.

In many cultures birth is treated as a transitional ritual to life for the child, and for the woman to motherhood. Our own urban industrial culture selects the second stage of labor as the high point of a ritual in which society forces its will on the laboring woman and struggles with her to overcome the barriers of the flesh. Expulsion is the occasion for energetic group activity as all those present in the room exhort, cajole, plead, and frequently threaten the woman and often participate to the extent of bearing down themselves. Tape recordings of action in the delivery room in the expulsive stage often sound as if a prize fight were in progress.

Yet labor is essentially a spontaneous physiological process. It is also a psychosexual experience. In the second stage the wave-like rhythm of expulsive contractions produces an urgent tempo remarkably similar in pattern and timing to rhythms of female orgasm. Masters and Johnson demonstrated that multiple orgasm is a normal female physiological sexual response and that it is not a matter of a woman reaching a climax, but rather of a series of waves of desire, each culminating in release. Exactly the same applies when there is co-ordinated psychophysical activity in the second stage of labor. Each contraction then produces mounting excitement and is spontaneously followed by relaxation, which restores and reinvigorates the woman for the next one.

The intrusive management of labor by those who act primarily as cheerleaders does violence to these spontaneous rhythms. Failure to understand the psychosexual nature of the second stage results in inappropriate encouragement. The woman is told to 'use every pain,' regardless of whether there is an urge to push with that particular contraction. She is also instructed to 'push as hard as you can'; but the uterus itself dictates the urge to push and the woman who is encouraged to 'listen' to her uterus, will be able, like an orchestra obeying the conductor, to follow much more subtle rhythms. The attendants tell her to 'push into your bottom,' yet birth is ultimately not an anal but a vaginal act, and it is essential that the

291

vagina open up to allow the passage of the baby's head. The whole emphasis is on the intensity of pushing rather than on the much more important release of soft tissues. As a result, many women are engaged in a battle between their own expulsive powers and rigid pelvic floor musculature and a tight perineum. When the stress is put on pushing rather than opening up, such a struggle is almost inevitable.

Women may be told to pull with their arms, fixing their hands in handgrips, at the sides of the delivery table, or grasping their own thighs. This involves a waste of energy and almost invariably leads to sore and aching shoulders postpartum. They are encouraged to strain so that they press down through their legs and feet and so get cramps. They are instructed to take deep breaths and hold it for as long as they can, which results in contracted throat musculature, groaning, a sore throat once delivery is completed, and broken blood vessels in the eyes and face.

Instruction to breathe heavily and to take deep breaths leads to marked over-breathing and symptoms of hyperventilation. The consequences of this, especially if it persists over a prolonged period, may be a decreased placental blood flow, fetal acidosis and fetal distress.

Women are frequently taught also to do heavy breathing in the second stage, as an integral part of a method of childbirth education. Pushing is synonymous with vigorous, accentuated inhalation and exhalation. Yet this is not at all what other mammals do in the expulsive stage of parturition. Animals such as dogs, cats, sheep and goats, for example, tend to take short, quick breaths in and out through the slightly open mouth. As the expulsive urge asserts itself, the breath is involuntarily held, just as it is in the laboring woman, and as soon as the animal can breathe again, it does so in the same light accelerated way. Such a model for breathing in the second stage is far less exhausting than that which is usually involved in the management of the second stage. I call it for convenience, and because I first learned it from a Cotswold ewe at lambing time who produced twins

292

with the minimum of fuss and with remarkable economy of effort—the sheep's breathing.

At the beginning of each contraction, the woman steadies herself, by one or two slow breaths. If one emphasizes the slowness rather than the depth of breathing, there is far less gasping and sucking in of breath than if a woman is trying to fill her lungs. As the contraction increases in power, the woman lifts her breathing to higher levels, until she is doing shallow, rapid breathing through her relaxed mouth so light that it is barely audible, but just loud enough for her to be aware herself of her own breathing rhythm. As the pushing urge asserts itself, the breathing spontaneously becomes accentuated and crisper, and then there is the dramatic moment when the breath must be held and she bears down, opening up below as she does so and 'leaning' on the contraction as she concentrates on actively giving birth and opening the vagina.

It is important that she focuses on this image of her body opening rather than on pushing. The pushing will look after itself provided she achieves full perineal release. As soon as she can breathe again she does so, in the same quick light way, until the next expulsive urge comes, and so on through the contractions.

The desire to push comes in waves, like the other rhythms of normal labor, and like defecation. Usually there are two, three or four urges to bear down with each contraction, interspersed by periods of a few seconds to about a third of a minute when the ligh breathing can be maintained and there is no overpowering desire to push.

As the contraction fades, the woman's breathing becomes deeper and slower and she finishes each contraction with a long, slow breath out, the 'resting' breath which allows her to achieve complete relaxation between contractions.

The woman, like the sheep, does not need to close her mouth and press her lips together in order to bear down effectively. In fact, there is much to be gained from keeping the lips soft and relaxed and the jaw dropped. It is an expression a woman spontaneously adopts as she focuses on vaginal, clitoral and pelvic sensations in intercourse, and the same pleasurable focus is helpful in labor. Mouth and vagina are so intimately associated in terms of body image that release of lips, tongue and muscles around the mouth can actively assist release of the perineum.

This relaxed approach to the second stage is one that demands relaxation also on the part of the attendants. Anxiety often expresses itself in the imposition of strenuous activity on the laboring woman, an activity which means that although there is more obvious haste, there is a good deal less speed.

The right time to start to push is when the woman can no longer avoid pushing, and there is much to be gained from waiting until the message conveyed by the uterus is clear and unequivocal and the desire to push is overwhelming and passionate. The woman who asks when she should push is not yet ready, and here the analogy with sexual intercourse and orgasm is also appropriate. Moreover, anxiety to have an urge to push, like anxiety to have orgasm, makes its attainment rather less likely.

A facilitating environment for the second stage of labor is similar to the environment which facilitates lovemaking. Although there are doubtless individuals who might enjoy intercourse on the narrow plank of the average delivery table, or in front of a crowd of casual observers, or with a time limit so that if they do not attain orgasm by 4:30 p.m., the act is completed without their participation, or in a stupefying haze of drugs which induce amnesia, confusion and vomiting; those too, who may actually like intercourse in a windowless, tiled cell surrounded by stainless steel equipment, or under the glare of arc lights or to receive enthusiastic applause throughout. However, many people do not appreciate such a setting for lovemaking and may actually find it so inhibiting that it hinders physiological function. We can assume that for most of us privacy, peace and comfort, the opportunity to select

294

whichever position is most convenient and to change position whenever one wishes, the absence of any urgency to complete the act within a specific time, and the knowledge that one shares the experience with someone loved, all contribute to a sense of well-being and to the ease and satisfaction with which the act is performed.

Few hospitals produce a setting for labor which corresponds in any manner to this, one in which the birth of the baby can be experienced with the same ecstacy in which it was conceived. But the challenge is there. Are there any obstetricians among us who will create that environment?

Reprinted with permission from *The Birth Center Newsletter* (Summer 1978 issue), published at 101 Tufnell Park Road, London, N7, England.

# *Perineal Massage Instructions*

*by Nan Koehler, 1984*

This exercise has 4 benefits;
1. It prevents tearing by helping you identify and relax-at-will your Kegel muscles. A relaxed muscle won't tear!
2. It decreases the length of the second stage because when the pelvic floor or Kegel muscle is loose the pelvis opens easily, allowing the baby to descend rapidly.
3. The oil massage strengthens the tissues and adds health-giving oil to the area which reduces the need for an episiotomy.
4. Daily contact with the vagina by your hands and/or your partner's hands reminds you where and how your baby will be released from your body. The goal is to be as casual about your vagina as you are about any other part of your body.

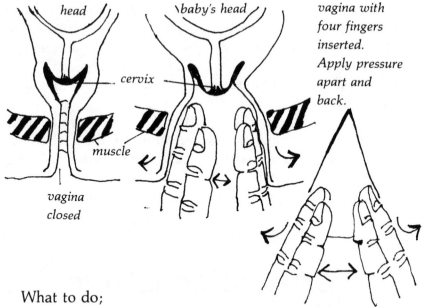

head / baby's head / vagina with four fingers inserted. Apply pressure apart and back.

cervix

muscle

vagina closed

What to do;

*For woman* — Rub the abdomen 2 times a day (morning and evening) with good quality olive oil clockwise, then counterclockwise (hard) ending with a sweep of the oil into and around the vagina and perineum.

*For men* — Beginning 4-6 weeks before birth, once a day wash hands and oil the two forefingers of both hands. Gently insert in the vagina to the 2nd knuckle (see picture) all 4 fingers, then slowly draw the two hands down and apart like a *triangle* until the woman feels a burning sensation and lots of pressure. Hold it there while she breaths and relaxes a little more. Relax your hold a moment and depress the perineum again. Do this 10 times. Each day you apply slightly more pressure until by the due date her vaginal opening can be stretched with ease to her rectum and she has complete control over relaxing that part of her body. Remember you work together. Make eye contact. Don't be afraid of discomfort and pain — you can't help her if it doesn't hurt. This is nothing compared to what it will feel like when the baby's head is stretching the muscles. Your goal is to make her as comfortable with that sensation as possible. *Any couple* who can do

296

this together will have no trouble giving birth. Please use this as a time of pleasurable closeness.

If you have any questions, contact your birth attendant.

A good book for those who really want to pursue this is *The Love Muscle* by Bryce Britton, The New American Library, Inc., 1633 Broadway, New York, NY 10019. 1982,

# Memo To Obstetric Staff

by *Penny Simkin, RPT*

FROM:_____ PHONE:_____

## Description Of Second Stage Techniques

This letter has been prepared to explain how this woman will be working during the second stage if she has no anesthesia. The techniques she has been taught are new and may be somewhat different from what you are most familiar with.

The differences you may notice are:

1. *Mother's position:* She has been encouraged to take whatever position is most comfortable to her and to vary her position during second stage until delivery: semi-sitting, sitting, sidelying, hands and knees, standing, squatting, etc. She has been discouraged from using the lithotomy or any supine position during descent of the baby, and for delivery unless and until forceps, vacuum extractor or episiotomy become necessary.

2. *Bearing down efforts:* Rather than prolonged breath holding and bearing down throughout the contractions, her bearing down and breath holding efforts will be spontaneous and in response to the strength and duration of her urge to push. Bearing down will be for a shorter period (5 to 6 seconds) than is usually encouraged. There may be

297

several moments between these bearing down efforts during which she will breathe without pushing.

3. *Pelvic floor relaxation:* This is of extreme importance. You can help the mother by:

1. suggesting that she try changing position if progress is slow;
2. reminding her to bear down with her urge, and not to push unless she has an urge;
3. reminding her to "let go" thereby relaxing the pelvic floor;
4. and, if spontaneous bearing down and changing position do not result in progress, asking her to bear down longer and more forcefully.

# *Rationale*

Prolonged breath holding and bearing down and the supine position are associated with fetal hypoxia and acidosis, maternal hypotension, and/or too rapid distention of the vaginal tissues, increasing the possibility of lacerations and the need for episiotomy.

Spontaneous bearing down efforts with breathing between results in better oxygenation of the fetus and gradual distention of the vagina. Second stage may last longer than with prolonged bearing down and breath holding, but the fetus remains in good condition throughout.

Varying the position according to the mother's choice may assist fetal descent and rotation, especially in prolonged second stages.

The mother has discussed the above with her physician or midwife and has his/her approval.

REFERENCES

*The Normal Second Stage Of Labour: A Plea For Reform In Its Conduct.* Beynon CL. *J Obstet Gynaecol Br Commonw 64(6):815-820, 1957.*

*The Influence Of Maternal Bearing Down Efforts During Second Stage On Fetal Well-Being.* Caldeyro-Barcia R. *Birth Fam J 6(1):Spring 79.*

*Alternative Positions For Childbirth—Part II: Second Stage Of Labor.* Roberts J. *J Nurs-Midwif* 25(5):Sep/Oct 80.

*Influence Of the Duration Of Second Stage Labor On Perinatal Outcome And Puerperal Morbidity.* Cohen WR. *Obstet Gynecol* 49(3):Mar 77.

*Obstetric Delivery Today: For Better Or Worse?* Dunn PM. *Lancet:*790-93, 10 Apr 76.

# *Avoiding Episiotomy*

## *Prenatally*

- Kegel or Pelvic Floor Contraction Exercise
- Pelvic Floor Relaxation and "Bulging" Exercise
- Practice various positions for second stage
- Perineal massage
- Education—what to expect during second stage
- Good nutrition to promote healthy tissues
- Treatment of vaginitis
- Pubic arch $> 90°$

## *During Second Stage*

- Reassurance and encouragement
- Relaxation of the perineum
- Spontaneous bearing-down (don't rush)
- Positions for comfort or to promote or slow progress
  Gravity-neutral positions for rapid descent
  sidelying, hands and knees
  Gravity-enhancing positions to promote progress
  semi-sitting or sitting
  squatting
  standing
  supported from above
- Use of mirror, touch of the baby's head to encourage efficient bearing down efforts
- Perineal massage and support (hot compresses)
- Cessation of bearing down when stretching and burning are felt in vagina. Pant or blow instead.
- Frequent monitoring of fetal heart rate.

299

*"PUSH" is a 4-letter word. Don't use it!*

# Management of Second Stage

| | Active Management | Physiologic Management |
|---|---|---|
| 1. | Dorsal propped position, then lithotomy for birth | Any of a number of positions (may try several) |
| 2. | Prolonged breath-holding with maximum bearing-down throughout each contraction | Spontaneous (usually short) bearing-down and breath-holding as urge demands. |
| 3. | Anesthesia (regional or local block). | "Natural anesthesia." |
| 4. | Loss of muscle tone in pelvic floor. | Conscious relaxation and bulging of pelvic floor. |
| 5. | Sterile field. | Mother encouraged to touch baby's head. |
| 6. | Episiotomy | Normal late surge of oxytocin increases softening of vaginal tissues and strength of urge to push, reducing need for episiotomy. |
| 7. | Forceps, for:<br>Fetal distress,<br>Lack of progress,<br>Persistent malposition of baby,<br>Inability of mother to push effectively. | Mother's pelvic floor muscle tone and relaxation, and-her bearing down, combine with contractions and gravity to descend and rotate the baby. |
| 8. | Delivery table | Bed, birth chair, other. |

© 1980 Penny Simkin, RPT, Penny Press, 1100 23rd Avenue East, Seattle, WA 98112.

*Handout Available:*

# Obstetric Tests and Technology A Consumer's Guide

by Margot Edwards, R.N., M.S., and Penny Simkin, R.P.T.

The expanded use of technology such as ultrasound, electronics, and biochemical analyses of amniotic fluid and fetal blood, makes possible an ever growing number of tests for pregnancy and labor: tests which assess the well-being or maturity of the fetus; tests which help predict hypertension that may develop during the mother's pregnancy; tests which give information on the size and placement of the fetus; tests for genetic abnormalities; tests which monitor the fetal heart rate; and tests which measure the oxygenation of fetal blood. Before consenting to a test, parents should know something about it, and whether its benefits exceed its risks. Tests are ordered to rule out and diagnose problems. Results of the tests may imply a decided action if problems exist. One means of deciding whether to have a test is to ask if the results will alter the physician's plan for care and/or treatment, or if his/her decision on how to proceed depends on the results of a particular test. If so, how? If not, then perhaps the test is not necessary. Parents are often asked to sign a consent or release form for certain tests, and signing should be based upon an informed consent.

The purpose of this pamphlet is to describe the tests and technology now in wide use in obstetrics: their rationale, accuracy, risks, benefits, and how the results might influence the doctor's management of pregnancy and labor. Thus parents may be helped to make informed decisions.

A list of references for this material is available from the publisher. Please send a self-addressed stamped envelope with your request. Copyright © 1980 by Margot Edwards. All rights reserved. No part of this pamphlet may be reproduced by any means without the written permission of the author. Additional copies of *Obstetric Tests & Technology—a consumer's guide* are available from: the pennypress, 1100 23rd Ave. East, Seattle, WA 98112. Single copy—$1.00; Bulk orders—$40.00 per 100 (includes postage & handling).

# *Summary of Development*

by *Kerry Mazzoni, Childbirth Educator, Novato, CA*
*Used by permission.*

| Calendar Mos. & Wks. Gestation | Ovum | Embryo-fetus |
|---|---|---|
| 1st mo. starts wk. 1 | | |
| 2 | | |
| 3 | Fertilization. | |
| 4 | CG secreted Implantation. Amnion forms Fluid collects. | Inner cell mass forms. Embryonic disc forms. Digestive system forming. Germ layers differentiated. |
| 2nd mo. starts 5 | CG secreted in quantity by chorionic villi. | Brain, nervous system forming. Heart developing and starts to beat. |
| 6 | 15-20 mm in diameter. | 405 mm long. Facial features form. Body flexed. Circulation starts. |
| 7 | Placenta taking shape. | 1/3 inch long. Arm & leg buds appear. Umbilical cord forming. |
| 8 | | 1/6 in. long. Wgt: 1 gm. Hands, feet, fingers and toes forming. |
| 3rd mo. starts 9 | Secretion of CG decreases. Placenta secretes estrogen and progesterone | Eyelids forming. Genital ridge visible but sexless in character. |
| 10 | | Human appearance. Respiratory activity evident. |
| 11 | | Eyelids fused. Sex distinguishable. Tooth buds forming. |
| 12 | | 3/6 inch; Wgt.: 1/2 oz. Skeleton becoming bone. Nails forming. |
| 13 | | Muscles contract occasionally and weakly. |

302

# Summary of Fetal Development

| Ovary | Uterus | Possible Maternal Signs & Physiologic Changes |
|---|---|---|
| | | Menstruation |
| | Length: 6.5 cm Capacity: 30 cc | |
| Follicle secretes Estrogen. | Restoration of mucosa. | |
| Ovulation. Corpus Luteum-Progesterone. | Mucosa thickens & becomes enriched by gland secretion. | Basal body temperature remains elevated. |
| Corpus luteum becomes C.L. of pregnancy. Secretion of estrogen & progesterone continues. | Mucosa invaded. Blood sinuses form. | Nausea. Fatigue. Breasts tense and tingling. |
| | | Amenorrhea. |
| | 1/18th of wall invaded by ovum. | Marked nitrogen loss. Blood sugar low. Basal body temp. constant. Endocrine tests positive. |
| | Mild contractions start. Cervix soft and blue. | Pressure on bladder. Frequency of voiding. Hegar's, Goodell's and Chadwick's signs. |
| | Mucus plug forming in cervical canal. | Profuse vaginal secretion, thick & acid. Nausea subsiding. |
| | | Salivation. Breasts larger & nodular. Montgomery's follicles appear. |
| Secretion of estrogen & progresterone decreasing. | | |
| | 1/3 of wall covered by placenta. | |
| | | Colostrum may be expressed from nipples. |
| | Size of orange. At level of umbilicus. | Nausea & vomiting rare. Plasma fat content increasing. |
| | Rising from pelvic cavity. | Bladder pressure less. BM minus 10. Blood sugar rising. |

303

# Artemis Speaks, Part III: Preparing the Body

| Calendar Mos. & Wks. Gestation | Ovum | Embryo-fetus |
|---|---|---|
| 4th mo. starts wk. 14 | Weight of placenta equals weight of fetus. | Nearly 4 inches long. Sex easily determined. |
| 15 | Placenta — estrogen & progesterone. | Lanugo appearing. Head hair forming. |
| 16 | | 6.4"; Weight: 1/4 lb. Muscles contract more vigorously. |
| 17 | | Skeleton visible on X-ray. |
| 5th mo. starts 18 | | Vernix caseosa forming on skin. Meconium collecting. |
| 19 | | Iron starts to be stored. Onset of rapid growth. Enamel and dentine deposited. |
| 20 | Placenta covers 1/2 uterine wall. | 10 " long. Weight: 3/4 lb. Fetal heart may be heard. |
| 21 | | Eyebrows & lashes visible. |
| 6th month starts 22 | | |
| 23 | | 25 mg. of iron stored. |
| 24 | | 12" long. Weight: 1¼ lbs. |
| 25 | | Skin red & shiny. Face wrinkled. Old man appearance. |
| 26 | Amniotic fluid 1.00–1.55000 cc | 15 inches long. Weight: 1½ lbs. Outline may be felt abdominally. |

304

# Summary of Fetal Development

| Ovary | Uterus | Possible Maternal Signs & Physiologic Changes |
|---|---|---|
| | Becoming an abdominal organ. | Blood volume starts to increase. Cardiac output greater. |
| | | Physiological anemia. Free HCl in gastric juice declines. Blood pressure lower. |
| | Contractions stronger but not palpable. | |
| | Uterine souffle. Fundus: 1/2 way between symphysis/umbilicus | |
| | Walls thin. | Decisive increase in blood volume starts. Nitrogen storage increasing. |
| | | BMR minus 6, rising. |
| Corpus L. begins to disappear. | 1/2 of wall covered by placenta. | Secondary areola appears. Internal ballottement may be felt. |
| | Height of fundus: at umbilicus. | Umbilicus flush with skin. Relaxation of smooth muscle, of veins, bladder, etc. |
| | | BMR minus 4, rising. External ballottement may be felt. |
| | | Urethral dilatation marked. Linea nigra appears. Chloasma may appear. |
| | Fundus above umbilicus. | Period of greatest weight gain starts (4–5 lbs. per month). Abdomen slightly distended. |
| | | BMR: Minus 3, rising. Striae gravidarium may appear. |
| | Fundus 2 fingers above umbilicus. | Period of lowest hemoglobin starts. |

# Artemis Speaks, Part III: Preparing the Body

| Calendar Mos. & Wks. Gestation | Ovum | Embryo-fetus |
|---|---|---|
| 7th mo. starts wk. 27 senile. Infarcts form. | Placenta progressively more descend (male). Subcutaneous fat stored. | Much iron stored. Testes |
| 28 | Placenta very thick; secreting estrogen & pregnanediol. | 14″ long; Weight 2 lb.=. Viable. Eyelids open. Fingerprints set. |
| 29 | | Weak cry. More rapid growth starts. |
| 30 | | Large amount of calcium starts to be deposited. |
| 8th mo. starts 31 | | Twice as much calcium is deposited as is retained by mother. 15.5 mg. nitrogen stored. |
| 32 | Amniotic fluid starts to diminish in amount. | 16″ long. Weight: $3\frac{1}{2}$ lb. Body rounding out. Presentation: usually vertex. |
| 33 | | |
| 34 | | |
| 9th mo. starts 35 | | 227.6 mg. iron stored. 3.16 gm. nitrogen stored. Largest deposit of calcium starts. |
| 36 | | 18 ″ long. Weight: 5+ lbs. |
| 37 | | |
| 38 | | 58.5 gm. nitrogen stored. High hemoglobin. Low $O_2$ tension. Cyanotic. Body well formed. |
| 39-40 | Placenta weighs 1/6 of fetal weight. Amniotic fluid 500–700 cc in amount. | 246.2 mg. iron stored. Lahugo shed. 20″ long. Weight: $7-7\frac{1}{2}$ lbs. |

306

# Summary of Fetal Development

| Ovary | Uterus | Possible Maternal Signs & Physiologic Changes |
|---|---|---|
| Corpus L. absorbed. | Wall soft and yielding. | Weight gain continues: 4 lb. per month. |
| | Fundus 3 fingers above umbilicus. Elastic tissue in wall thickening. | Period of lowest hemoglobin continues. BMR: Zero and rising. |
| | 1/6 of mother's total blood volume in uterine vascular system. | Marked protein storage starts. |
| | Braxton Hicks contractions palpable. | Blood volume highest. |
| | Height of fundus: half-way between umbilicus & ensiform cartilage. | Large amount of calcium lost. BMR: plus 2, rising. |
| | Limit of transverse widening reached. Longitudinal stretching starts. Pyriform in shape. | 3–4 lbs. gained during this month. |
| | | Striae gravidarum more marked. Pelvic joints progressively more relaxed. |
| | Braxton Hicks contractions stronger. | |
| | | BMR: Plus 4, rising. Large amount iron lost. Stomach flaccid on top of uterus. |
| | Height of fundus: at ensiform cartilage. | Umbilicus protrudes. Short of breath. Hemoglobin starts to rise. B.P. raises a bit. |
| | | BMR: Plus 5, rising. 2 lbs. gained during this month. Rise in free HCI. Cardiac output less. |
| | Engaged (nullipara). Height of fundus: slightly below ensiform cartilage. | Lightening (nullipara). Breathing easier. Varicosities. Ankle edema. Frequency of voiding. |
| | Weight: 2 lbs. Capacity: 4,000 cc. Length: 32 cm. | BMR: Plus 7, rising. May lose 2 lbs. BMR: Plus 10. |

# Labor Chart

| Phase of Labor | What You Might Feel | What You Can Do |
|---|---|---|
| *Stage I*<br>A. Early phase<br>0-2 fingers or<br>0-4 cm.<br><br>Contractions: 30-60 seconds long;<br>5 minutes or more apart. | Backache<br>Diarrhea or constipation<br>Abdominal cramps<br>Show<br>Ruptured membranes<br>Excited, impatient, talkative | EAT food and tea<br>Time contractions<br>Call Birth Team<br>Pelvic rock for backache<br>Slow deep breathing<br>Urinate every hour<br>Conscious relaxation<br>Get supplies ready<br>Go for a good walk in the fresh<br>air – walk while contractions are<br>coming on.<br>Take bath. |
| B. Mid-Phase<br>2-4 fingers<br>4-8 cm.<br><br>Contractions: 45-60 seconds long;<br>3-5 minutes apart | Stronger, more frequent<br>contractions<br>More serious concentration<br>Preoccupied<br>Dependent on companionship<br>Restlessness<br>Back and/or leg pain | Breathing: Deep or accelerated<br>chest<br>Effleurage (w/powder or corn<br>starch)<br>Ice chips or tea<br>Relax<br>Vary position of pillows and<br>laboring woman<br>Back rub<br>Concentrate on one contraction at<br>a time |

C. Transition
4-5 fingers
8-10 cm.

Contractions: 60-90 seconds long; 2-3 minutes apart or back-to-back and double peak

Leg cramps and shaking
Nausea and vomiting
Heavy show
Hot and perspiring
"Sleeping" between contrac-
tions
Total involvement and detach
ment
Apprehension
Increased pressure
Desire to push

Breathing: pant, pant-blow, and
blow
Coach—correct technique rate and
rhythm
Use eye-to-eye contact
Encourage to stay in present time
Thigh massage between contrac-
tions
Wake up in time for contraction
Make sure room is tranquil
Encourage other positions
Do not push until checked
DON'T PANIC

*Stage II*
Expulsion of Baby

Contractions: 45-90 seconds long; 2-5 minutes apart

Contractions may slow down
and change character
Urge to push
Pressure to rectum and perineum
Total involvement
Stretching sensation
Feel head moving down
Indian burn sensation (crowning)

Specific instructions for each
contraction
Relax perineal muscle
Push down and forward
Don't push hard
Physical support to woman
Be ready to stop pushing
Stop pushing when head crowns

*Stage III*
Expulsion of placenta

Slight contraction

Squat over bowl and push with
contraction

Reprinted with permission of Homebirth, Inc.,™ Box 162, Norton, MA 02766. Reprint 105, c. 1976.

309

# Medical Emergencies

*Emergency Back-Up Plan:* Most births occur without major complications. For that small percentage of births that do require immediate and decisive action, the most important factor to consider in addition to knowledge of first aid treatment is an emergency back-up plan. This plan must be well-planned, well-rehearsed and fool-proof.

A. Method of getting to the hospital:
  1. *Private car:* Have gas in the car; a driver familiar with the routes to both the hospital of your choice and the hospital with the nearest emergency room. The car should be of a practical size so that the woman in labor could lay down, if necessary. Have blankets for mother and baby. Plan how the woman could be carried to the vehicle: stretcher, board and blanket, coffee table, several strong people attending birth.

  2. *Ambulance, Police or Fire Dept., Rescue Units, Project Place:* Make arrangements for these services before labor begins. Alert them when labor begins and if services are not used, notify them of successful birth. Know their procedures — rescue units will sometimes only transport to the nearest hospital.

B. *Birth Team:* Each member should know the possible emergencies and appropriate treatment; each member should have specific jobs both for the normal birth and in case of an emergency. These jobs must be well understood, assigned and practiced in a birth rehearsal before labor begins. Possible jobs in an emergency:

  Calling doctor, hospital, emergency transportation unit — being specific as to situation and location

  Carrying mother to car

310

Carrying baby to car
Driver of car
Attendant to mother on trip
Attendant to baby on trip
Babysitter to other siblings or pets

C. *Phone Numbers:* These numbers should be posted near the telephone:
Members of birth team including medical professional who will attend birth
Doctor who has agreed to provide back-up at hospital—he/she should be alerted when labor begins
Hospital of choice
Nearest hospital with emergency room
Ambulance, Police and Fire Dept.,
Rescue Squad, Project Place

Reprinted with permission of Homebirth, Inc.,™ 89 Franklin Street, Suite 200, Boston, MA 02110. Reprint 107:1, c. 4/1976.

# *Possible Medical Emergencies*

This section should not be construed as a training program to teach lay persons how to deal with medical emergencies. It is merely to inform parents of the possible emergencies that can occur in childbirth at home and the steps which should be taken if they do occur. This information is necessary for them to make rational decisions and hence be responsible for their birth experiences. The subjects covered in this section are:

I. Hemorrhage
II. Prolapsed Umbilical Cord
III. Arm or Leg Presentation
IV. Fetal Distress
V. Respiratory Distress in the Newborn

If any one of these complications occurs, institute first aid measures and alert your medical backup team in order to get mother and/or baby to a hospital as soon as possible.

In addition to the medical emergencies listed here, there are other situations which would cause the birth to deviate from the normal. These situations, which include tight nuchal cord, shoulder dystocia, and previously undiagnosed breech presentation, are not considered medical emergencies as such since the ability to deal with them should be well within the realm of the medical professional in attendance.

For further information concerning management of the actual birth, we highly recommend Gregory White's *Emergency Childbirth* manual.

I. *Hemorrhage:* In a normal birth the amount of blood lost is one-half to one cup. Also a few spoonfuls of blood mixed with mucus (like red current jelly) lost before or during labor is normal. A blood loss of over two cups is not normal.

  A. *Signs* of Hemorrhage:
    1. Blood loss:
      a. *Before or during labor:* Loss of more than a few spoonfuls of blood
      b. *During and after delivery:* Loss of more than two cups of blood (total)
    2. Shock as indicated by:
      a. Pallor, cold sweat
      b. Feeling faint, dizzy, confused, apprehensive
      c. Falling blood pressure, rising pulse
    3. Abdominal pain (not present in all cases)

  B. *Treatment* of Hemorrhage:
    1. In all cases of hemorrhage:
      a. Take mother to hospital quickly
      b. Alert Emergency Back-Up Team
      c. Have mother lie down with lower half of body elevated

d. Keep mother warm with a blanket

e. Have mother drink water (salt water, if possible), one-half cup every 20 to 30 minutes

2. If hemorrhage occurs after birth, in addition to the above, also:

a. Have baby (or anybody) nurse to stimulate uterine contractions

b. Massage uterus gently, do not pull on cord

c. If placenta has been delivered and uterus does not contract with massaging, begin bimanual compression

II. *Prolapsed Umbilical Cord:* This means that the cord comes out of the cervix or vagina before or alongside the baby's head. Since the cord carries the baby's oxygen supply, compression of the cord by the aftercoming head would cause distress in the baby.

A. *If head is crowning:*

1. The woman must bear down and birth the baby as quickly as possible

2. Alert Emergency Back-Up Team

B. *If the head is not visible in the vagina:*

1. Transport mother to *closest* hospital emergency room as quickly as possible in the *knee-chest position*

2. Alert Emergency Back-Up Team, especially alerting hospital emergency room to the exact situation

3. The cord:

a. Do not compress or pull on the cord. As long as it is still pulsating, the baby is receiving oxygen.

b. If possible, while mother is in knee-chest position gently hold cord up in vagina

c. If unable to put cord back into vagina, wrap it in a clean, warm, moist cloth and hold close to vagina

4. Using sterile gloves, the presenting part may be gently elevated in the vagina

III. *Arm or Leg Presentation:* This is when an arm or leg appears at the cervical or vaginal opening before the head. Unless baby is very tiny, labor is a mechanically impossible one since baby is wedged crosswise in the birth canal.

    A. Transport mother to the hospital as quickly as possible

    B. Keep mother in knee-chest position

IV. *Fetal Distress:* This means that the baby's blood supply (and therefore its oxygen supply) has been interrupted. This is usually due to cord compression. The fetal heart rate is the best guide to how the fetus is faring. The normal fetal heart rate varies from 120-160 beats/minutes. Each baby's heart rate should not vary more than 10 beats/minute in either direction from its prenatal rate. Be familiar with your baby's normal heart rate.

    A. *Signs of fetal distress:*

        1. It is not unusual for the fetal heart rate to fluctuate during a contraction, but if it *does not return to normal after the contraction,* the baby is in distress.

        2. If the fetal heart rate goes *below 110 beats/minute* at any time, the baby is in distress.

        3. If the fetal heart rate goes *above 160 beats/minute* at any time, the baby is in distress.

        4. If the *amniotic fluid is not clear,* that is, colored yellow, green, or brown and/or is foul smelling, this indicates that the baby has passed some meconium which is a sign of fetal distress.

    B. *First Aid for Fetal Distress:*

        1. *If the baby's head is crowning:* Birth the baby as quickly as possible

        2. *If the baby's head is not visible in the vagina:*

            a. Transport the mother to the closest hospital emergency room quickly

            b. Mother should be in the position which bring

the fetal heart rate closer to normal such as knee-chest or side positions

   c. If oxygen is available, mother should breathe it deeply

C. *Precautions:*

   1. Always check the fetal heart rate after the membranes rupture

   2. Check the fetal heart rate periodically during labor and more frequently as labor progresses

V. *Respiratory Distress in the Newborn:* A normal newborn will initiate respirations as soon as the cord stops pulsating (usually within two minutes) if not sooner.

A. *Signs* of respiratory distress

   1. Baby's body (other than hands, feet, and presenting part) does not get pink after respirations have begun

   2. Difficulty breathing: Nasal flaring, retracting (with each inspiration the outline of the ribs is visible), groaning or grunting with each respiration

   3. Normal respiratory rate in the newborn is 40-60 respirations/minute. If respirations are quite slow and gasping, the baby is in distress.

   4. No spontaneous respirations

B. *First Aid:* To be instituted immediately and on the way to the hospital where the baby should be transported as soon as possible:

   1. Position baby in horizontal position with head turned on side on flat, hard surface.

   2. Using bulb syringe, suction mucus first from the mouth and secondly from the nostrils, if necessary. (Always squeeze the bulb before placing tip in mouth or nostril.) If no bulb syringe is available, wipe out the mouth with a clean cloth.

   3. Dry off baby and *keep warm*

   4. If the baby is breathing on its own and oxygen is

315

available, hold the oxygen mask near the baby's face.

5. If the baby is having slow, gasping respirations and is limp, or if there is no spontaneous respirations, begin mouth-to-mouth resuscitation

 a. The technique of mouth-to-mouth resuscitation is not difficult in itself, but should be studied by attendants *before* labor begins as part of one's prenatal preparation. An excellent source is the *American Red Cross First Aid Textbook.*

 b. *Steps* in mouth-to-mouth resuscitation:

   I. Clear any mucus from mouth

   II. Extend head slightly back—football hold is excellent way to hold baby

   III. Placing mouth over baby's mouth and nose, gently puff a small amount of air into the newborn (not more than a mouthful of air).

   IV. The chest should rise and fall with each respiration

   V. Breathe into the baby about 20 times per minute

   VI. Keep a hand gently placed on the infant's stomach to prevent it from becoming bloated with air

   VII. If the baby begins to breathe spontaneously at a normal rate, resuscitation may be stopped; if not, continue resuscitation on route to the hospital

 c. Any baby who requires resuscitation at birth should be taken to a hospital as soon as possible even if the crisis is apparently passed.

Homebirth, Inc.,™ 89 Franklin Street, Suite 200, Boston, MA 02110

316

# Emergency Instructions

by Kay Mathews

When you expect that labor will start soon or after it begins if you miscalculate, prepare the room where you expect to give birth. If the room is small and cluttered, please remove those things which might be in the way and won't be needed. Clear off a dresser, chest, or table and put out the supplies you have bought plus the towels, sheets, other supplies.

If you have a child under 5, please arrange for someone to be there whose sole duty is to be with the child and care for him/her in case the labor/birth is upsetting the child in any way.

Have phone numbers of attendants, doctor, hospital ER room and ambulance taped close to phone during the last month of your pregnancy.

If you get any *heavy* bleeding of bright red blood during the first stage of labor, go immediately to the hospital.

If the baby is coming very quickly and attendant is not there yet, do not be afraid. Everything is normal and OK if things are moving that fast. You can have the baby by yourself and do a beautiful job! When you feel that pushing is unavoidable, try a few tentative pushes. If it hurts, don't do it. Wait a few contractions and try again. You can pant or blow out (the slower the better) to keep from pushing.

Get comfortable, but do not lie flat on your back. If someone is with you, they should wash their hands and prepare to catch the baby. When you feel your perineum stretching and burning, try to refrain from hard pushing. The person with you can try to slow down the birth of the head so that the baby won't shoot out too fast.

If water bag is unbroken, break it when it is visible and see that none of it covers the baby's mouth and nose. Once the head is out, it will probably rotate by itself to one side. The rest of the body will come out with the next contraction. Do not push.

317

The baby's color may be bluish to purplish. This is normal; don't panic. If cord is around neck, unwind it. If baby's face is very mucousy and there seems to be much liquid in its mouth and nose, wipe the mouth with a thin, clean cloth. In an emergency, you can gently suck the mucous from the baby's nose if you have no syringe.

If it doesn't breathe right away, gently rub it's back, hold the head lower, tap the feet. If it doesn't breathe after 1 or 2 minutes, give very gentle mouth to mouth resuscitation, covering mouth and nose.

Put baby on mother's tummy and to the breast if the cord is long enough. Cover the baby with a blanket or towel.

Do not cut the cord or pull on it. WAIT

The placenta will probably come in 15 minutes to 1 hour. Put it in a bowl on the bed and leave baby attached to it.

There will be some gushes of blood during the birth of the placenta. Keep the towels for attendant to see blood loss.

If the mother bleeds excessively, such as over 2 cups (remember that the blood may be mixed with the waters and look like a lot more) AND shows the following symptoms: cold, clammy skin, sweating, paleness, extreme weakness, chills, severe chest pain, rapid pulse, put her in head down position and call an ambulance. Elevate the hips. Give no food or liquid.

If the woman is bleeding heavily but has none of the above symptoms, keep the baby at the breast or have someone else nurse. Give her strong tea (angelica, American Saffron and shephards purse are good for bleeding). If really concerned, give her 1 t. of cayenne pepper (capsicum) in 1 cup of warm water and have her drink it quickly.

318

# Parents' Emergency Birth Instructions

## (Author Unkown)

If the baby comes quickly, remember the following:

1. Don't be afraid; if the baby comes that fast then everything is OK.

2. Relax, let things move along, try to pant as you feel the baby's head stretching you. Get comfortable.

3. Attendant should (if possible) wash hands before handling baby. If you know how, slow down the birth of the head so it doesn't "pop" out. This will reduce the chance of tearing.

4. If water bag is not broken, break it as soon as it is visible on the outside. Make sure there is none of the membrane over the baby's face.

5. Baby's head will turn on own and with next contraction body will slide out. The baby's head will be bluish; don't panic. This is normal and necessary to stimulate breathing. If cord is around neck, unwind.

6. IF BABY SOUNDS MUCOUSY, WIPE MOUTH WITH TOWEL (NOT KLEENEX). IF BABY DOESN'T BREATHE, HOLD WITH HEAD LOWER THAN FEET, LIGHTLY SPANK FEET AND RUB BACK.

7. Put baby on mother's abdomen and to breast if cord is long enough.

8. DON'T cut cord. DON'T pull, WAIT.

9. The placenta will come away in about 15-30 minutes. There may be a gush of blood then. This is normal.

10. Keep everyone warm, give mother something to drink with honey in it. And you had better have some too!

Artemis Speaks, Part III: Preparing the Body
# The Question Of Silver Nitrate

*by Rosemary Wiener*

In nearly all American hospitals and most birth centers, silver nitrate drops are routinely put in the babies' eyes shortly after birth. Some home birth attendants also routinely use silver nitrate.

Why is this done? If the mother has gonorrhea, the germs in her vaginal tract could get in the baby's eyes during birth. Unless the baby's eyes are treated with a substance that will kill the gonorrhea germs, the baby's eyes can become severely infected. This can result in blindness. It has been estimated that approximately 5% of all women giving birth actually do have gonorrhea.

If the baby is born by caesarian delivery instead of vaginally, there is only a remote possibility that the baby could pick up gonorrhea germs from the mother's system. However, silver nitrate is still routinely put in the eyes of Caesarian babies.

Expectant mothers can be tested for gonorrhea. However, sometimes the test produces "false negatives." In other words, she could have the disease but it does not show up on the test. Usually testing for gonorrhea is not a part of routine prenatal care. If you have not been tested for it, and if there is any chance that you and your husband or partner may have gonorrhea, it is highly advised that you ask your doctor to test for it.

If both partners of a marriage or relationship began the relationship as virgins and have had no other sexual partners, it is impossible for either of them to have gonorrhea. If both partners of a marriage or relationship remain faithful to each other over a long period of time, and have not previously had gonorrhea, or have had it successfully treated in the past, the chances of their having gonorrhea is highly unlikely. People who have a number of sexual partners almost inevitably get gonorrhea at some time or other. Anyone who has a positive

320

test for gonorrhea should take the responsibility of informing his/her sexual partner(s). In some cases, just one partner of a marriage or relationship can give the disease to both. For example, a woman could contract gonorrhea even though she has been faithful to her husband or partner, if he has had sex with someone else.

Sometimes attempts to treat gonorrhea will not completely cure it. Gonorrhea germs do not survive outside the body. With extremely rare exceptions, the disease is only spread through sexual contact. (You cannot catch gonorrhea from toilet seats, dirty dowels, or public restrooms.)

Most lay midwives attending home births do not routinely administer silver nitrate. In practice, it has been extremely rare for midwives to encounter any difficulty with babies' eyes because of this. However, occasionally it has happened that a mother did have gonorrhea, gave birth at home, and silver nitrate was not administered. In cases like this it has been learned that there is **time** to treat the baby's eyes before permanent damage takes place. Apparently the baby does not instantly go blind from the gonorrhea. Within the first day or two after birth, the baby's eyes will ooze and become irritated, and if this happens it can be treated. If you are giving birth at home, if your birth attendant does not administer silver nitrate or other type of prophylactic ointment for the baby's eyes, and if there is any possibility that you may have gonorrhea, it is of utmost importance that you be alert to this, and get the baby to a doctor immediately to have his/her eyes treated if this should occur.

Individual couples know their own personal choices, values, and sexual behavior. Today many parents are becoming concerned about routine administration of silver nitrate into their baby's eyes, especially if they are certain that they do not have gonorrhea.

**What is the concern about silver nitrate?** Normally a newborn baby's eyes are very clear and beautiful. Usually the healthy newborn who was born without medication is alert and aware and will look around at his/her environment, and most importantly make eye contact with his/her parents.

Silver nitrate is a caustic, burning substance which causes the baby a great deal of pain. After it is administered the baby's eyelids become swollen and puffy and remain that way for several days. The drops appear to cause temporary blindness. Many people are becoming concerned that silver nitrate can interfere with bonding because the baby cannot see his/her parents. In some cases the baby's eyes may ooze and be irritable for many weeks after the silver nitrate is administered. Adults who have had other experiences with silver nitrate have verified that it causes a painful, burning sensation when applied to the skin. There is no doubt about the fact that this is painful for the baby.

Frequently people think that babies' eyes are naturally "puffy little slits" at birth that "do not open" for several days. This is not true. What they have observed is the effects of silver nitrate. They have never seen a baby whose eyes were clear and untraumatized from birth on, and therefore they do not know the difference.

**What are the legal requirements about silver nitrate?** In each of the states of the U. S. there is some type of state regulation about treatment of the newborn infant's eyes shortly after birth for prevention of "infectuous conjunctivitis of the newborn." The exact wording of this law varies from state to state, but in most states it is **not the law** that the preparation that is to be put in infants' eyes **has** to be silver nitrate.

In the Washington State Administrative Code (WAC 248-100-295) opthalmia neonatorium) the regulation on this matter reads as follows:

"Prevention:

(1) Instillation of a one percent solution of silver nitrate into the conjunctival sacs of the eyes of all infants shortly after birth.

(2) Upon request of the medical staff of a hospital, the use

of some other effective and suitable preparation in lieu of silver nitrate solution may be authorized by the state director of health, providing the name and concentration of the prophylactic agent is recorded on the birth certificate of the infant."

If you are living in a state other than Washington and are concerned about silver nitrate, it is highly advised that you find your own state's regulations about this matter. State legal documents are available to the public in most major public libraries. The page with the regulation in question can be xeroxed if desired.

**What is being done about alternatives to silver nitrate?** Some parents who have questioned silver nitrate have met considerable resistance on the part of the medical profession. Silver nitrate has been routinely administered to all newborns in hospitals for such a long time that many doctors and hospital personnel simply assume that it is the law. Perhaps they have never before heard anyone question its practice. Frequently it takes repeated attempts at questioning a medical practice before changes can be made.

If you wish to question the pactice of routine silver nitrate at your local hospital or birth center, your most effective "tool" will be a copy of your state's regulation about this. (Remember that even if you are planning a home or birth center birth, need for hospitalization may arise. It is highly advised that you investigate the practices of your local hospital in case you or the baby need to go there.) Knowledge of your state regulations, combined with a "professional" attitude on your part, and preferably discussing the matter well in advance of the baby's birth, will be more likely to be listened to and respected. Angry "ranting and raving" will more likely result in your being dismissed as a "fanatic."

Because of people's questioning of the matter, some hospitals and birth centers are now allowing parents who do not want silver nitrate to sign a waiver to this effect. (People who do not believe in certain medical practices, such as Jehovah's Witnesses who do not believe in blood transfusions, have been signing similar waivers for years.) In some cases the hospital or birth center personnel will not put anything in the baby's eyes if a waiver is signed. In other cases they prefer to administer another type of ointment such as penicillin or erythromycin. These ointments are generally clear, vaseline type substances. They are still unnecessary in the 95% of babies whose mothers do not have gonorrhea, but they do not burn or cause pain as does silver nitrate.

Allowing the baby's eyes to be clear and untraumatized after birth is one thing which can help give him or her a more peaceful beginning in life. If you are concerned about this and will be giving birth in a hospital or birth center, question them about this procedure. If you will be giving birth at home, make sure you know your birth attendant's policy on this. Write letters about it. Talk with your doctor or birth attendant about it. Perhaps your efforts in this area will cause them to be open to less painful alternatives to silver nitrate.

Copies of this article are available at the following rates: Single copy—15¢ plus self-addressed stamped envelope (business size), 50 copies—$5.00 plus $1.00 postage, 100 copies—$9.00 plus $2.00 postage. Order from: Rosemary Wiener, 4521 Fremont Street, Bellingham, WA 98226. © June 1981

# The Placenta

### by Martha Serrie Benedict

The placenta for mammals is one natural way to replenish the energy and nutrient requirements of the mother post partum.

After delivery of the placenta and examination for any abnormalities, it should be washed in cool running water to rinse the blood and stored in a clean, air tight container till ready to be prepared (preferably later that same day).

There is nothing unusual about the taste of placenta. It may be likened to an organ meat comprised of sinew and soft parts inter-meshed. It may taste most closely to liver—but not quite. It is a little difficult to cut so use a sharp knife and cut into small (1/2" cubes) pieces. Do not include the umbillicus. This can be saved for future use. The taste is a little strong so until a taste for it is developed, it may be good to include cooking ideas from the following tried recipes.* The rejuvinating effects will be felt from ingesting even small quantities of placenta.

1. 1 placenta cut into 1/2" cubes
   2 diced onions
   3-4 cloves garlic mashed
   olive oil
   vegetable seasoning
   pinch of cayenne

   Saute the onions in olive oil till limp (10 minutes). ADD vegetable seasoning/garlic and placenta. Cover and cook till done—about 8-12 minutes. ADD pinch of cayenne. Serve with hot brown rice.

2. 1 placenta cut into 1/2" cubes
   l diced onion
   10-12 cloves garlic mashed
   olive oil
   vegetable seasoning
   vegetable water

   Saute onion in olive oil. ADD garlic and placenta. Cover and cook 8-12 minutes till done. Stir in vegetable seasoning to taste. If dry add vegetable water. Serve with boiled parsley potatoes.

3. 1 placenta cut into 1/2" cubes
   1 sliced onion
   3 tablespoons curry powder
   olive oil
   1/4 cup fruit juice
   apple slices/raisins/coconut shreds/chutney

   Saute onion in olive oil. ADD garlic/apple slices/

raisins/coconut shreds and placenta. MIX in 3 tablespoons curry powder (or to taste). Pour fruit juice over all. Cover and simmer 8-12 minutes till done. Serve with chutney and brown rice.

*Note: if eaten fresh, it is not strong or wierd tasting. I recommend it — it's very delicious. *Nan Koehler*

Martha Serrie Benedict, Certified Acupuncturist, 427 Locust St., Santa Cruz, CA 95060. (408) 425-4977.

Note to be placed on the front door after your baby's birth — designed by Melissa Johnston, Camp Meeker, 1981.

*Thank you for your visit. Please limit it to 10 minutes as we need our REST. If you wish to stay longer, please do one of the following:*

_____ Wash dishes

_____ Prepare some food or tea

_____ Tidy up and/or sweep

_____ Water the plants

_____  _____

Mother Care

326

# After Birth Instructions

*by Nan Koehler, 1977*

1. Check the fundus (top of the uterus) every 15-30 minutes for the first 2-3 hours after the birth. Then taper off to every 1-2 hours until 12 hours later. The fundus should be below the navel and hard as a baseball. With nursing, the mother might feel the uterus contracting. These are called after-birth pains. The more the baby sucks on the breast, the more the uterus contracts, the less the mother bleeds, and the sooner she recovers from the birthing experience.

2. Check the umbilical cord of the baby every time you change his/her diaper. Dab around the base with alcohol 2-3 times a day. Check for redness and/or tenderness around the belly button.

3. Drink 2-3 pots of Comfrey leaf or root tea. This will accelerate the healing of the placental site in the uterus. When making the tea use no metal with the herb. Boil water, pour over the comfrey (1/3 cup to a pot of water), steep for about 10 minutes. If you are using the root, simmer in an enamel or glass pot for about 15 minutes.

4. If the Mother is sore or tore in the birthing do a sitz bath as needed. One time/day for no tears until soreness is gone — usually 2-3 days; 4 times/day for tears or stitches. Make the tea, pour in a shallow dishpan and squat over the pan with the perineum in the hot comfrey water as long as possible.

5. Bedrest until the bleeding has stopped altogether — about one week. The better the mother stays down right after the birth, the quicker she'll recover in the long run and the easier her task of caring for the new baby. Keep visitors away until the baby is older.

6. Don't let anyone but the mother handle the baby — especially visitors. The father or close relatives can handle

327

the child, but not for long. This keeps the baby centered and mellow.

7. The family needs a lot of quiet time hanging out with the baby. They need to get acquainted with each other. The more time put into the child at first in satisfying its basic needs, the less time the child will demand later. The first three months are the most important in establishing the child's basic personality. If the parents want to make any influence on the child, this is the time. There are many interesting books written around this theme. A three month period of isolation with the baby insures a good bond between mother and child which lays the foundation for their whole life together. Read *Birth* by David Meltzer.

# *Mastitis — Catch It Early!*

*by Nan Koehler, February 1979*

Many women, during their time of breastfeeding, get an infection in the breast. This condition is very easy to treat at home with home remedies, especially when caught early. When it's out of hand, then one needs to resort to antibiotics. I have had mastitis repeatedly. (I feel as though I've been nursing a baby for ten straight years. Now I'm working on my fourth child who is a year and a half and still mostly nursing.) Here is the regime I've developed that works really well for me.

At the first sign that your breast feels different — itchy, achy, sore, lumpy or extra full — wear a bra and keep it on until your breast feels normal again. (You probably will have to continue wearing a bra until your nursing days are over.) Second, make yourself some apple cider vinegar tea (2 Tsp. of apple cider vinegar in a quart of warm water) and sip that while fasting and resting the rest of the day. Drink 3 quarts of the tea in one day if you wake up with sore breasts, or one quart if you get sick in the evening.

If you have a fever, go to bed right away and stay there (sipping the tea, nursing your baby on the sore side, *keep it empty*, and placing a heating pad on your breast when the baby is on the other side or not at the breast) until you have a "healing crisis" (a good sweat). Then you know the worst is over. Rest the next day because you'll probably feel pretty weak for several days. Mastitis is like getting a cold. If you weren't nursing, you'd get a sore throat instead. Fatigue, stress, poor diet (especially sugar or overeating), nursing a child with a runny nose, sleeping on a full breast or wearing tight straps over the breast will all set you off.

If your mastitis is very advanced, then you might like to put ice on your breast instead of heat until the redness and swelling go down. Also, herbal poultices on the sore spot are wonderful for drawing out the infection. Once it's red on the outside, you know it will get better soon. Mullien, comfrey, and lobelia are my favorites. Onions or potatoes (grated raw) work well also.

To summarize:
1. wear bra
2. keep breast empty
3. apply heat or cold
4. rest
5. This is most important:
   Fast and drink apple cider vinegar tea until you feel all right again — usually takes 24 hours.
6. apply herbal poultice

If your condition isn't improved within 24 hours with this regime call your local MD for some antibiotics. (But I know you won't need to if you follow the steps listed above.)

# Proper Nursing

The position of the nipple in the baby's mouth.
A. and B. are wrong in that the nipple is being chewed.
C. is correct — the nipple is well within the baby's mouth.

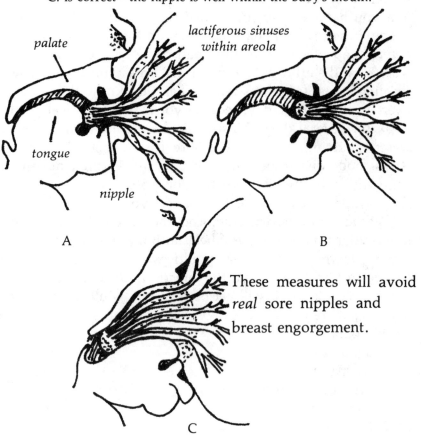

palate

lactiferous sinuses
within areola

tongue

nipple

A

B

These measures will avoid *real* sore nipples and breast engorgement.

C

Thus to maintain successful lactation, the necessary requirements are:

1. An adequate intake of food and fluid by the mother.

   *carbohydrates and water*

   *2-3 quarts of water/day (In California and other dry areas, drink 6-8 quarts of water/day.)*

2. Nurse baby very frequently.

330

# After Birth Information

## The Baby:

The baby may suck right away — the baby needs to be held and to be in skin-to-skin contact with its mother and family whether or not it is sucking. Even if the baby is not into it, put him/her to the breast every few hours to try again so that he/she gets use to it.

The baby is not dirty and does not need to be washed — any vernix (white creamy stuff on the baby) can be rubbed into the baby's skin and meconium (baby's first stool) can be washed off with warm water, or dissolved with vegetable or vitamin E oil and wiped off. If you want to wash the baby, wait at least until the cord has fallen off (usually four days to a week after birth) and then sponge bathing works fine.

The cord should be kept out of the diaper and the diaper folded down enough in front to keep the belly button free of it. You can apply alcohol to the end and base of the cord several times a day until it drops off. If any blood is coming from the cord, you should re-tie it and keep an eye on it to make sure it is not bleeding any more. If the belly skin around the navel looks red or infected, if any pus or foul smell is around the cord or navel, you should consult a doctor.

Sometimes when you have fed and changed your baby, he/she will still be fussy. Sometimes this can be gas in his/her stomach (sometimes relieved by rubbing his/her back while he/she is lying on your lap) or sometimes he/she just wants to be held and rubbed, or the energy in his/her environment has become too hectic for his/her comfort. Look for a quiet, calm space for you and he/she to be in when you feel this happening.

If the baby is bleeding anywhere (besides a tiny spot of blood with the first urine, or with a girl a small amount of blood coming from the vagina soon after birth), you should consult a doctor.

If the baby has not urinated or passed meconium after twenty-four hours, consult a doctor.

If a baby becomes at all jaundiced (yellow-looking skin or whites of eyes), especially within the first twenty-four hours of life, consult a doctor. To prevent jaundice, give a sunbath, 15 minutes on each side two times a day. After your milk has been in for a day or so, you may take your baby to a clinic or doctor for a PKU test. This test may determine whether or not your baby has a disease which interferes with protein metabolism and which, if left undiagnosed, can lead to mental retardation. When diagnosed, it may be treated through diet.

If the whites of the baby's eyes look irritated or have a discharge, consult a doctor.

Leave the baby on his/her stomach or propped on his/her side to sleep so that if she vomits any mucous or milk it will drain out of her mouth and not choke him/her.

If the baby's body feels warm, hands and feet feel cool (not cold), the baby is not too hot or cold. If baby's armpit temperature is 100° or more, contact the doctor.

In general, the baby's breathing will occasionally be irregular or gasping once in a while. Coughing, sneezing and crying all help clear out the baby's lungs the first few days. However, if the baby has a fever and is continually gasping and grunting with each breath or breathing over 60 times a minute, see a doctor. When awake, the baby should have good muscle tone (flexed arms and legs, grasping hands) and not be extremely laid back. If the tissue around the eyes seems dried out or the eyes begin to look more protuberant, or if the skin, when you pinch it between your fingers feels un-elastic or stays pinched, then the baby may becoming dehydrated for some reason and you should definitely consult a doctor. If the baby has less than six wet diapers per day, he/she may becoming dehydrated.

At first a newborn's stool is the color and texture of tar. Within a few days, a breastfed baby's stool changes to a very loose, creamy textured, mustard yellow. The frequency of

332

bowel movements in a breastfed baby varies a great deal from many times a day to once every week or ten days. Both are normal if the baby is eating only breastmilk.

Be careful in choosing commercial baby products. Mineral oils will absorb vitamins from the skin, vegetable oils will not. Some baby powders have Zinc Stearati which will harm baby's lungs. Cornstarch is a natural alternative. It is normal for baby's skin to peel the first week.

## The Mother

Learn to check for the hardness of the uterus and you should continue to feel for it every so often to make sure it feels firm. If it is not hard, or you cannot seem to feel it where it was before, you should gently rub up a contraction. Firm but gentle. Getting the baby to nurse will also help to stimulate the uterus to contract.

Whenever you stand up, any blood that has collected in the back of the vagina will come out. When nursing makes your uterus contract you may have a gush of blood. *If two or more pads are completely soaked during any half an hour period you should call a doctor*, and save the pads in case he wants to look at them.

If you have a 100° temperature for more than 12 hours or so in the week following birth, this could indicate infection. Your lochial discharge (watery bleeding) should smell like a period. If it smells foul, or if there is any pus in the discharge, you may have an infection and you should consult a doctor.

Your whole vaginal area should be kept clean, since even if you don't have any tears, the whole birth canal is slightly open and traumatized. Many women find that soaking in a clean warm shallow (3-4" deep) "sitz" bath several times a day eases the discomfort of abrasions or stitches. A cold pack applied after birth will help ease the swelling. If it burns when you urinate, you can pour lukewarm water over yourself as you urinate, or sit in warm water to urinate. Try to keep your bowels loose. Always wipe front to back.

Some women feel that both local application of, and inclusion in the diet, of vitamin E helps promote faster healing. Also, the application of warm herbal compresses (ginger, for instance) to the outside of the vaginal area are felt by many to help. Exposure of the area to air and sunlight is good for healing.

To get your body in shape and for a good nursing experience, you need as much or more protein in your diet as when you were pregnant. A diet high in protein and iron will help you feel better and will be good for the baby too.

Labor is equal to a 50 mile hike, so rest well the first week after birth and then gradually increase your active hours each day. Many women have found that if they don't rest at first that they end up having to do it later.

Exposure to sun and air is good also for your nipples when you are beginning to nurse, especially good if your breasts tend to be sore. Your breasts do not need to be washed more often than the rest of your body; they secrete antibodies which should not be washed away, as well as important natural lubricants. It is much more important to wash your hands after going to the bathroom or before handling your breasts.

When your milk comes in, your breasts may feel uncomfortably full and hard. Sometimes a hot towel applied to the breasts will speed the let-down of milk. If you feel hard lumps or hot red-painful areas in your breasts, warm compresses, bed rest, and keeping the baby (or someone) sucking seems beneficial.

If you have any problems or questions on breastfeeding, or would like support for it or mothering in general, call or attend the meetings of your local La Leche League.

Many people find that after birth their urge to make love seems completely dormant for varying periods — some people for as long as they are not ovulating, whether that is two months or two years. It seems that this is based on some hormonal balance and happens to many people. If it is not understood for what it is, this change in a relationship can lead to hard times. Many women feel all their energy going out to the baby, and the man feels rejected. Touching and affection are often forgotten, or the woman feels that since she does not feel like getting into making love, that they better stay away from the whole physical affection trip. If both partners know what to expect, and can understand it, this fear can be removed, and both people can be free to express their affection for each other in whatever way is comfortable for both of them.

Reprinted with permission. Homebirth, Inc.,™ 89 Franklin Street, Suite 200, Boston, MA 02110.

## *Great Handout Available:*

# *When Your Baby Has Jaundice*

## What Can Parents Do?

There are some things parents can do to help avoid jaundice in their babies, and much they can do if the baby has jaundice. Following are some pointers that can help both parents and baby through this difficult time.

1. *Avoid drugs known to be associated with newborn jaundice, if at all possible.* See earlier discussion.

2. *Breastfeed your baby as soon as possible after birth and frequently thereafter.* This gives the baby colostrum, an excellent laxative, which speeds the passage of the baby's first stool — meconium. Meconium is laden with bilirubin which is reabsorbed by the baby's blood stream. In addition, early, frequent breastfeeding helps bring in the mother's milk faster, providing more fluid to promote ex-

335

cretion of bilirubin. Do not rush feeding. Relax and let the baby suck as long as he/she wants. This will help get lots of fluids into the baby to "wash out" the jaundice.

3. *Keep yourselves informed of bilirubin levels, treatment plans, and other items related to your baby's condition.*

4. *See if the baby can be treated at your bedside while in the hospital.* This will enable you to have more contact with your baby.

5. *If the baby remains in the hospital after you go home, spend a lot of time visiting your baby.* This is sometimes discouraging, as phototherapy causes a listlessness and sleepiness in the baby. In addition, many newborn nurseries are not really set up for parents' visits and the nurses and other staff may not welcome your presence for long periods. The baby needs voice and touch stimulation and his or her mother's and father's loving presence. Be as cooperative with the staff as possible, but remember that your baby is far more important to you than the staff, and time with your baby is very important to your later relationship with your baby.

6. *Please be reassured about the long-range outcome.* Most jaundiced babies recover completely within a few days or weeks, and although the time during treatment can be frightening and exhausting for you and stressful for the baby, it will pass and your family will be a loving whole shortly. If the jaundice is severe, and your baby is quite ill, these pointers will help you do as much as possible for your baby, and give the love and care essential during the illness. You can be sure that your role is a most important one in your baby's recovery and your future relationship.

For a more detailed discussion of this topic, including extensive references, see the Spring, 1979 issue of *Birth and the Family Journal*, available from BFJ, 110 El Camino Real, Berkeley, CA 94705. The article is entitled, "Neonatal Jaundice," by Simkin, Simkin, and Edwards.

336

# Jaundice of the Newborn: Physiologic, Pathologic or a Symptom of Maternal Neglect?

by Nan Koehler, 1983

Predicting and preventing the occurrence of neonatal juandice has perplexed birth attendants for some time. (1) This is also a phenomenon that I have been thinking about. My perspective on this issue is not that unorthodox, but one for which there is little support currently in the medical profession; yet it has proven invaluable in helping women overcome this potential problem.

When I first began observing childbirth (in 1968), the occurrence of juandice seemed in the hands of fate. There was always a convenient explanation: the woman was oriental, the baby a little early or a poor nurser, etc. None of these explanations seemed to make much sense. Since then, a number of factors have influenced my thinking. First, the birth of my second child was in late October, coinciding with Indian summer. I couldn't refrain from catching the last few hot days and took him outdoors. His color was never tinged bronze like my first child's, and his health and vigor were markedly better. (This was in Pennsylvania, and needless to say, all my family criticized me severely for this recklessness!)

Second, I was impressed when I read that demand feeding, particularly the concept of using the breast as a pacifier, had beneficial results. (2) This affirmed my own personal experience with my babies.

337

Third, seeing many mothers who had engorged breasts, sore nipples and babies with faulty nursing techniques again impressed upon me how important it is to advise mothers to nurse their newborns a lot. (3)

Fourth, the clincher for me was in observing that postpartum women who were up, dressed, with dishes washed and house cleaned more often than not were the ones with the jaundiced babies. It also amazed me to watch a potentially yellow baby become pink and juicy looking after instructing the mother in how to nurse laying down and admonishing her about putting her attention to her baby—not to the house.

Fifth, women who can keep their urine clear and water—colored instead of straw-colored by maintaining their fluid intake during the days after the birth, have clear colostrum instead of dark yellow colostrum, and their babies have no problem with jaundice. The medical rationale for this is that both the mother and baby have expanded blood volumes, so that the possibility of jaundice is diluted. (4) In the same vein, recent work by DeCarvalho et al, reaffirms the laxative effect of breastmilk in stimulating the elimination of meconium, which is the vehicle for bilirubin excretion.

In summary, there are six factors which reduce the occurrence and severity of "normal-physiologic" jaundice of the newborn:

1. *Hydration.* The mother needs to drink 3-4 quarts of water/day.

2. *Sunlight.* Expose the baby to sunlight either outdoors or through a window twice a day for the first 3 days after birth—before any jaundice appears. Hold in lap about 10-15 minutes with baby naked. Beware of burn.

3. *Frequent nursing.* This means putting the baby to breast whenever it is awake whether or not it "acts hungry." Keep the baby in bed with the mother or on the mother's body so that she is aware of the baby's arousal. Newborn babies can sleep for hours and hours, rouse up and fall back

asleep again with no one noticing if they are stashed in a cradle or crib. After a week or two (when the natural endorphines are metabolized) the baby won't sleep so long or go back to sleep so easily.

4. *Number of defecations.* This is influenced by the relaxation of the baby and its environment, the sucking reflex response, ingestion of colostrum, and touch contact and stimulation by the mother. (5)

5. *Stimulus.* This is constant closeness, cuddling and touch stimulation by the mother. (6)

6. *Using the breast as pacifier.* See #3. This will establish a good milk supply. It is helpful for the mother to visualize her breast as the external umbilical cord, or IV, to the baby.

REFERENCES

1. DeCarvalho, M., et al. "Frequency of Breastfeeding and serum bilirubin concentration" *Am. J. Dis. Child,* 136 (8): 737, Aug 82.

2. Shiela Kippley, *Breastfeeding and Natural Childspacing.*

3. Carol Mikusa L'Esperance, Pain or Pleasure: The Dilemma of Early Breastfeeding. *Birth and The Family Journal.* Vol 7:1 Spring 1980, pp 21-26.

4. Nelson, *Textbook of Pediatrics, 11th Edition,* pp 442-443.

5. Simkin, Simkin and Edwards, "Physiologic" Jaundice of the Newborn, *Birth and the Family Journal.* Vol 6:1 Spring, 1979, pp 23-40.

6. Ashley Montegue, *Touching.*

# *Postpartum Exercises*
by *Mary Weiner*

## *From Day of Birth:*

1. Kegel—hold 5 to 10 seconds. Do 10 times, 3 times daily.

2. Deep abdominal breathing: inhale deeply, expanding abdomen. Exhale slowly, drawing in abdominal muscles strongly. Do 5 times, twice daily.

3. Lie on abdomen, pillow under abdomen and one under head and shoulders if necessary to prevent discomfort to full breasts. Pillows usually are not needed until milk comes in.

## From Day After Birth:

4. Lie on back with legs crossed at ankles: contract Kegel, buttocks, squeeze thighs together, lift head—hold; relax. Do 5 times twice daily.

5. Lie on back, legs straight: raise one knee slightly, reach toward it with opposite arm. (Do *not* touch knee.) Hold to count of 3. Do with alternate knee and arm. Do 5 times twice daily.

6. Lie on back, knees bent, hands on lower abdomen: contract buttocks and lower abdominal muscles, tilting pelvis so small of back meets floor or bed; then lift head until abdominal muscles contract firmly. Do 5 times twice daily.

## From 3 or 4 Days After Birth:

7. Frog position: do 3 times a day for several minutes each time. After milk comes in, do this after instead of before feeding baby so you won't spray milk all over everything.

8. For comfort and to increase circulation to your breasts—Lactation exercise: sit tailor fashion, arms crossed, hands touching alternate knees; raise arms over head on inspiration, bring arms down behind your back with palms facing out on exhalation; swing back of hands toward each other behind your back six times breathing in for the first three swings and out for the second three

swings; place hands on knees (left on left, right on right), shrug shoulders way up on inspiration, relax them down on exhalation.

*Do take the time to do these exercises.*
*It takes only a few minutes a day.*
*You will look and feel better.*

# Physical and Emotional Aspects of Sexuality in Pregnancy and Post-Partum

*Summary by Joan Lashbrook*

FIRST TRIMESTER:

1. Fatigue and/or nausea tend to decrease interest in sex.
2. Tender, enlarged breasts may become uncomfortable during sexual excitement.

SECOND TRIMESTER:

1. Engorgement of genitalia due to pressure from growing uterus leads to:
2. Increasing interest in sex, usually exceeding pre-pregnant levels.
3. Increased vaginal lubrication.
4. Capacity for multiple orgasm increased.

341

THIRD TRIMESTER:

1. After orgasm, uterus sometimes goes into tonic spasm instead of contracting rhythmically.
2. This sometimes produces cramping and discomfort.
3. Post-orgasm resolution phase lasts longer.
4. Orgasm may fail to relieve sexual tension.
5. Slight risk of air embolism if air blown into vagina.

NEAR TERM:

1. Fetal head low in pelvis: shallow penetration best.
2. Orgasm *may* induce labor if cervix is ripe.

POST-PARTUM:

1. Vaginal walls thin, lubrication sparse, especially in nursing mothers.
2. Breastfeeding sometimes produces sexual stimulation (occasionally orgasm!).
3. Interest in sex variable: may be higher or may be lower than pre-pregnancy.
4. Intercourse may be resumed 3-6 weeks post-partum, depending on episiotomy, etc.
5. Breast milk may leak during stimulation, may spurt out at orgasm.

Emotional conflict and guilt may play a large part in psychosexual responses:

- Guilt, if sex is felt to be primarily for procreation.
- Conflict between sexuality and developing mother role.
- Heightened eroticism may be upsetting (or fantastic!).
- Men, too, may have strong conflicts: e.g. hurting the fetus, overtaxing tired partner, possible jealousy of the fetus, confusion over partner's changing role, or changing shape. Or

this may all be very exciting!

- Later in the pregnancy, women may feel awkward and ugly, and probably need much reassurance.
- Alternate sexual positions and practices may create anxiety.
- Women may tend to focus attention inward instead of on partner as pregnancy progresses, and men may feel rejected.

Postpartum: Fatigue, crying baby, sore bottom, leaking nipples — not great for sex, but great for opening up to one another emotionally, deepening communication. You're in this together. . . .

BIRTH AND THE FAMILY JOURNAL, v.1:A, "Sexuality in Pregnancy and the Puerperium," Nancy Dendrick, R.N.

# *Herpes in Pregnancy*
*by Carla Reinke*
*An excerpt from an excellent pamphlet, available from The Pennypress.*

## *Decreasing the Number of Flareups*

L-LYSINE

- Increase the amount of lysine in the diet, and decrease arginine.
- Lysine is available in health food stores (be sure to buy only lysine and L-Lysine).
- Dietary sources of lysine: fish, chicken, beef, meat, cheese, brewer's yeast, soybeans, eggs, milk.
- Dietary sources of arginine: nuts, peanut butter, coconut, brown rice, whole wheat bread, oatmeal, raisins.

343

DECREASING STRESS
- Cut back on work hours.
- Get adequate rest and exercise.
- Eat a balanced diet.
- Practice relaxation/yoga, meditation.
- Don't overwork.
- When possible, postpone major life changes (i.e., moving, changing jobs, etc.).

Improving body's immune response:
- Quit smoking.
- Take Vitamin C*.

Avoid intercourse when partner has sores if it frequently causes you to have sores.

Practice good hygiene.
- Bathe frequently.
- Wash hands after going to the bathroom, handling the genitals, or engaging in sexual activity.

## Relieving the Pain from Sores

- Take warm baths or sitz baths for comfort.
- Dry areas heal faster. Air dry sores thoroughly; you might use a hair dryer.
- Xylocaine spray or ointment, Campho-phenique.
- Milk of Magnesia — use the settled white particles, dab on with cotton for pain relief.
- Burrow's Solution — use as cool compresses, 2-3 times daily.
- Vitamin E — apply directly to herpes sores.

- Bathe or soak affected area in baking soda in water.

*Take 10 grams of Vitamin C throughout the day and 300 mg. Vitamin B.

## SUGGESTED ADDITIONAL READING

*Planning Your Baby's Birth*, by Penny Simkin and Carla Reinke. Pennypress, Inc., 1980 ($0.50).

*Cesarean Birth — A Special Delivery*, by Kathy Keolker, Pennypress, Inc., 1981 ($0.50).

*The Herpes Handbook*, by Terri Gunn and Mary Stenzel-Poore. V.D. Action Council OHSU — L220A, Portland, OR 97201 ($2.00).

A list of references used in the preparation of this pamphlet is available from Pennypress, Inc. Please enclose a self-addressed stamped envelope with your request.

Carla Reinke is a childbirth educator, past President of the Birthplace, an out-of-hospital birth center,and is presently completing her studies in nursing.

Copyright © 1982 by Carla Reinke. All rights reserved. No part of this pamphlet may be reproduced by any means without written permission of the author.

*Herpes in Pregnancy* is published by and available from Pennypress, Inc., 1100 23rd Avenue East, Seattle, WA 98112. Price: 1 to 5 — $0.50 each (including postage). For quantity prices, write for our flyer.

Send away for this helpful handout.

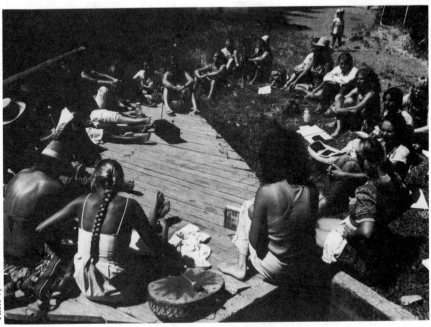

Photo by David Burns

Rainbow's End Study Group

345

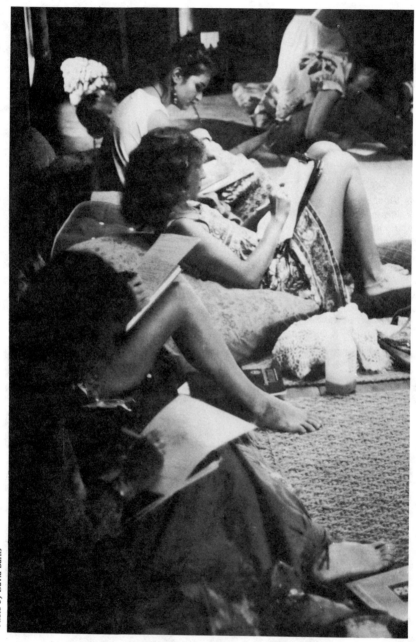

Photo by David Burns

*Rainbow's End Study Group*

346

# PART IV

# Preparing the Mind

*What is normal?*
*Gathering a repertoire of possibilities.*
*Learning to relax the mind.*

# Class Outline – Preparation for Childbirth and Parenting

*by Nan Koehler*

*Review Class.* For those having their 2nd, 3rd, etc., baby. Film showing and discussion.

*Class 1.* Orientation to pregnancy, birth and childrearing. Introduction to each other. Couples who have birthed most recently will share their experiences and show off their babies.

*Class 2.* Preparing the body for pregnancy and birth. Nutrition, herbs, exercise, rest. Prenatal yoga, body awareness and relaxation.

*Class 3.* Stages of labor. First stage. The mother's pelvis, the baby's head, the path through the pelvis, presentation and lie, the mechanics of labor and delivery. Bradley Method. Relaxation.

*Class 4.* Second stage of labor. Positions for labor and delivery. Role of husband or support person. Role of guests at birth. Review of Bradley Method and relaxation.

*Class 5.* Third stage of labor. Placenta formation, function and birth. Examination of used placenta. Lamaze method and relaxation.

*Class 6..* Kegel muscle preparation. Communication skills. Birth drama. Dealing with grief in childbearing. Review of Lamaze method and relaxation.

*Class 7.* Complications of labor and birth. Dealing with unexpected problems; emergency birth instructions, medical considerations and backup, dealing with hospitals and birth technology. Having a good birth experience in spite of problems. Your role as a medical consumer, giving feedback to MAKE CHANGES. Slide-show of Cesarean birth.

*Class 8.* The baby; newborn exam, appar score, head molding, umbilical cord care, genitalia, eye drops, PKU and others tests, jaundice, things to watch for. Feeding the baby; breastfeeding, solids, supplements (vitamins, fluorides). Immunizations, circumcision. Post-partum, visiting, rest. Slideshow on bonding.

*Class 9.* Films: bring guests and relatives who will be at your birth. Review of normal birth. Discussion.

*Class 10.* Birth visualization, relaxation techniques, breath control.

TIME TO BE ANNOUNCED:

*Class 11.* Fertility Awareness with emphasis on Natural Birth Control.

*Class 12.* Postpartum. Bring your new baby and share with others. See class #1.

PARENTS HAVE THE OPPORTUNITY TO BE WHAT THEY WISH THEIR CHILDREN TO BE.

# *Physiology of Labor Relaxation*

*by Carol Shattuck*

What happens when a woman in labor is fearful and tense and tight? A look at the physiology of the uterine muscles will show just what happens.

Look at the diagram of the three uterine muscle layers. The *long up and down layer* of muscle fibers is the one a woman feels in action during contractions. When it contracts, it both pushes the baby down into the cervix, and pulls up and opens the cervix around the baby's head.

*Long Muscle Layer*
*Fundus*

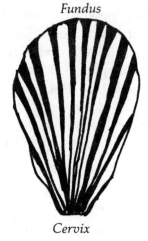

*Cervix*

The *circular muscle layer*, you will notice, is rather sparse in the fundus of the uterus and quite dense in the cervix area. This circular layer holds the cervix closed and resists the long muscles. Gradually it gives away and thins out with contractions and allows the baby's head through the cervix.

*Circular Muscle Layer*
*Fundus*

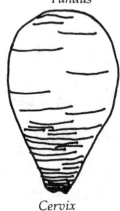

*Cervix*

The *criss-cross layer* intertwines with the blood vessels that supply the uterus. Their action effects the blood supply to and from the uterus, brings oxygen and food to the uterus and takes away the waste products of muscular action.

350

## Criss-Cross Muscle Layer
### Fundus

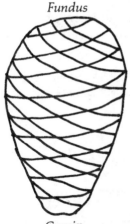

*Cervix*

Now let's link up these three muscle layers with the nervous system. When a person is frightened or anxious, her sympathetic nervous system is activated. You are probably aware that when this happens, the person experiences the sensations of the "fight or fright" pattern: the heart rate and respiration rate and blood pressure all go up, the skin sweats, the digestive system shuts down, and the liver increases its sugar output.

In the labor process, this sympathetic system also effects the *circular* muscle layer of the uterus. It contracts and tightens and thus resists very strongly the action of the long muscles. So you have two muscles working against each other and the result is that the woman feels pain and her labor time increases. Also, the *criss-cross* muscle layer that affects the blood supply is constricted. When those criss-cross muscles remain tight between contractions, the large veins are partially constricted and the blood can't carry away all the waste products. Furthermore, the arterial blood supply is hampered in bringing food and oxygen to the uterus, because, in general, the sympathetic nervous system shuts down the blood supply to all the abdominal area.

This is the classical "Fear-Tension-Pain Syndrome" which Grantly Dick-Read described 35 years ago. When a woman is anxious and fearful about labor, her whole body is tense and

351

tight; then the labor contractions are felt as labor pain. Thus, the super-most-important actions that a woman can learn in preparation for labor are to find and alleviate any sources of fear and anxiety, and to RELAX.

Reprinted with permission of Carol Shattuck.

# The Psychological Issues of Childbirth

by Tonya Brooks

*... The woman who is happy, prepared, educated, and confident will have little trouble with her birth...*

In the seven years that I have done research in childbirth and infant-mother relationships, it has become clear that the psychological issues are universally important to women and are virtually ignored by the medical establishment.

Over the last two years I have counseled more than 100 women who were interested in childbirth at home, and the following topics have emerged as being of great concern. It is from these topics that the third meeting of the ACAH series called "Psychological Issues" was evolved. The meeting is concerned with the mother and the baby as Spiritual Beings rather than as bodies, and with what things Beings can do in childbirth to make it a safe, esthetic experience.

It is significant that medical science has not studied relationships between obstetrical difficulties and psychological problems. It is very clear from our group's experience that the better a person's psychological well being, the easier and less complicated her labor.

# Fear

Anxiety and, to a lesser extent, fear are common in a pregnant woman. There is the fear of pain, fear that "the baby won't be all right," fear of not "doing well" in labor ("I might have to ask for something [drugs]."), etc. A woman who is afraid will not labor well because her fear is based on conscious or unconscious inability to confront what is happening. Such a woman's labor could be prolonged (uterine inertia), difficult, or could even stop cold. Conversely, the woman who is happy, prepared, educated, and confident will have little trouble with her birth, whatever it may be like. Her pain threshold will be higher, and her ability to confront contractions will be greater.

# Intuition

The real basis of confidence is the knowing and the decision by the mother or both parents that things will go well. Doctors and society are fond of trouncing on intuitive knowingness because it supposedly is not based on objective and testable data. (I know because I *know* is not acceptable to them.) Most people know more about their own bodies than anyone else. For instance, a pregnant woman in most cases will be the first to know that "something's wrong." One must learn to listen and trust her own intuition and learn to differentiate it from fear, counterpostulates, or thinkingness (*knowing* is different from thinking).

# Responsibility

Basically responsibility has to do with making things go right. I believe emphatically in the integrity and the power of Beings themselves; if a person makes the decision that things will go right, then he will do those things in the physical universe necessary to make that happen. To begin with, the responsibility for making childbirth safe is primarily the responsibility of the parents and secondarily that of the doctors. A woman can easily get into trouble the minute she relinquishes the responsibility for her own body and that of her baby to anyone else. This responsibility may be shared with another who has greater knowledge, but final decisions should rest with the person involved.

There are several areas in which an expectant mother and her husband can take responsibility for their own children's births. The mother should get good prenatal care in which every possible problem is explored and resolved. The parents need to have enough knowledge and intuition to judge medical competence and to see that those present at the birth are experienced and intelligent enough to handle the unexpected and are unobtrusive to the laboring woman. A pregnant woman must be responsible enough to eat well. She needs a good deal of rest, particularly as her due date draws near, because pain tolerance goes down proportionately to how tired the body is. She should regularly practice her labor techniques so that when the birth time comes she can handle each contraction instead of being overwhelmed by pain, and can actively work to give birth to her baby.

The father's role in birth is significantly greater at home and gives him a much more active involvement in it. It is his responsibility to make sure medical trade-offs are as few as possible. That is, trading the good vibes of home for the disjointed ones of the hospital, but not sacrificing valid medical knowledge. While the woman is involved with her labor, her husband should make sure the labor room is as clean as possible, that the attendants are clean and are wearing clean clothes, that there is a phone available, that an alternate emergency plan exists and is well understood by attendants, that the hospital and the routes to it are known, that there is available transportation and extra people to carry the mother to the car if need be, and that all attendants know what to do whether the labor is normal or not.

354

Lastly and most importantly, it is the husband's responsibility to see that no one upsets his wife, to coach her so that she does her job perfectly, and to see that the environment is quiet and calm.

## Pain Threshold

Contractions themselves are the longest part of labor: they take place over a period from a few to many hours, and each can last as long as two minutes or more at the peak of the labor. One can easily be overwhelmed by the pain as indeed many of our mothers were. (In these cases, drugs, however harmful they are, once seemed like a Godsend.) There are several things that can be done, however, to raise a laboring woman's pain threshold so that she can control her labor contractions. First, as I have already mentioned, a pain threshold will drop significantly if a woman is tired, so that rest in the last months of pregnancy is of great importance. The pain threshold will be higher on a confident, well-prepared mother. But the most important tool a woman has in confronting and handling pain lies in the concept called "staying in present time." When overwhelmed by pain, one tends to experience a diminishing of analytical awareness, and the subconscious mind takes over. One begins to subsconsciously associate the present pain with all similar pain which one has experienced in the past, and one has a much more overwhelming feeling than just the sensation actually experienced in the present.

## Trauma

Trauma prolongs labor significantly because it upsets the Being and interrupts the body rhythms of labor. This is why a ride to the hospital and hospital routines and procedures are so damaging to the laboring woman. First there is the ride itself. Then she must be admitted (which might cause her to worry about the money). Next comes the "prep"; she is shaved, given an enema, and showered. Next she goes to the

355

labor room where she may be plugged into a fetal heart monitor (two electrodes are placed up the vagina and skewer the baby's head to monitor its heart beat and the strength of the contraction). Then she is taken to the delivery room where she is placed on a small table with her legs strapped in stirrups. After the delivery of the baby, the woman is brought to the recovery room where she is watched if she is recuperating from drugs or not watched if she has delivered "normally." Finally, she goes to her own room, where she might get to see her baby, depending on how long the doctor and hospital separate the mothers from their babies for the "observation period."

Any upsets should be avoided during labor because psychological or physiological upset can cause the body to react and sometimes labor will stop — cold turkey. This happens so often in hospitals that they may give routine doses of pitocin, a synthetic pituitary hormone which speeds up the body and causes the uterus to contract. This hormone also often puts the baby into acute stress (thus the medical justification for the fetal heart monitor) and forces doctors to use forceps to yank the baby out fast.

Psychological upsets do not only occur in hospitals. They can happen at home as well, pehaps caused by something as simple as a loud noise or an unsupportive remark by an attendant. Antagonistic, non-supportive, or fearful people should never be allowed at any birth because they undermine confidence. Every effort should therefore be made to make the home a quiet, safe place filled with good and loving vibrations.

Lastly, it should be reiterated that upsets, however small, interrupt the physiological rhythms of the body, thereby prolonging labor. The evidence that bears this out is that the average length of labor for a first baby in the United States is 12 to 24 hours (not using pitocin) while the average length of labor in 51 mothers from ACAH has been 5½ hours!

# Control of Contractions

If a woman is overcome by pain during labor and particularly during birth, she will probably not experience the ecstasy of the birth and she may even be unable to relate emotionally to her child. If this happens, a dreadful guilt will often ensue. This sequence of events is relatively common and frequently causes post-partum depression. It is more likely to happen in an undrugged birth. Therefore I would like to emphasize that the laboring woman stay on top of the contractions so that she is not overcome by pain. She should ride the contractions like waves and use Lamaze or Reed breathing techniques as if she were exercising or lifting weights. She should keep her attention focused outward on what she is doing so that she stays in present time. This is her biggest asset, and it is her husband's responsibility to see that she does so.

Women should also be aware of the fact that babies in the posterior or unusual positions cause much harder labors and require the mother to have an even better confrontation of the pain, because when the contractions let up, the pain often does not stop.

# Separation Trauma

Separation trauma is upset which is experienced by mother and baby when the baby is removed from its mother for an "observation period" in the hospital. The big danger for the mother is post-partum depression (a conservative estimate is that about 65 percent of the women in this country experience it), difficulty accepting the baby, and guilt.

Separation trauma is a very big issue because so much is involved. First, there is a physical loss of mass (baby, water, and placenta) and the body's corresponding shock which is physiological in origin. Second, the psychological trauma of separation to mother and baby is usually devastating to them both. Dr. Ashley Montagu describes it beautifully in *Touching: The Human Significance of the Skin*. Dr. Lee Salk's studies of premature babies showed that even the ones who

357

had medical justification for being in an incubator responded better when their mothers were allowed to take them out to feed and fondle them.

## Sexuality and Childbirth

I noticed after several meetings of ACAH that the most often discussed subjects were episiotomies and circumcision, even though they were not, by any means, the most important subjects. This seems to indicate everyone's great concern with their own sexuality. The sexual issue takes on even greater importance when the metaphysical issues are considered.

The following thoughts have been taken from the combined experiences of the participants at our meetings and are valuable because they are based on common sense and are practical. In regard to lovemaking, expectant couples can make love as long as the woman feels physically able and so long as there is no vaginal bleeding. Lovemaking should be gentle because tissues in pregnant women are softer and often more tender than usual.

Sexuality during pregnancy is sometimes a problem because pregnancy and nursing occasionally extinguish sexual desire. This is attributed physiologically to increased hormonal activity, but I believe it to be psychological in origin. A woman can let herself make love if her husband wants to and she is understanding and patient, and quite often she will be glad she did, but both partners must be tolerant, reasonable, and patient.

Communication is always the key to working out sexual problems, but people must be willing to tell each other what is happening, and each must be willing to accept what the other is saying without being defensive.

One of the reasons sexuality is emotionally difficult for the pregnant woman is social conditioning about vaginal size. As evidence, there are dirty jokes and songs, Germaine Greer's

358

idea of "Cunt Hatred," and doctors' "humor," i.e., "I'm going to sew you up nice and tightly and hubby will really like that," or (as was said to me) "Let me sew you up so you won't flap in the breeze." If her husband can understand these thoughts, it will be easy to see the reservations about making love which many pregnancy women or new mothers may have.

Women should know that sagging, loose muscles, both vaginal and abdominal can *always* be exercised into perfect original shape, and that cotton underwear facilitates post-birth healing because of increased air circulation. Stretch marks and other body alterations after pregnancy can be big ego deflators. The only thing one can do is consider stretch marks as stretch marks, and make no associations. Would an appendectomy scar be an ego deflator? I don't think so.

I don't think there is any doubt that lovemaking can tran-scend the physical plane. Birth should be looked at as a beau-tiful, productive end to the conceiving union as well as the beginning of a new family.

## *Family Considerations*

In home birth, the father has a great deal of responsibility and actually makes it possible for his child to be born safely. It is much easier for him to meet his new child at home where in-tegration into the family is not interrupted by hospital stay. The ecstasy of childbirth is not an ending, but a beginning. Likewise for siblings, new babies are more accepted if they know where the baby comes from of course at home the mother is not separated from her older children. They can ac-tually watch the birth if they are mature enough to be still and quiet.

The greatest psychological issue is that a small new body is animated by a spiritual Being, and as such birth welcomes that Being into a new existence. The optimum place for the baby to meet his family and begin life anew is in the home where the environment is quiet, not traumatic to mother and baby, and controlled by the parents.

Copyright © *The East West Journal*
Reprinted with Permission. August 1974, Vol. IV, No. 7. p24.

# Touch Relaxation

Touch relaxation is a method of learning relaxation and body awareness which is done through touch between partners. The helping partner rests his or her hand over the part of the body which is contracted. The helper's hand is relaxed. The relaxing partner responds to the warmth and pressure of the helper's hand by releasing the tension of the contracted part in the direction toward the touching hand. The exercise is a mutual releasing, the released helper's hand and the released body part of the relaxer. One partner is not the subordinate pupil. The method is promoted by Sheila Kitzinger, a well-known English childbirth educator and social anthropologist who wrote *The Experience of Childbirth*.

For best results, practice about four times a week as partners and two other times a week when the relaxer is alone imagining the helper's touch. When partners practice together, better relaxation awareness is obtained with the relaxer nude or lightly clothed so the helper can feel the relaxation of the muscles. A semi-reclining position allows the partners to see each other's faces. Make the relaxer's body comfortable by using pillows to support the head, shoulders, back and knees. Discuss how firm the relaxer wants to be touched and adjust accordingly for different body areas. Relaxer concentrates on the body sensations of being tense and relaxed.

Relaxation is important as a tool for labor ease, as it allows the uterus to contract more efficiently, provides more oxygen for the baby, prevents excessive tiredness and fatigue and promotes an easier recovery after birth. It is very helpful in coping with the tensions of being a mother and father, too. Lastly, relaxation promotes longevity and, once learned, can enhance the enjoyment of life.

Body awareness is necessary in labor to access which body parts are tense and need relaxing and to understand the various labor sensations coming from the uterus, cervix, birth canal, and back, so the reaction is not one of complete hysteria but one of comprehension and knowledge of the

360

parts working in labor and their action. The body and mind can then sort out a reasonable response and reaction to the incoming sensations.

To begin the practice session, get comfortable and do the Mabel Fitzhugh total body relaxation exercise several times. Sigh out and relax completely. Listen to the sound of your own slow breathing. The relaxer tells the helper when to begin.

H - helper    R - relaxer

ABDOMEN
R - Pull in the abdominal muscles toward the spine.
H - Place both hands over the lower curve of the abdomen, palms toward the pubic bone.
R - Relax the abdomen in the direction of the helper's touch.
H - Notice the feeling of the relaxed and tense abdomen.

SHOULDER
R - Press shoulders together like angel's wings; pull shoulders back towards the center of the back. (Women in transition sometimes look like this which can lead to overbreathing and hyperventilation.)
H - Hold hands firmly on the front of each shoulder.
R - Release towards the touch.
H - Hands should mold to the shape of the shoulders and touch with the whole hand, not just fingers. Can be done in transition if relaxer is tense.

HEAD
R - Frown, wrinkle up the eyes. Hold position for a while to gain awareness of the feeling.
H - Rest the first two or three fingers on the brow over the bridge of the nose and stroke upwards over the brow resting with light pressure at the sides of the

361

temples, then go back and do it again. Repeat several times. Each time, lift the hands off the temples and go to the center of the brow to stoke again.

R - When relaxed, the brow should feel broad with plenty of space there.

SKULL

R - Shoot eyes toward the top of the head; notice tension in the skull muscles.

H - Rest hands over the top of the head. When relaxer releases the skull feels warm to the touch.

R - Release towards the touch.

JAW

R - Grit teeth, tense jaw. "I will do this my own way, will not let anyone interfere with my labor" is perhaps the thought when the jaw is tense in labor.

H - Rest hand on either side of the jaw, just underneath the ears, palms toward the ears. The relaxer's jaw will drop into helper's hand.

R - Releases towards the touch.

LEGS

I R - Point heels, toes towards the ceiling and tense one leg.

H - Place hand firmly over the instep and the other hand over the front of the foot. Work foot muscles a bit, then move up to the muscles on either side of the leg (not over the bone) with a firm squeezing, kneading movement. Reach the top of the leg and finish with a long stroke down to the ankle to remove any residual tension.

R - By the time helper reaches the top of the leg it should be completely relaxed.

H - Put one hand behind the knee, one behind the ankle. Slowly lift the knee towards the abdomen and draw a slow circle with it, then draw a circle the other way. The leg should feel very heavy and joints loose.

R - Let helper move leg, keep relaxed.

*Repeat with other leg.*

II  H - Lift both feet with hands, holding feet, not ankles. Swing legs from side to side slowly.

R - Feel full release of legs.

H - Slowly lower legs, don't drop them.

III  H - Massage the upper leg on the outside from the knee up to the top of the thighs, up and down.

R - Roll out thighs towards the touch, knees fall out.

H - Massage the inside of the thighs up and down with fingers pointed towards the floor; use the whole palm for massage. Every now and again, let the hands sweep over to the outside of the thighs. Useful during transition when the legs can't relax, are cold, or start to shake.

R - Relaxes thighs. Position of legs should remain rolled out to the side to be relaxed. When helper massages the inside of the leg, think about relaxing the pelvic floor, opening the door.

HANDS

R - Clinch up hand.

H - Both hands work muscles.

R - Let all tension flow to the helper's hands; let hand drop.

*Repeat with other hand.*

ARM

R - Raise the whole arm; make it stiff like a board.

H - Touch wrist from above; support wrist underneath with the other hand.

R - Let hand drop.

H - Keeping one hand on the wrist, move up the muscles

on the inside of the arm to elbow with a squeezing movement.

R - Whole forearm relaxes.

H - Release support under the wrist, support solely under the elbow.

R - Arm drops inward, biceps are still tight.

H - Move up over biceps with one hand, continuing to support under the elbow until hand reaches the top of the arm, then press firmly on the shoulder. Finish by a firm squeezing, stroking movement down the arm, finishing at the wrist.

R - Now arm is like putty in the helper's hand.

H - Take fingers in hands and shake arm to make sure the arm is relaxed all the way down. Finish by holding the wrist, because holding the hand causes the hand to contract. Lower arm gently. Exercise with the arm can be used in labor.

*Repeat with other arm.*

## BACK

R - Turn on side with a well-rounded back. The side position helps to release the shoulder muscles during labor. Hunch up the shoulders, positioning toward the ears almost like a fetal position.

H - Rest a hand on each shoulder with the palms on the top and thumbs behind the shoulder, hold hands still.

R - Release toward the touch, unfold.

## SACRUM

R - Remain on side. Hollow back as if having a bad backache, shoulders back, buttocks out. This is a position in back labor, or a backache during labor.

H - Place palm of hand firmly on the sacrum. Move flesh on the bone, not just the skin, which creates friction. Massage with a rotary movement, every now and then sweep over the buttocks, then come back to the sacrum.

R - Release toward the massage.

## BUTTOCKS

R - Squeeze buttocks together like holding a $5 bill which someone is trying to take away.

H - Place one hand firmly over each buttock. Get close to relaxer's body at right angles so helper can use the weight of own body through arms, rather than using all the energy with your own arm muscles or helper will get tired. Get low enough. Use a firm kneading motion, but not so hard relaxer rolls off bed. Can be used during transition and pushing when the baby's head is descending and creates rectal pressure. Almost impossible to tighten the pelvic floor muscles when this massage is done.

## NECK AND THROAT

R - Position is on back with pillow under shoulders.

H - Hold head. It's cupped comfortably in both hands and pick it up holding full weight, shoulders only are supported by pillows, don't cover ears.

R - Let lips go soft, moist, loose as if glossy new expensive lipstick were applied. Helps release throat muscles.

H - Gently, with minimal movement, start to roll the head in hands. Rotate in small circles and slowly lower to pillows.

R - Relax and enjoy.

This handout is reprinted with permission from the author, Margaret B. Foley, RPT. For copies, including revisions, contact Read Method, Preparation for Childbirth, 1300 So. Eliseo Drive, Suite 102, Greenbrae, CA 94904. (415) 461-2277.

# Breathing Techniques

## Slow Chest Breathing

1. Take an organizing breath (a deep lateral chest breath) when contraction begins. Focus on focal point.
2. Slowly inhale through your nose and exhale through your mouth, 6 to 10 times per minute.
3. Inhale quietly and let your exhalation be audible to those close by, keeping your mouth slightly open and relaxed.
4. As you breathe, expand and relax your chest, keeping your shoulders and abdomen relaxed.
5. When contraction ends, take a deep relaxing breath — exhale as if sighing.
6. Completely relax.

PRACTICE SESSIONS:

Practice every day, fifteen to twenty minutes a session. Be able to use this pattern for 60 seconds. Try to make the breathing physically effortless, it should not tire you. Practice in different positions, sitting up, lying down, standing up and in the car. Remember to think about the breathing pattern and to relax totally. Think of blowing off tension with each breath out.

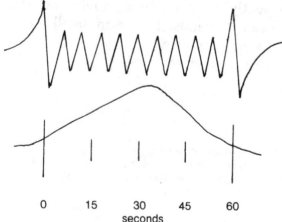

0     15     30     45     60
seconds

366

# Accelerated Breathing

1. Take an organizing breath when contraction begins. Focus on focal point.

2. Inhale through your nose and exhale through your mouth, gradually accelerating your breathing as the contraction increases in intensity. Keep your mouth and shoulders relaxed.

3. As the rate increases toward the peak of the contraction, breathe in and out through your mouth. This is shallow breathing with movement in the upper chest. The rate should not exceed 1 to 2 breaths per second.

4. As the contraction decreases in intensity, gradually decelerate your breathing.

5. When contraction ends, take a deep relaxing breath — exhale as if sighing.

6. Completely relax.

PRACTICE SESSIONS:

Add this breathing pattern to your daily practice session. Be able to use this pattern for 60 to 90 seconds, in several body positions. Find a rhythm that is comfortable and effortless for you. Practice varying the breathing pattern, reaching the peak breathing rate at various points in the contraction. In labor some contractions peak earlier than others, some have double peaks, etc. By practicing variations, you are better able to adapt your breathing as necessary in your own labor.

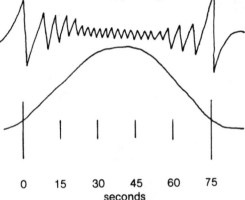

0    15    30    45    60    75
seconds

367

# Transition Breathing

1. Take an organizing breath. If the contractions are peaking sooner, this breath should be quicker than before. Focus on focal point.

2. Breathe through your mouth in shallow, even breaths at a rate of 1 to 2 per second, throughout the contraction.

3. After every third or fourth breath, blow out quickly with a "puh" sound. Find the pattern you are comfortable with, then keep it constant throughout the contraction. Count to yourself — "One, two, three, four, puh" etc. You may want to practice more complicated patterns which require greater concentration to deal with the more difficult contractions of transition: e.g., 1, 2, puh; 1, 2, 3, puh; 1, 2, 3, 4, puh; 1, 2, puh, etc.

4. When contraction ends, take a deep relaxing breath.

5. Completely relax.

PRACTICE SESSIONS:

Add this breathing pattern to your daily practice session. Transition contractions may last 2 to 3 minutes. Be able to use this pattern for that length of time. Practice in various body positions. Relax for 30 seconds between practice contractions to prepare you for the brief rest period between transition contractions in labor.

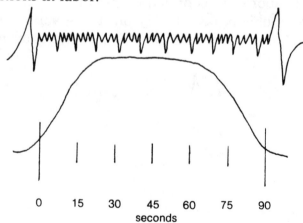

0    15    30    45    60    75    90
seconds

368

# Controlling the urge to push:

The urge to push is an instinctive reaction to the pressure of the baby on the pelvic floor. It is characterized by a feeling of pressure deep in the pelvis, a feeling like wanting to move one's bowels. The mother either holds her breath, makes grunting sounds as she breathes, or has a catch in her breath. She should begin bearing down and pushing if her cervix is fully dilated, but she should not bear down if her cervix is not yet fully dilated. If she should push or bear down during a premature urge to push, it is usually a wasted effort and it can bruise the cervix.

To control a strong premature urge to push, to bear down or to hold your breath, lift your chin and use the "puh, puh, puh" breaths of the transition breathing pattern, until the urge subsides. Then use the transition breathing for the rest of the contraction.

PRACTICE SESSIONS:

Each day practice the transition breathing two or three times, incorporating an imagined "urge to push." When the coach says, "Urge to push," lift your chin and "puh, puh, puh" until he says, "Urge passes." As a variation, and to keep your coach on his toes, try occasionally holding your breath or grunting in the middle of a practice transition contraction. This should signal him to coach you to "puh, puh, puh."

# Pushing — the second stage of labor

Time to change gears — many women feel a very strong urge to push during these contractions. As the baby moves down the birth canal the mother wants to "join in with her uterus," and push the baby out. If you have had no medications which dull your feeling this urge to push, let your body be your guide in giving you signals of when and how to bear down. Between contractions you should try to relax completely.

369

# Body positions for pushing:

You can push effectively in various positions. Most women and most physicians seems to prefer a semi-reclining position, supported by pillows, a back rest or the delivery bed adjusted to support her. Some women hold their legs, pulling them back and apart; others let them relax and fall to the sides; others use the stirrups or footrests attached to the delivery bed or table.

Another popular position is side-lying, with the upper leg supported by the father, partner or nurse. During contractions, the mother curls her upper body over her uterus while bearing down. If the semi-reclining position is uncomfortable due to back pain or leg cramps, try the side-lying position; it usually helps.

A squatting or kneeling position, with the mother being supported is often an excellent position, especially when the baby is coming very slowly.

Another position which may be both comfortable and effective is the all fours or hand-and-knees position. This position allows the mother to arch her back, rock forward or backward, up or down as she feels the need.

The position you choose will depend on how you feel at the time of birth, on your surroundings, and on your attendant's (doctor or midwife) preferences. You should discuss the possibilities with attendant and practice pushing in the possible positions.

Practicing pushing is more difficult than practicing breathing techniques, because the way you push will depend on the character of your contractions, and how strongly you feel the urge to push. Practice according to the descriptions below, however, and adapt your pushing as necessary when in labor.

# Expulsion Breathing (Pushing)

1. Contraction begins.

370

2. Breathe deeply and slowly, letting the contraction guide you in accelerating as necessary to stay on top of the contraction. When the urge to push is really strong, hold your breath, tuck your chin on your chest, and curl your body over your uterus, pull in your abdominal muscles, and RELAX YOUR PELVIC FLOOR. You might let out a bit of breath as you bear down, making a "grunting sound." When necessary, let all your breath out and quickly breathe in and bear down again; continue as long as you feel the urge.

3. Contraction ends — slowly lie/sit back and take two relaxing breaths.

4. This routine continues for each contraction until the baby's head is almost at the point of crowning. At this point the doctor or midwife will tell you to stop pushing to allow slow passage of the baby through the vaginal opening. At the attendant's direction, immediately relax and let all the air out of your lungs. If the urge to push is still strong, raise your chin and pant or "Puh, puh" as lightly and rapidly as you can. Continue the panting until the urge goes away or until you are able to push again.

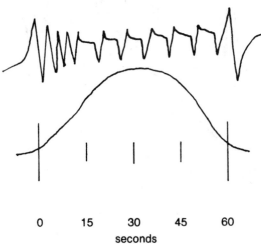

0    15    30    45    60
seconds

371

If you do not feel the contractions or the urge to push, due to medications or some other factor, follow this routine:

1. Contraction begins.

2. Take 2 or three quick deep breaths, hold the last one in, tuck your chin on your chest and bear down, pulling in your abdominal muscles. Think of *releasing your pelvic floor muscles*. Bear down for a slow count of 9 or 10, release your air quickly, take another breath and repeat the routine until the contraction eases off.

3. Contraction ends — slowly lie/sit back and take two relaxing breaths.

4. This routine continues for each contraction until the baby's head is almost at the point of crowning. At this point the doctor or midwife will tell you to stop pushing to allow slow passage of the baby through the vaginal opening. At the attendent's direction, immediately relax and let all the air out of your lungs. Pant, if necessary, to keep from bearing down.

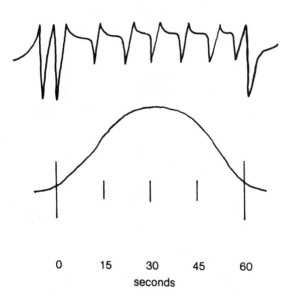

0    15    30    45    60
seconds

PRACTICE SESSIONS:

Practice pushing in various body positions and be able to continue this pattern for 60 to 75 seconds. Practice taking 3 or 4 breaths before holding your breath for 9 or 10 seconds. The coach may count slowly up to 9 to help you know when to take another breath. Remember to practice pushing and panting with your eyes open, as you will want to see the birth of your baby. Do not bear down with all your strength in practice — only enough to feel relaxing and slight bulging of the perineum. During the birth, let your body tell you how hard to bear down.

Reprinted from pp. 47–50 in *Becoming Parents*, Childbirth Education Association of Seattle.

# Pregnancy as an Altered State of Consciousness

*by Arthur D. Colman, M.D.*
*Libby L. Colman, Ph.D.*

Two and a half years ago we wrote the book *Pregnancy: the Psychological Experience.*[1] As the title implies, our approach was largely experiential — what is it like to be pregnant? We used objective data, but our stance was subjective, too, for we were expecting our third child while we were writing. We were inside the experience. Inevitably (since pregnancy can not last forever) our point of view has shifted. We are outside the experience. We have gone beyond the observations in our book to attempt an evaluation of pregnancy as a pivotal moment in the total life cycle. Is it as special as it feels while you are in it? Does it have a lasting influence on personality development? What is its impact on life style? We have chosen to approach these questions by looking at pregnancy as an altered state of consciousness, a term chosen because of its current association with psychological theories and treatment procedures which are oriented toward human growth, for we see pregnancy as the epitome of positive growth experience.

An altered state of consciousness (ASC) is defined by Charles T. Tart as "qualitative alteration in the overall patterning of mental functioning such that the experiencer feels his consciousness is radically different from the 'normal' way it functions."[2] The term is helpful although the entire notion of altered states of consciousness is simplistic, since the human mind does not necessarily function in distinct categories. Furthermore, there is no one state that can accurately be labeled "normal." Rather, a wide band of experienced states all of which seem more or less to represent everyday conscious functioning are taken to be "normal." Variations from this are "altered states." Thus dream states, trance states, religious ecstacies, peak moments of bliss, sudden highs and acute depressions are all "altered states of consciousness." The labels are imprecise, but the attempt to understand the fluid and complex workings of the human mind is both intriguing and beneficial, as it brings us closer to an awareness of our human condition and helps us deal with life.

The ASC's that have been most often studied recently have been those which show up clearly on EEG changes: sleep, alpha wave states, and occasionally hyonogogic, hypnopompic, and other transitional sleep states. Alcohol and marijuana intoxication, meditation, possession, autohypnosis, and psychedelic drug states have also been explored. These are all time limited states in which the subject is quite aware that something "different" is happening. There are certain other states of consciousness which are quite altered from the normal waking consciousness which are part of the life process, but not daily like sleep states, nor chemically induced, like intoxication. We are thinking of orgasm, labor and the act of dying, three extraordinary phenomena that are difficult to study, but which appropriately fall into the area of of altered states of consciousness. There are other life process states that also entail a significant change in the consciousness of the subject, but which are not as time limited and intense as orgasm, labor, and the act of dying. These include fetal consciousness, adolescence, intense grief states, psychosis... and pregnancy.

During the nine months of pregnancy, a woman passes through her usual wide range of consciousness states. She sleeps, wakes, laughs, cries, has orgasms, becomes intoxicated, works, plays, continues her life as a person. But, as repeated studies have shown, she is undergoing profound physiological and psychological changes. Some women change more than others, but all enter into the special state to one degree or another. Characteristically, they become more intensely emotional than usual and rapidly swing from one mood to another, a phenomena known as emotional lability. They are unusually prone to anxiety, depression, insomnia, crying spells. In a typical study, 84% of pregnant women describe themselves as having "the blues" in contrast to only 26% of the control group; 68% of pregnant women and only 5% of the controls experienced "unexplained crying."[3] It is not unusual for a pregnant woman to think she might be "going crazy" when she realizes that she is over-reacting to the world around her. She may become obsessed with dreams and symbols, become suddenly superstitious, feel extraordinarily vulnerable, or become phobic to cars, to small spaces, or to strangers.

The psychological changes of pregnancy can not be exclusively attributed to hormonal changes, because pregnant fathers frequently undergo a parallel set of psychological changes. They gain weight, experience nausea and vomiting, have abdominal bloating or experience intestinal distress and toothaches at a rate far greater than non-pregnant men. Furthermore, these symptoms go away after the baby is born.[4] We must presume that these changes take place because of the intense meaning that pregnancy has for an individual and because of the profound identification of the man with his

375

woman. In other words, pregnancy is not an "altered state of consciousness" only because of altered chemical balance. It is also a special state because of the content of the pregnant consciousness.

Pregnancy involves us in a confrontation with our uncontrollable biological states and with irreversible change. Furthermore, it shatters the illusion of our separateness and reminds us of our interconnectedness with others. We tend to define growth through separation and individuation. We use terms like "cutting the apron strings" in the assumption that the goal of living is individual autonomy. "Grown up" is synonymous with being "on your own." Being mature means to "know who you are." The process of emerging from the womb into the arms, from the arms to lap, from lap to yard to school and finally to leaving home is indeed a continuous progression of increasing individuation. The illusion, however, is that this pinnacle reached in adolescence is a stable condition that we achieve on our own. Pregnancy may then seem like a throwback to infancy, for a pregnant woman is never alone. From the inside, the mother has the baby with her always as part of her body consciousness. From the outside, she needs the emotional and economic support of her husband to help her through the child bearing and rearing. Suddenly she is not independent, not on her own. She may become confused about who she is and what is happening.

The pregnant parents are now the outside components of an experience they had before from the inside. Because of the frequency with which the fetal position and fetal memory occur in adult life, it is hard to ignore the possibility of trace memories, of subjective ties to our earliest experience as a source of these phenomena. We have experienced union, the merger of our "self" in another being, from the very beginning of our existence. It should not be surprising that we might want to return to such a state at other points in our lives. During pregnancy we are most sensitive to this possibility. First, we can feel the baby move and may be stirred by profound, unreachable feelings about our own time in the womb. Second, as part of a pregnancy, we are literally involved in a union, in a merger with another being, which can be experienced as a mystical, transpersonal state. The "I" is no longer alone. It is submerged in a larger and more meaningful system. And third, as a pregnant woman or man, our physical and psychological status may predispose us to ideas and confusions which we would not feel at other times.

We know that pregnant women often do become confused about who is the baby and who is the mother. This complicated and basically irrational identity confusion is generally quite normal. In fact, it seems to be a part of a healthy psychological progression through pregnancy. The first psychological task of a pregnant woman is to believe that she is pregnant and to incorporate the fetus into her body image. At about the time that the mother feels the fetus move, she begins to realize that, although the fetus is within her body and is real, it is not simply a part of her. It is a separate, complete being with its own boundaries and its own identity. Naming often reflects the attempts by the parents to identify the baby as a distinct entity, a Sam or a Mary.

After the mother has differentiated the baby's being from her own, she must prepare for the physical separation, the delivery. As in all aspects of pregnancy, there are various responses to this issue. Many women are eager to have the baby on the outside. Some were frightened by the intrusive intimacy of having it within. Others, however, don't want to let go. They may dream of "losing" their baby, or of having it delivered in some bizarre and frightening way. The idea of loss may actually bring on depression. It is necessary to prepare for this, for ultimately, every fetus is lost at the moment a baby is gained.

The process of separating from a fetus and letting a baby grow up is a process of losing a part of one's own being. Love is the experience of being merged with another. In pregnancy, this love is a concrete reality. It often provides a sense of

377

ecstatic completion, of wholeness, of transcending the usual limited boundaries of the individual, of the "I". Pregnancy is an altered state of consciousness largely because it plunges the individual's awareness from its usual secular pursuits into profound involvement in universal processes. It breaks through the barriers of our aloneness and unites us in a primordial love.

Pregnancy is the original experience from which our notions of love and ecstasy derive. It is that state in which each of us began, warm, protected, merged with another system whose reassuring rhythms, whose very life blood, sustained us. As we emerged into a consciousness of self over the years of our childhood and adolescence, the enveloping, protecting maternal figure faded into a reality, merely a person with whom we had to learn to relate. We have profound residual feelings about this person who is always "mother" for us. As we enter pregnancy, we become one with "mother" — not necessarily with the person we know now as "Mom" but with our primitive memory of the omnipotent being who nurtured us. We are in the process of becoming "mother." That is a magical and awesome task. No wonder pregnant women typically undergo some identity confusion in relation to their mothers and to other women.

Pregnant fathers are faced with watching their wife/lover become transformed into "mother" simultaneous to their own confrontation with themselves as "father." They may become irritated with their wife's frequent phone calls to mother. Fairly typically, however, the pregnant woman moves beyond her obsession with "mother" and begins to evaluate the "father" in her husband. This is a frequent source of conflict in a relationship. The wife characteristically starts criticising her husband's driving, or his hair style, his income, or his hobby. She may make unusual demands on him to test his loyalty and devotion (will he make breakfast if I have morning sickness; will he go out for pickles and ice cream in the dead of night?).

Pregnancy may be the first occasion in a marriage when the

378

partners realize the extent to which they are interdependent, psychologically, socially, and economically. The baby is literally a representation of the physiological union of the two into one. As such, it is a mystical symbol of their love. Life, however, has to be lived on a practical as well as a mystical plane. The merger may feel like a trap. One of the main tasks of pregnancy is to reconcile the identity confusions and prepare for the smooth functioning of the family after the birth.

---

### Transactional Analysis of a Pregnant Couple

| MAN | WOMAN | |
|---|---|---|
| lover | lover | — adolescent, cultural overlay |
| husband | wife | — adult give and take interacting |
| father | mother | — primitive ideas from childhood |

While interactions and confusions of these three levels are inevitable, there may be a dynamic tension rather than an irresolvable conflict. The role/person dichotomy can productively be worked on during pregnancy, when new roles are emerging and a new identify is being forged.

---

After pregnancy, the members of the family seem to become more distinct, more separate. The process, however, is not as sudden and total as it may seem. In the post partum weeks the family emerges only gradually from its earlier fusion. The subtle inter-connectedness of the mother-infant relationship is only beginning to be recognized by scientists. Lee Salk's article in *Scientific American*[5] and Marshall Klaus' work at Stanford and Cleveland[6] remind us that mothers who are with babies during the first hours, days, and weeks after birth behave differently towards them than mothers who are separated. Some of these behaviors may seem petty and incidental — is it important that a woman keep her head aligned with her baby's in an *en face* position or that she hold him on the left, not on the

379

right? We must hesitate before we answer these questions. We may have a nice set of answers we *think* are right, just as left handed mothers *think* they hold their baby on the left to keep their right hand free. We simply do not have all of the answers to our own behavior. Our motivations often lie beyond our linguistic comprehension, particularly in the primitive areas of pregnancy, childbirth, and parenting. People *need* each other in more profound ways than they realize. When bonds are formed, they can reach beyond social interaction to levels of biological need and interdependence—into the altered states of consciousness experienced as union and merger in love.

We have not touched on the phenomena of labor and delivery as altered states of consciousness because they, as the dramatic climax of the pregnancy experience, have received more attention than the longer, less precise stretch of gestation. There is increasingly good literature reminding us that the events of childbirth have been sacred to most cultures, that birth is a moment in which we are closer to the meaning of existence than to our day to day routine. Now the implications of this attitude are spreading beyond a desire for dignified, even ecstatic, childbirth rituals. We see that our other rites of passage, our special moments in the life cycle when we move from one phase of our selfhood to another, have become sterile, replaced by external events and holidays celebrated with intoxicants or vicarious experience. The move toward "natural" childbirth, toward having women awake and aware of the difficult transitional moment of birth, has led to a deepening realization that other involving moments in our inner, personal lives can be celebrated with meaning. Modern technology does not have to turn us into automatons. It can liberate us from certain fears, provide us with certain sheltering conveniences. But only we can choose to seize our lives and make them meaningful, to dare to experience the altered states of consciousness that are part of our biological heritage.

380

## Pregnancy as Altered Consciousness

It is possible to view each moment of our lives as a new beginning. This is the mission of mystics like William Blake who said that it is one thing to compare the sun to a golden guinea, but quite another to see it as a heavenly host singing hossanas to the Lord. It takes exceptional exertion to make daily moments sacred, to imbue the mundane with metaphor and universal meaning. The ecstatic states of consciousness that so many strive towards through religion, drugs, or encounter groups is potentially presented in a remarkably pure form in pregnancy, where merger is not only a subjective experience but a physical reality. The union of two beings creates the undifferentiated dyad of mother-fetus. This blending is unique to pregnancy but related to other altered states of consciousness in which the individual experiences himself at one with something or someone other than himself. If we bury this potential in banal routine and in technology which has no meaning to the subject, we will be turning our backs on the prototype of profound human experience.

Arthur D. Colman received both his A.B. and his medical degree from Harvard. His psychiatric training was at Langley Porter in San Francisco. He is the author of over 30 articles and 2 books and is currently associate clinical professor of psychiatry at the University of California Medical School. He is also in private practice of psychiatry in Sausalito.

Libby L. Colman received her B.A. from Wellesley and her M.A. from San Francisco State in English and American Literature. Her doctorate is from George Washington University in Shakespearean Literature. She is co-author with her husband of *Pregnancy: The Psychological Experience* and author of three children's books.

Reprinted with permission of *Birth and the Family Journal*, VOl. 1:1, 110 El Camino Real, Berkeley, Ca. 94705.

## BIBLIOGRAPHY

1. Colman, Arthur D., M.D. and Libby Lee Colman, Ph.D. *Pregnancy: The Psychological Experience.* Herder and Herder, 1971.

2. Tart, Charles, T. "Scientific Foundations for the Study of Altered States of Consciousness," *Journal of Transpersonal Psychology*, II (1971), 93.

3. Parks, J. "Emotional Reactions to Pregnancy." *American Journal of Obstetrics and Gynecology*, LXII (1951), 339.

4. Trethowan, W.H., "The Couvade Syndrome," *British Journal of Psychiatry*, CXI (1965). 57-66.

5. Salk, Lee. "The Role of Heartbeat in the Relations Between Mother and Infant," *Scientific American*, CCXXVIII (May 1983), 24-29.

6. Klaus, Marshall, et al. "Maternal Attachment — Importance of the first post-partum days." *New Engl. J. Med.* 286:9 (1972).

381

# Birthing Normally

Figure 1

**Weights represent risk factors, including**

A. Affective content
B. Beliefs
C. Character type (body structure)
D. General physical health
E. Emotional stress
F. Physical stress
G. Biochemical risk factors
H. Physical risk factors

$\left\{\begin{array}{l} \text{Relative} \\ \text{contribution} \\ \text{of individual} \\ \text{factor} = \beta \text{ weight} \\ \\ \text{Amount of} \\ \text{given factor} \end{array}\right.$

### GENERAL OUTCOME OF BIRTH
(Dependent variable in our multiple discriminant function)

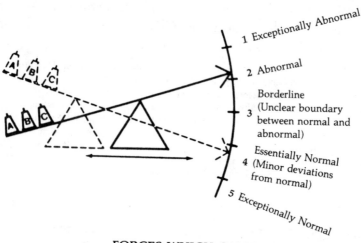

1 Exceptionally Abnormal

2 Abnormal

3 Borderline (Unclear boundary between normal and abnormal)

4 Essentially Normal (Minor deviations from normal)

5 Exceptionally Normal

### FORCES WHICH CAN MOVE FULCRUM:

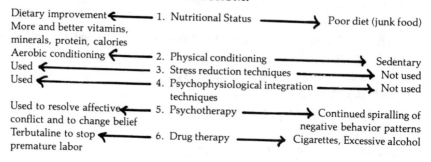

Dietary improvement ← More and better vitamins, minerals, protein, calories    1. Nutritional Status → Poor diet (junk food)

Aerobic conditioning ←    2. Physical conditioning → Sedentary

Used ←    3. Stress reduction techniques → Not used

Used ←    4. Psychophysiological integration techniques → Not used

Used to resolve affective conflict and to change belief ←    5. Psychotherapy → Continued spiralling of negative behavior patterns

Terbutaline to stop premature labor ←    6. Drug therapy → Cigarettes, Excessive alcohol

382

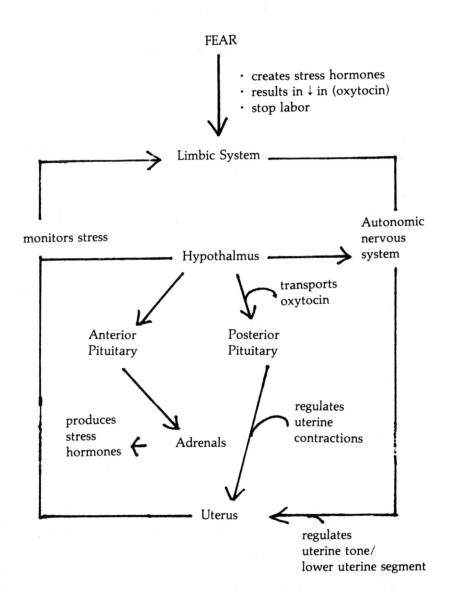

FEAR

- creates stress hormones
- results in ↓ in (oxytocin)
- stop labor

Limbic System

monitors stress

Hypothalmus

Autonomic nervous system

transports oxytocin

Anterior Pituitary

Posterior Pituitary

produces stress hormones

Adrenals

regulates uterine contractions

Uterus

regulates uterine tone/ lower uterine segment

Reprinted with permission of Gayle Peterson, *Birthing Normally: A Personal Growth Approach to Childbirth*, Mindbody Press, 1981, Berkeley. Appendix 11, Page 189-190.

# Affirmations

### by Nancy Wainer Cohen

WOMAN:

*I am a strong and capable woman.*

*I do not need to recreate my last birth.*

*My pelvis will release and open as have those of countless women before me.*

*I accept my labor and believe that it is the right labor for me, and for my baby.*

*I feel the love that others have for me during the birth.*

*I treat my mate lovingly during the birthing.*

*I have a success consciousness.*

*I have a beautiful body. My body is my friend.*

*Contractions are an effortless way to assist my baby into the world.*

*I can see my last birth as a learning experience, from which I am growing and changing.*

*I embrace the concept of healthy pain.*

*I have enough love to go around.*

*I can be strong, confident, assured, and assertive and still be feminine.*

*My baby knew how to "get in" and it knows how to "get out"!*

*I help my baby feel safe so that it can get born.*

MAN:

*I take care of myself during this pregnancy.*

*I see my wife as a strong and capable woman, and this does not threaten me.*

*I support her during her labor, even when she is in pain.*

*I express my love to my wife easily and frequently.*

*I accept the labor that is meant for us.*

*I accept feelings of helplessness.*

384

*I am sensitive, tender, open, and trusting, along with my "manly" qualities.*
*I feel the love that others have for me when I need support.*

Put stars(*) by the affirmations that feel right for you. Write the affirmations many times during the course of a week. Say them aloud, too, and use your name in the sentences. Then use the second and third persons also. Add other affirmations that would be helpful to you personally.

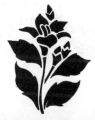

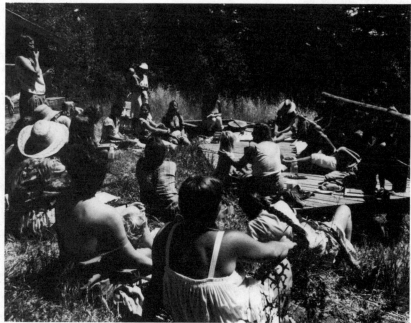

Photo by David Burns

Rainbow's End Study Group

385

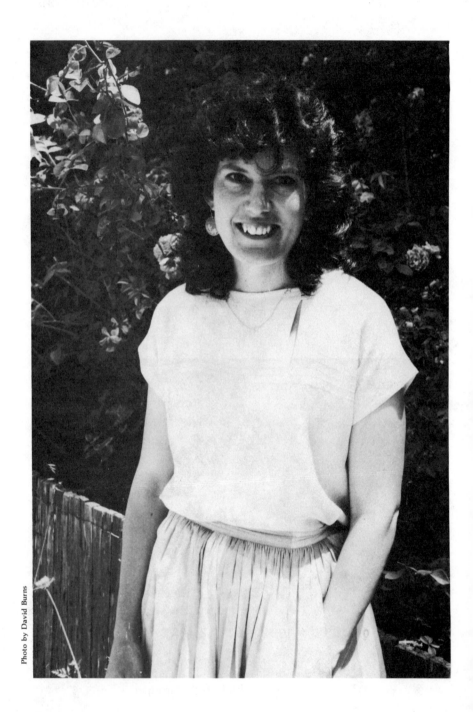

Photo by David Burns

*Patricia Natalini (See page 71)*

386

# PART V
# *Preparing the Spirit*

*Opening to the love/truth around us, surrendering to the power of mother nature, or whatever you call it. Learning not to complain is another way of saying the same thing. Trust the process; our bodies have their own wisdom which is beyond our capacity to understand.*

# Ina May Gaskin
# *Spiritual Midwife*

### by Linda Solomon

Adair Neumann labors in a softly-lit room at the Farm, the spiritual community of 1,500 near Summertown, Tennessee. Her body steadily opens to the explosion of new life. She feels intensely awake. No drugs dull her pain.

Ina May Gaskin, her grey-streaked hair in waist-length pigtails, climbs the stairs of the large communal house to where Adair labors. Ina May, the midwife who founded and directs the Farm's birthing program, joins the three midwives surrounding the naked woman on the bed. Watching Adair, who has traveled from New Mexico to have her baby at the Farm, the midwives merge their breaths, focusing their energy on the mother-to-be.

"How's it going?" Ina May asks, covering Adair's hand with her own.

"Great," Adair answers, her face flushed and perspiring.

The contractions come too slowly, so Ina May asks Adair to rise. She stands, her belly hanging huge from her small frame. Soon, Adair's upright pose works, and the contractions speed up.

When Adair feels the baby coming, the midwives help her lie down, stroking and caressing her. She pushes with all her might, and a head appears, the first patch of hair glistening wet, then the little face, and he's out.

"You did it," says Ina May. "It's a beautiful, six-and-a-half pound baby boy."

She swaddles the infant in blankets and places him on Adair's chest. Adair smiles at Ina May in response. It is the only payment the midwife will receive for her services. "It was just the way I wanted it to be," Adair says. "It was wonderful."

A stream of shared respect flows between mother and midwife. With courage and grace, Adair has completed what Ina May believes to be one of life's most challenging and important

388

passages. She has struggled, endured, and shown her feminine strength in brilliant colors. She is life and she knows it. These are qualities Ina May Gaskin can respect.

Ina May Gaskin did not go to nursing school to learn the art of midwifery. She became a "lay-midwife," gaining her skills through experience and by reading all the books on obstetrics and gynecology she could get her hands on. Unlike certified midwifes, who become registered nurses and go through two years of nurse-midwifery school, lay-midwives learn through apprenticeship and independent study. Ina May trained herself to deliver babies at home, modeling herself after self-trained female healers who, ever since Eve, have assisted women during birth.

By the standards of the American medical establishment, Ina May's training was unconventional and her orientation unsafe. Warren Pearse, president of the American College of Obstetricians and Gynecologists, the major trade organization or obstetricians in the United States, called parents who choose to have their babies at home "child abusers," and said the home birth environment was unsafe.

However, Ina May believes the dehumanizing methods of delivery favored by male establishment obstetricians like Pearse help create attitudes that can contribute to mothers or fathers abusing their children. She believes the rising rates of divorce, child abuse, incest and rape reflect America's poor system of handling birth.

"Birth is one of the natural ceremonies that is available to the family and society to hold things together," she says. "If you have a family that's bonded with trust and love, it helps them stick together. That helps the society function together. When you put birth in the hands of an elite, especially a male elite that can't possibly understanding giving birth, having never experienced it, you wind up with a crazy system."

Changing a "crazy system" has been at the forefront of Ina May's mind since the 1960s, when she married Stephen, the dynamic idealist who rose to counterculture fame preaching from a soap box in the Haight-Ashbury district of San Francisco. A philosopher and writer, Gaskin developed a large, loyal following with his sharp ideas and his easy-smiling charm.

Ten years ago, his charisma and beliefs motivated a group of 250 people to travel around the United States in a bus caravan looking for a good place to buy some land and do nothing less than start a new society. The society would grow out of the principles evolved by "flower children" during the peace movement in general, and out of Gaskin's ideas in particular.

During the odyssey, the caravan stopped in Evanston, Illinois, and there, in a school bus parked on the Northwestern University campus, a woman bore a child. Coaching the woman was Ina May Gaskin, then 31. She had no training in obstetrics. The baby came out easily and began to breathe by himself.

"I was in a state of complete amazement for several days," Ina May says. "I felt a definite calling to be a midwife, but my English major in college hadn't prepared me for anything so real-life as birthing."

Although her studies had not prepared her for a career as a midwife, her personal experiences had. Ina May was born in Marshalltown, Iowa, to a father who worked in the farm loan business, and a mother who was a home economist and the daughter of farmers. She was close to her grandmother, who liked to give her biographies of powerful women, women who made their names as innovators, healers and political organizers. The collection included the lives of Elizabeth Cady Stanton, Susan B. Anthony, Elizabeth Blackwell and Clara Barton. The stories of these pioneers of suffrage and women's rights inspired the young girl and by the age of 12, Ina May knew she wanted to be like them. "They put their lives on the line," she said. "They fought slavery. They were moral leaders. When I hear the word 'feminist,' I think of them."

Ina May wanted to accomplish. She knew women possessed inner power and strength, but she did not see American society drawing their power out. Were bravery and wit only for little boys who became men and went to war?

390

No, she decided when she became pregnant with her first child in 1965. For a natural childbirth she would need all the bravery, wit, courage and strength she could muster. But when she entered the hospital to give birth, "there they came with the drugs," she said. She was anesthetized, shaved, and given an episiotomy. "The event went from being natural and interesting to being rather terrifying," she recalls. The experience left its marks.

The drugs removed the physical pain, and left emotional pain in its place. After the birth she had a hard time showing her baby "full affection." She felt duped and depressed.

"Now," says Ina May, who has four children ranging in age from six to 17, "I'm careful never to treat anyone in the detached, professional, almost disgusted manner that is so common in the hospital world. When I'm being a midwife, I'm treating a woman exactly the way I would like to be treated. I know that if a woman has a beautiful time having her baby, she will carry the experience with her for the rest of her life. She will pass her good feelings about childbirth on to her daughters and sons. Her daughters and sons will pass it on to theirs, and the good feeling will be passed on through the generations."

"Birth is holy," Ina May says, "and if we treat every childbirth with that kind of value, then we will start doing something to make changes that will be far-reaching and permanent for the whole society."

Changing the society was on her mind as she crossed America with the caravan from San Francisco in 1971. When the group reached Tennessee, they bought land in the middle of the state and settled down to work.

Pooling their resources and living communally, the small group grew into what is now a thriving village of families and old people. They opened their doors to unwed mothers, emotionally disturbed children and Guatemalan refugees. They gave them shelter and incorporated them into their tightly knit society.

The group developed their own method of natural birth control and started a solar energy construction company, a book publishing company, and an international service organization with bases in Guatemala, Africa and Ireland. Last year they began providing money and volunteers for a free ambulance service to the residents of New York's South Bronx. Because Farm members are vegetarians, they created a soybean manufacturing company that sells "ice bean," an ice cream substitute, to health food stores nationwide.

To maintain their health, the group developed a health care system that provides free service to Farm residents, and because they needed to deliver their own babies, Ina May began to study midwifery. She attended births and soon was training other women to be midwives.

Ten years and more than 1,300 births later, Ina May had built a home birth system with statistics on safety that outscore national averages. She provided an example to an increasingly technological medical establishment of how simple, safe and (at $25 a delivery) cheap childbirth can be.

At the Farm, where midwives deliver all normal pregnancies, the neonatal mortality rate was 7 per 1,000 live births, compared to the national neonatal death rate in 1978 of 9.5 per 1,000 live births, according to the National Center for Health Statistics. Neonatal deaths include babies who die in the first 7 days of life.

In 1979, in the United States, 16.4 percent of the children born in non-military hospitals were delivered Caesarean section, with the numbers rising to 17.7 percent of births in the Southeast in non-military hospitals. This compares quite poorly to the 1.8 percent, or 24 of the Farm's 1,300 births, that have been delivered by Caesarean section.

Some doctors dismiss the statistics at the Farm, saying they come from a highly selected population of very healthy women. One of these doctors is Allen Killam, a professor of obstetrics and gynecology at Vanderbilt University, who questions the safety of home birth in general.

"I think these statistics are somewhat biased," Killam says, "but again, everyone has their own pet statistics, and there haven't been very well-controlled studies done by anyone. But after 21 years of experience, I believe I can do a much better job in a hospital situation than I, or anybody else, can do at home."

Dr. C. Arden Miller, former chairman of the Department of Maternal and Child Health at the University of North Carolina, has a different point of view. After completing a study of home birth in North Carolina, he concluded that it provided "individualized, personalized, and non-oppressive, family-oriented care," at a lower cost than hospital births.

Testifying before Rep. Albert Gore (D-Tenn.) at his congressional hearings on midwives, Miller said, "the record of safety and favorable conclusion of pregnancies at the Farm has been impressive — no maternal deaths and an infant mortality rate substantially better than for the rest of Tennessee."

Dr. Marshall Klaus, author of *Maternal and Infant Bonding,* said that "in the Farm's society, medical care is more than just medicine. It's peace of mind. They are thinking about the complete person."

Dr. David McMillan, professor of psychology at the Center for Community Studies at the Kennedy Center, Peabody College of Vanderbilt University, had this to say in his testimony about the Farm, which he visited frequently:

"The Farm culture uses the birth experience effectively to build and promote a spiritual sense of family and community. Birth at the Farm is an important occasion that can be shared by the couple and their community of friends. It is an important memory in their relationship bonds."

Unlike the Farm, McMillan said, "Our culture often anesthetizes the mother, excludes the father and tells friends to stay away. Often new parents become more distant and hostile with each other and isolated from friends who don't understand the magnitude of what has just happened to them. The Farm maximizes the community's opportunity to share the joy and the excitement of the miracle of birth."

Margaret A. Emrey, a nursing consultant with the California State Department of Health, who helped start the first midwifery program in a San Francisco hospital, said, "Ina May does a beautiful job. She and the midwives she has trained have a very highly developed intuition. They sense what is going on with people."

The Farm does provide for the non-routine delivery too. Two doctors live and work full time at the Farm and assist the midwives if complications occur during childbirth, and the community has its own pharmacy, laboratory, a neonatal intensive care unit and 40 paramedics. Because of its state-approved ambulance service, no woman bears her baby more than two minutes from transportation to a hospital.

In contrast with hospitals, which routinely administer IVs and episiotomies to women in labor, only 26 of 1,300 women who gave birth at the Farm took anesthesia and 22 percent received episiotomies. Ninety-nine percent of the women who bore their babies at the Farm breastfed them successfully afterwards.

Yet, though the care is so much more personal than at a hospital, each birth costs the Farm only $25.

Ina May has spread her ideas to health practitioners and consumers throughout this nation and Canada through her book, *Spiritual Midwifery* (which sold 130,000 copies last year) and speaking engagements, at which she attempts to communicate a respect for the process of birth, a process she calls a "sacred event."

"Don't have an abortion," she tells women at the end of her book. "You can come to the Farm and we'll deliver your baby and take care of him, and if you decide you want him back, you can have him."

Two hundred women have taken her up on this offer. After bearing their babes at the Farm, only 11 gave their children up. Ina May explains this by saying that after experiencing a pregnancy and natural childbirth, women feel bonds with their children, which only the worst of circumstances can break.

394

"You change your concept about yourself when you have a baby," she says. "There's a power in you that wasn't there before. If you're knocked out, you don't get the benefit of the experience."

Ina May is a midwife of ideas as well as habits. Believing fervently that birth is best handled and understood by women, especially women who have borne children, Ina May tells her audiences that returning "the major responsibility for normal childbirth to well-trained midwives, rather than having it rest with a predominantly male and profit-oriented medical establishment, is a major advance in self-determination for women. The wisdom and compassion a woman can intuitively experience in childbirth can make her a source of healing and understanding for other women."

Though Ina May approached her second labor infinitely wiser about childbirth, she was dealt another emotional blow. The child was stillborn. "A person can get well from anything," she says, "as long as they're still alive." She recovered from her deep sense of loss with the birth of her next child, a healthy baby—a birth Stephen Gaskin attended. Except for the two Farm doctors, Gaskin is the only man who lives in the community to hold the respected title of "midwife."

When asked about feminism, Ina May's answer swings to midwifery. "Without midwifery, the feminist movement could not exist," she says, "because midwifery is too central to women. People are going to have children and the help of women is crucial at that time. The intelligence women have needs to be shared. Midwives in the society create trust and cooperation among women, instead of setting them against each other."

The United States suffers from an "appallingly bad" system of sex education, according to Ina May. "Young women feel they have nothing to offer but their sexuality," she says. "That was the teaching of the 1930s, 1940s and 1950s. This attitude results in abortions, broken marriages, child abuse, and fear and loathing of childbirth and childbearing."

At the Farm, children learn about sex from the farm animals and insects as well as from their teachers, parents and the midwives. "We don't have to tell them a lot," Ina May says. "They know people aren't that different from all the other animals running around."

Farm children respect sex more than children outside the community, Ina May believes, because they understand the result of sex. "We don't have much teenage pregnancy," she says, "because the kids know exactly what causes it. They have seen people get pregnant young. They know that when a girl gets pregnant, she gets taken out of action, and when a boy becomes a father, he has a lot of responsibility. Our kids don't want to get tied down."

"Abortion," says Ina May, "is necessary on some occasions, but it is not something women in a sane society would do casually. In an insane society that does not support its women, like ours, abortion happens on a mass level."

Ina May has lectured at Roosevelt Hospital in New York City, San Francisco General Hospital, Case Western Reserve, the State University of New York at Stony Brook and Tuskegee University in Tuskegee, Alabama. She has appeared on NBC's "Today Show" and on "The Phil Donahue Show." She is now writing a book on breastfeeding.

At a conference of the American Society for Psychosomatic Obstetrics and Gynecology in San Antonio, Texas, Ina May addressed a group of physicians. According to the "Obstetrics and Gynecology News," some physicians in the audience were skeptical, until the speech changed their attitudes. One physician remarked that the women in the films seemed to be treated like "prima donnas" by the Farm staff. Another, who said he had been biased against the Farm before the film, said it convinced him Ina May's procedure was well-planned and provided good backup, laboratories and transportation.

"I'm trying as hard as I can to spread a consciousness that midwifery is something we need," Ina May says, "and that the United States, however unconsciously, set out on the wrong path when it discouraged midwifery.

"The United States ranks 16th in the world in infant mortality, yet we put more dollars into obstetrics than any other country. I try to let people know there is a different way of doing things."

In the communal houses around the Farm, families prepare for dinner. Adair breastfeeds her baby. Ina May says good night to the new mother and heads home.

It is dusk. She rides her bicycle over the dirt road. The fields look green against the pink sky and the air smells of an afternoon rain. Going home, the midwife feels renewed.

Linda Solomon, formerly a reporter for the Tennessean in Nashville, Tennessee, is now writing a book about the politics of childbirth.

Reprinted from *Yoga Journal*, May-June, 1982.

# *Avoiding Stress*

1. Plan some idleness every day.
2. Listen to others without interruption.
3. Read books that demand concentration.
4. Learn to honor food.
5. Have a place for retreat at home.
6. Avoid irritating, overly-competitive people.
7. Plan leisurely, less structured vacations.
8. Concentrate on enriching yourself.
9. Live by the calendar, not the stop watch.
10. Concentrate on one task at a time.

On the wall in Will Well's (Chiropractor) Office, Forestville, California.

397

# The Emotions of Pregnancy and How to Deal with Them

*by Karen Shultz*

In childbirth handbooks and classes, a great deal of emphasis is placed upon diet, exercise and hygiene. While these matters are of paramount importance, I feel that the radically transformed emotions of the pregnant female are *not* put into an essential perspective.

Not only should the woman herself be prepared for these emotional changes, but the people closest to her should be ready to deal with her new fluctuations in personality. And it must be remembered that the unborn child also absorbs the patterns of the mother's feelings which, through her chemical changes, can affect the child before and after birth. Chemicals and hormones related to her states of mind pass through her circulation into the placenta of the fetus, and then onward into the baby's bloodstream.

"A pregnant woman's health has certain manifestations, but first and foremost, she must be happy . . ." was the astute observation of natural childbirth pioneer, Dr. Grantly Dick-Read. "This demands companionship (on the part of the husband) and interest in her baby if her husband shares her hopes and anxieties, her laughter and her waves of fear. He alone can be the safety valve of her unpredictable emotions and accept unmoved the explosions of her love, hate, jealousy, and anger. The storms are usually followed by warm sunshine . . . A disturbed mind will upset the circulation of blood to certain organs of the body. It will cause serious deprivation of oxygen supply and some of the vital substances from the glands within the body which are essential for the well-being of the small fetus in the womb." (From the classic book, *Childbirth Without Fear*).

Psychiatric studies have shown that pregnancy can create a deviant, borderline mental state somewhere between neurosis and psychosis. This may sound so very heavy, but many women will read this with a knowing smile. (Husbands, too!) But it is comforting to realize that these states can usually be alleviated by the "outside" influence of family love and understanding, in conjunction with certain common-sense practices on the part of the expectant mother.

A good friend, who always seemed so vivacious and gay throughout her pregnancy, later confided to me that she had a crying spell every day. Having experienced four pregnancies, my husband and I both know what to expect from my "pregnant" emotions: very high highs and very low lows! And it happens every time — I hardly feel like the same person I used to be in the pre-pregnant state. And I can always feel myself subtlely returning to a stronger sanity *after* childbirth!

Spiritual Midwifery offers a fine descriptive statement: "Hormones are as heavy consciousness-changers as psychedelics . . ." And they (the midwives) have some good advice: "Your emotions are very close to the surface and you might feel like laughing or crying for no reason at all . . . Do something with an older child, or cook something nice for the family. These emotional whirlwinds are short-lived, and you can keep it together until they pass."

Dr. Robert Bradley points out in *Husband-Coached Childbirth* that the "pregnant" brain may swell as do other parts of the pregnant anatomy, and this phenomenon, complete with alterations in circulation caused by the contracting uterus in the last trimester, can cause sudden bizarre outbursts of emotion and peculiar dreams. While this may sound a bit superstitious, it seems that a full moon is especially capable of teasing the waters of the brain, thereby causing even *more* erratic behavior! Yogically speaking, mood changes in the eighth month are attributed to circulation of *Ojas* (subtle energy) between mother and child.

What are (assuming you are in good health and already eating an adequate diet) the two greatest offenders of the pregnant woman's emotions?

WORRY AND FATIGUE!
Both of these seem to be the main external triggers of negative emotional states.

With daily family living, there will always be everyday worries, small and large, that come and go. During pregnancy, however, the various concerns can become magnified out of normal proportion. And somehow, pregnancy seems to go hand-in-hand with extra money problems. Everyone's situation is a little different, but money is usually the number one worry of most pregnant women that I have known. Try to arrange for payment of medical care as early in pregnancy as you can, so as to lessen that aspect of prenatal tension!

Good advice from Helene Ellis, pertaining to all kinds of worries, from *A Birth Book for my Friends* "Work it out together. (To the husband — ) Listen for serious complaints and lesser complaints (they may both appear in the same velocity) and seek solutions to complaints calmly."

It is vital to have a sympathetic husband with whom to discuss all your fears. But also, the trusted feminine ear of a good friend or relative is a valuable resource. This lady can help you to look at your problems rationally and can give you additional encouragement.

When things *do* become too much for you, get a change of scenery *fast!* It really helps. Whether you live in the city or the country, choose a route that you can walk every day in the fresh air. It will do wonders for you. Or, husbands, take your wives out to a good film if you can afford it (she'll love the diversion), to a pleasant natural setting, or to the home of a good friend. Her temporarily confused world will regain its usual sense and energy. Maybe she *has* been staying around the house too much!

Spiritual well-being is of prime importance in pregnancy. A transcendent positivity is more beneficial to the psyche than anything else. Whatever your religious background or beliefs, take advantage of spiritual group gatherings. You'll feel yourself rising higher, and your baby will love it, too!

Arrange to do things for yourself and your family beside housework. Easy-going sewing projects, reading, light

400

gardening, etc., are all very good. Birth books (and there are so many good ones out) make the coming baby more of a reality and will add to the understanding of yourself. Find out about the growth of the fetus and share this knowledge with your older children.

And you must realize that your physical energy is much lower — don't push yourself. Your body is hard at work in the creation of a new human being! You'll experience a kind of inertia in the first three months, with a reasonable amount of energy in the mid-months, and on the homestretch your body will be heavy and tired. Nap if and when you can, don't skimp on nighttime sleeping, and get off your feet 10 minutes an hour in the last couple of months. Fatigue can quickly give rise to tension or depression, so don't be afraid to take it easy when you need it. Surely, somethings just might not get done, but you'll have to re-orient yourself completely to a slower-paced lifestyle. You'll be happier and so will your family!

This article was not intended to portray the pregnant condition as an emotional nightmare! It serves only to prepare you for changes that will most probably come your way. But you'll also experience incredible joys — unique realizations of the miraculous nature of Creation as Life Itself grows within you. Probably at no other time in your life will you have such a direct link with the Cosmos. Just tune into it!

## Harmless Treatments for Prenatal Mood Fluctuations

Homeopathic remedies can be an effective aid in alleviating certain emotional states during pregnancy. 30x potency pellets are available from Standard Homeopathic Co., P.O. Box 61067, Los Angeles, CA 90061, for $3.50 per 1-oz. bottle. (Add $1.50 postage). Take 2-3 pellets 4 times a day until improvement is definitely noted. *DO NOT* take them for more than one week.

*Sepia:* indifferent, depressed, fear of being alone, faint feeling.

*Pulsatilla:* easy weeping, changeable moods, craves sympathy, mild personality.

*Ignatia:* Contradictory, *much sighing,* sometimes hysterical, wide mood swings, wants to be alone.

*Natrum Muriaticum:* irritable, headaches, worse with sympathy, weepy.

*Aurum Metallicum:* deepest depression, suicidal, quarrelsome, has nightmares.

Published courtesy of *MOTHERING PUBLICATIONS,* vol. VI, P.O. Box 2208, Albuquerque, New Mexico 87103.

# *Yoga Instruction for Self-Control*

*Words of wisdom from "The Doctrine and Practice of Yoga" by Swami Mukerji, published in 1922 by the Yogi Publ. Society, Chicago.*

## *Will-Power*

Will-Power grows by faith in one's ability by exercise; by devotion to the UNCONDITIONED SPIRIT.

In your efforts to develop Will-Power, be not afraid that your health will break down. in fact, Perfect Health is the result of a perfect Will. Deny the power of disease and weakness over yourself. *"I can never be ill. My body is my slave. It shall always manifest perfect health."* Convince your passive mind—which has charge of your body—of this by repeated commands, demands and assertions. Always think of your body as being as strong as adamant. Never talk of

402

either health or disease or weakness. You must be above caring for these. They are your Natural rights. Only when you lower yourself they have power to trouble you. Go beyond the lower self. Your business is to care for the Higher-Self — that in which "You" live, move, and have your being. Also teach and train your Will to move along negative lines of self-repression as well as along positive lines of Self-Expression. Balance both. The former precedes the latter. Now I will pass on to the subject of SELF-CONTROL, with the distinct understanding that Self-Control and Will-Power are inextricably bound up in each other. You get the real "practical work" in the endeavour for Self-Control.

## Self-Control

Rightly has it been remarked that it is easy to talk of and write upon this subject but most difficult to possess it. Perfect Self-Control means infinite power. Only the Buddas and the Christs of this World manifested Perfect Self-Control. "Anything short of the absolute control of thought, word and deed is only sowing wild oats," said Vivekananda. It is with no little diffidence that I approach this subject as whoever handles this subject is rightly culpable as being a "Do-as-I-say-and-not-as-I-do" individual.

## Preliminary Steps

"The first requisite," says Mr. Atkinson, "of concentrating is the ability to shut out outside thoughts, sights and sounds; to conquer inattention; to obtain perfect control over the body and mind. The body must be brought under the control of the mind; the mind under the direct control of the Will. The Will is strong enough, but the mind needs strengthening by being brought under the direct influence of the will. The mind, strengthened by the impulse of the will, becomes a much more powerful projector of thought vibrations than otherwise and

403

the vibrations have much greater force and effect.

The first four exercises are meant to train the mind to readily obey the commands of the mind. Take them in the privacy of your own room and never talk of them to others. Also do not let their apparent simplicity lead you to neglect them. If you are one of those empty-brained men who go about talking of their exercises hoping in this way to win praise, you will never succeed. Be serious, earnest and sincere in your work. Give up, once for ever, all fickle-mindedness and learn to accumulate Power in silence and through work. Prayer gives you strength to "work"—the answer comes from your Larger Self—which is the Spirit of God "brooding" over all and pouring strength into all. But do not fly in the face of DEITY by expecting it to "do the work" for you while you go about loafing after offering your prayer. Nonsense. That man prays who works constantly, silently, patiently, unceasingly and intelligently.

EXERCISE 1.

Sit still; relax your body all over and then neck, chest, and head held in a straight line; legs crossed one under the other and weight of the body resting easily upon the ribs; right hand on right leg, left hand on left leg. There should not be a single movement of the muscles in any part of the body. Mind, you must avoid all rigidness and tension of the body. There should not be the least strain on muscles. You should be able to "relax" completely. Start with 5 minutes. Continue till you can accomplish the 5 minutes sitting without any conscious effort, increase to 15 minutes which is about all you need. The aim is to give you absolute dominion over all involuntary muscular movements. It is also an ideal "rest-cure" after fatiguing physical and mental exercise or exertion. The principal thing is "STILLNESS" and you can, if you like, practice it even sitting on a chair or anywhere else; the idea is one of "relaxation" and physical and mental quietude. Let not the apparent simplicity of this exercise deceive you. It is not so very easy after all. You will find that by concentrating the mind upon a

404

particular train of thoughts or ideas or by joining the mind to the Larger Self, you can easily lose all idea of the body and thus maintain this stillness for a considerable length of time. Genius, inspiration and intuition are more or less the scientific and psychological results of self-forgetfulness. "When he sits down to meditate," it was said of Vivekananda, "in 10 minutes he becomes quite unconscious of the body although it may be black with mosquitoes." Do you understand now? Absolute physical self-forgetfulness is essential to deep concentration. Dr. Fahnestock called it the "STATUVOLIC" condition or that state in which the Will-Power is really active and the 'outer-self' is totally in abeyance and forgotten.

EXERCISE 2.

Cultivate a self-poised attitude and demeanour in your everday life. Avoid a tense, strained, nervous, fidgety manner and an over-anxious appearance. Be easy, self-possessed and dignified in your bearing. Be courteous, thoughtful and quiet. Mental exercise and Will-Culture will enable you to acquire the proper carriage and demeanour. Stop swinging your feet and moving your hands or rocking your self backwards in your chair while talking or sitting. Stop biting your nails, chewing your moustache, rolling your tongue in your mouth or any other unnecessary movement such as may have become "second nature" with you while studying, reading or writing. Never twitch or jerk your body. Never wink your eyes or look blank. Train yourself to stand sudden and loud noises with equanimity and composure. Such things betray lack of control. Do not let anything outside (or even within you) disturb your composure. When engaged in conversation let your speech be calm and measured and your voice well-controlled and even. A certain degree of reserve should always be observed. In short, keep yourself well under control on all occasions. You can acquire this poise by always carrying the thoughts of "Firmness," "Self-Control," and "Self-Respect" in your mind and letting these express themselves in your outward bearing. Avoid bluster, self-assertion, gossip, levity or light talk, too much laughter, excitement and so forth. Too much laughter weakens the will. Be a quiet, earnest-thinking being. Be serious. Regard "solitude" as the greatest medium of self-development.

EXERCISE 3.

Fill a wine glass full of water and taking the glass between the fingers, extend arm directly in front of you. Fix your eyes upon the glass and endeavour to hold your arm so steady that no quiver will be noticeable. Commence with one minute exercise and increase until the 5 minutes limit is reached. Alternate right and left arms. Increase to 15 minutes.

EXERCISE 4.

Sit erect in your chair, with your head up, chin out and shoulders back. Raise your right arm until it is level with your shoulders, pointing to the right. Turn your head and fix your gaze on your hand and hold the arm perfectly steady for one minute. Repeat with left arm. Increase the time gradually to 5 minutes. The palms of the hands should be turned downwards.

The following exercises are meant to aid you in getting under control, such mental faculties will produce voluntary movements.

EXERCISE 5.

Sit in front of a table, placing your hands upon the table, the fists clinched and lying with the back of the hand upon the table, the thumb being doubled over the fingers. Fix your gaze upon the fist for awhile and then slowly extend the thumb, keeping your whole attention fixed upon the act, just as if it was of the greatest importance. Then slowly extend your first finger, then your second and so on, until they are all open and extended. Then reverse the process, closing first the little finger and continuing the closing until the fist is again in its original position, with the thumb closed over the fingers. Repeat with left hand. Continue this exercise 5 times at a sitting, then increase to 10 times. Don't forget to keep your attention closely fixed upon the finger movements. This is the main point.

EXERCISE 6.

Place the fingers of one hand between the fingers of the other, leaving the thumbs free. Then slowly twirl the thumbs one over the other, with a circular motion. Be sure to keep the attention firmly fixed upon the end of the thumbs.

*N. B.* Exercises Nos. 3, 4, 5 and 6 have been culled (with slight modifications by me) from the works of Yogi Ramacharaka.

# *The Care and Feeding of Wives, Husbands and Ummers*

*By Ronald Steelman*

I come to this subject from two subjective idea centers. One is negative and reflects my law practice, with its rites and jargon, like "dissolution of marriage" and "partnership agreement." The other is my own limited experience in marriage, which has been as pleasant and rewarding (give or take a few bad scenes) as my professional experience in this area has been disgusting. From this vast reservoir of prejudice, and unencumbered by any pretense of scientific method or moral or religious validity, I am happy to provide these maxims:

407

## 1) IF YOU'RE GOING TO HAVE CHILDREN, GET MARRIED.

Many alternative relationships have evolved over the years, and this evolution has been busier than ever recently. It has produced, in the words of a good Friend of ours, the "ummer."

An ummer is a person who enjoys an intimate relationship (something more than a "friend" but less than a spouse) with your relative or close friend. The name "ummer" derives from the term used to introduce this person to your own associates, e.g. "I want you to meet Cynthia (or Fred, etc.), Ralph's umm . . . er . . ."

Contemporary mores sanction the ummer relationship even when the parties live together in a state which, in earlier times, would have been labeled "sin" if not certified as marriage by the County Clerk. I personally feel that ummerhood is okay, and that if two people enjoy a relationship which is mutually supportive and constructive, enjoyable, and not harmful to themselves or their close associates, then the extent of their physical, spiritual and intellectual intimacy is no one else's business.

On the other hand, if one wishes to adopt or bear children, the ummer relationship is really inadequate. It is not fair to the mother, father or child to embark on childrearing without a commitment to a permanent relationship. Fatherhood should mean more than a support check and reasonable visitation, if any; motherhood should mean more than a burdensome task to face alone, and childhood should mean more than passing time. Childhood should mean growing up in a complete, stable family unit and being free to form one's own relationships. Ironically, this freedom appears curtailed in children from "broken homes," who seem fated to repeat their parents' patterns of unstable alliances.

## 2) IF YOU'RE NOT GOING TO HAVE CHILDREN, IT MAY BE BETTER NOT TO GET MARRIED.

408

This is, of course, the converse of maxim no. 1. While the rules are not completely reversible, there is some validity in this permutation. Being an ummer may have its drawbacks, but it's not nearly as dreadful as being, or even feeling, locked into a bad situation. More of this in maxim:

## 3) BE CAREFUL WHOM YOU MARRY.

I am constantly appalled at some of the people people marry. Many of the pairings which pass my view might have looked great in central casting, the tennis tournament ladder, or the nominating committee report, but ye gods! One does really choose a mate, or at least one surely exercises some choice; yet amazingly, many choose mates who are incompatible emotionally, culturally and spiritually. It is the young who seem most compelled to make these horrible mistakes, and I suspect it has a lot to do with confusing a desire for experience, physical intimacy and peer status with choosing a complementary partner, all of which may be another good argument for ummerhood.

## 4) DON'T BEAT YOUR WIFE OR NAG YOUR HUSBAND (OR YOUR UMMER EITHER) AND VICE VERSA.

Wives, husbands and ummers don't like being beaten or nagged, and they will react every time, or if they don't seem to react, even worse may be in store. If you feel the need to strike out with hand, club, or tongue, reflect on your anger. It may be sufficient to resolve your feelings merely to express them, but do so honestly, so that you and your mate will be able to understand them and deal with them. Say, "I feel," not "you are." If you are tired of coddled eggs for breakfast, say "I am tired of coddled eggs for breakfast," *not* "You're a terrible cook!" Better yet, why don't *you* cook breakfast for a change and shut up about the coddled eggs? This leads to the next maxim:

409

## 5) BE METICULOUS ABOUT SHARING THE BENEFITS AND THE BURDENS.

No marriage will work unless there is an equal sharing of assets and obligations, expenses and profits, and unless both parties agree and believe that there is in fact such an equal sharing. This may, but need not, mean an actual division of the various tasks and joys, or it may mean a mutually agreeable exchange and accounting of the jobs and rewards. This may seem unromantic and mechanical, but I have never seen a good marriage without a mutual desire to share both work and rewards, and a strong mutual effort to keep things fair.

## 6) IF YOU'VE BEEN MARRIED THREE YEARS OR HAVE CHILDREN, DON'T GET DIVORCED.

Divorce is fine for beginners, but for old marrieds or parents it creates problems which surpass its benefits. Except for a few people who have made a drastic mistake and have realized their error early on, no one has ever found happiness through divorce. The economic and emotional cost of divorce is catastrophic, and the gain nonexistent. Divorcing persons seek peace, freedom, fulfillment, liberation, etc., and find loneliness and penury. The exciting new relationships, either before or after divorce simply turn into a new set of problems, and all the years of loving, caring, sharing and security are down the tubes. Therefore:

## 7) IF DIVORCE THREATENS, INSIST ON COMMUNICATION AND COUNSELING.

(Even if it doesn't work, communication and counseling never hurt anyone.) It may be late, and you should have started sooner, but don't give up. Think of your errant spouse as a victim of emotional disease, and insist on immediate diagnosis and therapy, and don't forget you need it, too. Drag him or her, even screaming and kicking, to progressive stages of intense aid until the cure takes. The spouse will insist he or

410

she really wants out, and may have been planning, consciously or not, for years, but be firm and simply do not permit it.

I realize that this maxim is contrary to current belief that it takes two to save a marriage. In fact, one can do it, and I have seen it done. It requires a firm belief that divorce is not a viable solution, a suppression of one's natural pride, resentment and bitterness, and a strong commitment to discovering a new dimension in the relationship which needs to be found. It also helps to be extremely lovable and indispensable.

Incidentally, lawyers and courts are of no help at all in reconciliation, and in my opinion actively oppose it.

## 8) KEEP YOUR OWN IDENTITY AND LET YOUR MATE HAVE HIS OR HERS.

Avoid the connubial "we." You may live at the same address, be parents of the same children, and have a lot in common, but if you think and act alike and agree on everything, one of you has a problem. Give yourselves time and space to grow, and share the growing.

## 9) CHOOSE A SUPPORTIVE ENVIRONMENT.

To make your marriage work, avoid role models like Hugh Hefner and Elizabeth Taylor. Don't take six-month consulting contracts in Las Vegas or Morocco where the family can't go along. Go to Meeting. Reflect: If there is that of God in every person, then I am closest to God when I am closest to my spouse. Or Ummer.

Ronald Steelman is an attorney, a member of Orange County (CA) Monthly Meeting, a member of College Park Friends Educational Association and a writer of "scurrilous limericks" for the Orange County Bar Bulletin and the Harvard Law School Bulletin.

Reprinted with permission of *FRIENDS JOURNAL*, Volume 23, number 20, copyright 1977.

# Life Processing Center

## Mental Equivalents for the Central Body

### by Carol Bridges

The central portion of your body is where your life is physically processed. The organs, muscles, nerves, and vessels of this area work to digest all of the experiences you put your body through as you go about your daily living. The central body houses the etheric center known as the Solar Plexus, your point of individual power. This chakra once connected you with the body of your mother through the navel. Through this cord you were unfailingly nourished by her. But once the cord was cut, you were on your own. Ever since then, you have been perfecting your individual way of getting the world to meet your needs.

Unfortunately for our body's health, we have often learned to meet our needs by being ill, thus calling our "mother" back once again to nourish us. We have found ourselves at a loss, for a certain period of time preceding illness, as to how to fully satisfy our worldly goals and desires. So, we want to go "home," to return to that all-nurturing womb, and let someone else take care of us for awhile . . . until we feel strong again. As we mature, however, we come to realize that our biological mother can no longer serve us in the same capacity (even though many try). We begin to see that we have a much larger mother who is the Earth herself. This new mother, once we attune ourselves to her, is able to provide for us once again. If we plant a few seeds, she gives us the foods of our choice. If we save wild space in which to forage, she provides life-giving treats. If we refrain from paving over her with concrete, she provides woods for homes and heat. If we are careful with our trash, her water is always clean enough to drink. It's so simple with Mother Earth.

412

The more we stray from her simplicity, the more likely we are to encounter disease and dissatisfaction. If you pick and eat wild greens, you can almost taste the vitality. Of course, if your usual diet consists of super-homogenized, chemicalized, over-processed foods, she may bring about a cleansing to bring you back home. Home, you might say, is not only where the heart is, but where the tummy lives. Your body shows the emotional condition of your homelife. Do you need to stuff it with extra sweets? Is there a feeling of emptiness? Do emotional struggles get processed well at home? How hard do you have to work to keep things in shape? These are multi-level questions for the multi-level work your stomach area does. You have only to look down to see the answers.

If your digestive system is in good order, let's examine the reproductive system. The main food here is self-acceptance. Each day you should have a healthy dose. The world is always (through ads, parents, mates, teachers, religions) attempting to tell you what to do with your sexual energy. It is such a powerful force, everyone wants to make sure it is going in a good (or profitable) direction. If you are not giving your energy to their cause, they may try to elicit some guilt. Guilt is perhaps the second most driving force, but, in the long run, is very debilitating. Your healthiest sexual expression is doing what makes your soul happy. And only you know what that is.

You may want a child right now when all conditions seems to say, "No you can't afford it." Or you may NOT want a child when everything seems to suggest that this is the time. WITHIN YOURSELF, you know the course you must take. Your soul has manifested in earth TO LIVE, not to deny itself life's experience. Sometimes you may need to do "hard" things, just to acquire the experience, and therefore knowledge, so your soul can grow. The reproductive systems says "create." For you that may mean babies, or it may mean works of art or communities or businesses or crocheted hats. But you must reproduce "yourself." You must make real your ideas. Make real your dreams. This is healthy reproduction.

If you are not fulfilling the purpose of your bodily systems, they will definitely rebel. But the cure is always simple. Go home. Touch earth. Create. The farther you are away from this simplicity, the more you may have to struggle to return. Just remember, Mother needs you now more than ever. And you need Mother Earth.

*Breasts* — Represent nurturing, mothering.

*Tumors in Breasts* — Frustrated desires for growth within the family or home.

*Milk Allergy* — Need to separate from being over-mothered.

*Ribs* — Represent close family structure

*Broken Ribs* — A feeling of separation from close family.

*Back* — Represents one's support system.

*Upper Back* — Relates to holding on/letting go of others.

*Lower Back* — Relates to balance in giving and receiving male and female powers.

*"Get Off My Back"* — A feeling of having to take care of someone else more than you feel you should.

*Stomach* — Distribution center of food and thought. Symbolizes home.

*Stomach Ache* — Need to feel loved or need to feel your service is appreciated.

*Stomach Problems* — Incapacity to assimilate ideas; fear of new ideas.

*Ulcers* — Need to feel babied, eat soft foods of babyhood. Anxiety; something eating away at you.

*Colitis* — Guilt, oppression, defeat. Needs affection.

*Vomiting* — Wanting to return to the state immediately preceding something that just happened.

*Overeating* — Not sure of tomorrow's supply.

*Overweight* — Padding from the world.

*Sensitive Stomach* — Too open to seeing negativity in the world or in people.

*Appendicitis* — Fear of life. Blocking the flow. Afraid to go ahead into that which you intuitively feel you must.

*Gas Pains* — Undigested ideas. Gripping an experience that should be passing.

414

*Indigestion* — Dread, anxiety.

*Gall or Kidney Stones* — Feelings of irritation. Collecting stones to "hit back." Hard thoughts you cannot seem to dismiss.

*Bladder Ailments* — Anxiety, holding on to old ideas.

*Kidney Ailments* — Hoarding. Criticism, disappointment, frustration.

*Mononucleosis* — Feeling pressure by those in authority.

*Bedwetting* — Fear of father or authority figure.

*Hepatitis* — Fear, anger, hatred.

*Liver Problems* — Depression, repression, chronic complaining, anger.

*Hernia* — Strain, mental load. Self-punishment. Anger. Incorrect creative expression.

*Pancreas Ailments* — Holding on to regret.

*Hip Problems* — Fear of going forward in major decisions. Unable to reproduce. Not acknowledging life's power. Out of touch with earth.

*Constipation* — Desire to slow up or stop a condition or experience in your outer world or to hold on to people or property or money. Holding on to hurts.

*Diarrhea* — Wish to get something over with, especially duties, obligations, or a visit you don't expect to be pleasant.

*Hemorrhoids* — Burden, pressure, tension; afraid to let go.

*Menstrual Cramps* — Tension, gripping, holding on.

*Menopause Problems* — Self rejection. Fear of aging. Fear of no longer being wanted.

*Impotence* — Sexual pressure, guilt. Spite against a previous mate.

*Prostrate Problems* — Giving up. Defeatism. Sexual pressure and guilt. Belief in aging.

*Vaginitis* — Feeling of loss of something or someone loved. Sexual guilt.

*Venereal Disease* — Belief that genitals are sinful and dirty. Need for punishment to overcome guilt.

415

## *Let us affirm in ourselves:*

*I am nurturing.*
*I live in harmony with the universal male and female forces.*
*I accept the love my close family offers.*
*I have a strong system of support.*
*I digest and assimilate all experiences, creating health,*
*    wealth, and success within a balanced life.*
*I am at ease with my world.*
*My home expresses me and nurtures me.*
*There is always plenty of everything I need.*
*I am secure in each moment.*
*I flow gently toward a better and better life.*
*I let go of all that interferes with my good and move*
*    enthusiastically into my emerging well-being.*
*I joyfully fulfill my earthly work.*
*I forgive the past and give myself to the present.*
*The food I provide for my body is assimilated efficiently*
*    and completely, releasing into my system all of the*
*    nutrients and energy I need.*
*I resolve all difficulties easily and quickly, bringing love*
*    through myself to others.*
*I am creative.*
*I am attractive.*
*I am radiant.*
*I am loved.*
*And from this point of perfect power, I give my total self*
*    to life.*

This article is the third in a series of Mental Equivalents for bodily ailments. The Affirmations, when said each day, begin to subtly realign the body with its perfect image, restoring harmony.

Reprinted by permission of Carol Bridges from *Earth Nation Sunrise*, published by Church of the Earth Nation, RR3, Box 507, Nashville, In. 47448.

416

*Consider the consequences of your name and please give your child a name carefully — read this interview.*

# On the Path

by Earl Nickel

*The people who offer their services through "Common Ground" tell the story of how they got into their work and what changes have come to them along the way.*

One day while searching for meaning in my life, I came upon the study of astrology. As soon as I was told the "basics" of my chart, the Leo in me was hooked. I had to know more. The flame ignited (Leo is a fire sign), I leapt into the study full force. As my understanding and appreciation deepened with research and application, I found that beyond the curiosity of my own chart, I was profoundly interested in the psychological underpinnings of people. I began to appreciate the intricate complexity of each individual as well as the relationships that bind people together.

I continued my metaphysical and spiritual explorations, touching upon such areas as Tarot, Numerology, Palmistry, Tai Chi, Meditation, Sufism. During this period I happened to read a "children's" fantasy series called The Earthsea Trilogy by Ursula LeGuin. I was spellbound by this story about a willful young boy who sails across the seas to a school of magic to become a wizard. One part of the book that grabbed my attention was the idea of a "true speech" which contained the inner true names of each thing in the world. Once one knew the true name of a person or thing, s/he had power over it.

Strangely enough, the next year, out of the blue I was drawn to attend a school of esoteric learning. It was in England, so I had to "sail" across the sea; it was a school that focused on the mysteries (magic) of creation; the main building, including the inner court, could have come right out of the book. Coming to the Bay Area afterwards, I began getting involved with things here. One day last November a psychic healer friend of mine who works with sounds asked

417

me "Can you pick out a person's unique sound from the astrology chart?" I was intrigued. We talked. After she left, my thoughts crystallized around the concept of our names being the focus of our identity and how we express our uniqueness. I immediately flashed to the Earthsea Trilogy. A person's individuality is their "signature," their true name. This name operates on many levels; for example, each name has a particular sound quality and internal phonetic structure. Earl is soft, gentle and connotes to me the openness of a bluish sky at dusk. Nickel is more solid (the *ck* is hard), is two syllables and feels earthier. As an astrological correlation, I am an air sign rising which corresponds to the name Earl (first name is personal as is the rising sign). My sun sign is Capricorn, earth, which matches well with my earthier last name. Each name also has a visual/symbolic association and this is reflected in recurring dream symbols, favorite pictures and, for some, in a produced logo (as I use in my astrological ads). The letters themselves have meaning (the Sufis have a well developed science on this), as does the whole spelling in a numerological sense. For example, I have a lot of 9's in my numerological name chart which shows my need to develop a universal perspective and to learn how to see things through to completion (arrghh!). How we sign our names as well as the colors we choose all tell us more about the patterns of our uniqueness. It is said that others are a mirror to us but sometimes their names can be a pointer also. From 1973-77, I was intimately involved with 6 women who were *all* named Susan and who were, incredibly, all Cancers! Alright, I'm listening.

Many sophisticated ancient cultures had a well developed science of Naming and I believe that the main reason that there is the disharmony in the world today is that we have lost our true names. Hence, the project — and hopefully a book to come from it.

Reprinted with permission from *Common Ground Directory,* 2418 Clement St., San Francisco, CA 94121.

*"On the spiritual path, one always falls forward."*
— *Irine Nadel*

418

# A Long-Overdue Attack on Natural Childbirth

*by Dave Barry*

Let's just take a quick look at the history of baby-having. For thousands of years, only women had babies. Primitive women would go off into primitive huts and groan and wail and sweat while other women hovered around. The primitive men stayed outside doing manly things, such as lifting heavy objects and spitting.

When the baby was born, the women would clean it up as best they could and show it to the men, who would spit appreciatively and head off to the forest to throw sharp sticks at small animals. If you had suggested to primitive men that they should actually watch women have babies, they would have laughed at you and probably tortured you for three or four days. They were real men.

At the beginning of the 20th Century, women started having babies in hospital rooms. Often males were present, but they were professional doctors who were paid large sums of money and wore masks. Normal civilian males continued to stay out of the baby-having area; they remained in waiting rooms reading old copies of Field and Stream, an activity that is less manly than lifting heavy objects but still reasonably manly.

What I'm getting at is that, for most of history, baby-having was mainly in the hands (so to speak) of women. Many fine people were born under this system. Charles Lindbergh, for example.

Things changed, though, in the 1970s. The birth rate dropped sharply. Women started going to college and driving bulldozers and carrying briefcases and freely using such words as "debenture." They just didn't have time to have

419

babies. For a while there, the only people having babies were unwed teenage girls, who are very fertile and can get pregnant merely by standing downwind from teenage boys.

Then, young professional couples began to realize their lives were missing something: a sense of stability, of companionship, of responsibility for another life. So they got Labrador retrievers. A little later, they started having babies again, mainly because of the tax advantages. These days you can't open your car door without hitting a pregnant woman. But there's a catch: *Women now expect men to watch them have babies.* This is called "natural childbirth," which is one of those terms that sounds terrific but that nobody really understands. Another one is "pH balanced."

At first, natural childbirth was popular only with hippie-type, granola-oriented couples who lived in geodesic domes and named their babies things like Peace Love World Understanding Harrington-Schwartz. The males, their brains badly corroded by drugs and organic food, wrote smarmy articles about what a Meaningful Experience it is to see a New Life Come Into the World. None of these articles mentioned the various other fluids and solids that come into the world with the New Life, so people got the impression that watching somebody having a baby was just a peck of meaningful fun. At cocktail parties, you'd run into natural-childbirth converts who would drone on for hours, giving you a contraction-by-contraction account of what went on in the delivery room. They were worse than Moonies, or people who tell you how much they bought their houses for in 1973 and how much they're worth today.

Before long, natural childbirth was everywhere, like salad bars; and now, perfectly innocent civilian males all over the country are required by federal law to watch females have babies. I recently had to watch my wife have a baby.

First, we had to go to 10 evening childbirth classes at the hospital. Before the classes, the hospital told us, mysteriously, to bring two pillows. This was the first humiliation, because no two of our pillowcases match and many have beer or

420

cranberry-juice stains. It may be possible to walk down the streets of Kuala Lumpur with stained, unmatched pillowcases and still feel dignified, but this is not possible in American hospitals.

Anyway, we showed up for the first class, along with about 15 other couples consisting of women who were going to have babies and men who were going to have to watch them. They all had matching pillowcases. In fact, some couples had obviously purchased tasteful pillowcases especially for childbirth class; these were the trendy couples, wearing golf and tennis apparel, who were planning to have wealthy babies. They sat together through all the classes, and eventually agreed to get together for brunch.

The classes consisted of sitting in a brightly lit room and openly discussing, among other things, the uterus. Now I can remember a time, in high school, when I would have *killed* for reliable information on the uterus. But having discussed it at length, having seen actual full-color *diagrams*, I must say in all honesty that although I respect it a great deal as an organ, it has lost much of its charm.

Our instructor was very big on the uterus because that's where babies generally spend their time before birth. She also spent some time on the ovum, which is near the ovaries. What happens is the ovum hangs around reading novels and eating chocolates until along comes this big crowd of spermatozoa, which are tiny, very stupid one-celled organisms. They're looking for the ovum, but most of them wouldn't know if they fell over it. They swim around for days, trying to mate with the pancreas and whatever other organs they bump into. But eventually one stumbles into the ovum, and the happy couple parades down the Fallopian tubes to the uterus.

In the uterus, the Miracle of Life begins, unless you believe the Miracle of Life does not begin there, and if you think I'm going to get into that, you're crazy. Anyway, the ovum starts growing rapidly and dividing into lots of little specialized parts, not unlike the federal government. Within six weeks, it has developed all the organs it needs to drool; by 10 weeks, it

421

has the ability to cry in restaurants. In childbirth class, they showed us actual pictures of a fetus developing inside a uterus. They didn't tell us how these pictures were taken, but I suspect it involved a great deal of drinking.

We saw lots of pictures. One evening, we saw a movie of a woman we didn't even know having a baby. I am serious. Some woman actually let moviemakers film the whole thing. In color. She was from California. Another time, the instructor announced, in the tone of voice you might use to tell people they had just won free trips to Hawaii, that we were going to see color slides of a Caesarean section. The first slides showed a pregnant woman cheerfully entering the hospital. The last slides showed her cheerfully holding a baby. The middle slides showed how they got the baby out of the cheerful woman, but I can't give you a lot of detail here because I had to go out for 15 or 20 drinks of water. I do remember that at one point our instructor cheerfully observed that there was "surprisingly little blood, really." She evidently felt this was a real selling point.

When we weren't looking at pictures or discussing the uterus, we practiced breathing. This is where the pillows came in. What happens is that when the baby gets ready to leave the uterus, the woman goes through a series of what the medical community laughingly refers to as "contractions." If it referred to them as "horrible pains that make you wonder why the hell you ever decided to get pregnant," people might stop having babies and the medical community would have to go into the major-appliance business.

In the old days, under President Eisenhower, doctors avoided the contraction problem by giving lots of drugs to women who were having babies. They'd knock them out during the delivery, and the women would wake up when their kids were entering fourth grade. But the idea with natural childbirth is to try to avoid giving the woman a lot of drugs, so she can share the first, intimate moments after birth with the baby and father and the obstetrician and the pediatrician and the standby anesthesiologist and several nurses and the

422

person who cleans the delivery room.

The key to avoiding drugs, according to the natural-childbirth people, is for the woman to breathe deeply. Really. The theory is that if she breathes deeply, she'll get all relaxed and won't notice that she's in a hospital delivery room wearing a truly perverted garment and having a baby. I'm not sure who came up with this theory. Whoever it was evidently believed that women have very small brains. So, in childbirth classes, we spent a lot of time sprawled on these little mats with our pillows while the women pretended to have contractions and the men squatted around with stopwatches and pretended to time them. The trendy couples didn't care for this part. They were not into squatting. After a couple of classes, they started bringing little backgammon sets and playing backgammon when they were supposed to be practicing breathing. I imagine they had a rough time in actual childbirth, unless they got the servants to have contractions for them.

Anyway, my wife and I traipsed along for months, breathing and timing, respectively. We were a terrific team. We had a swell time. Really.

The actual delivery was slightly more difficult. I don't want to name names, but I held up *my* end. I had my stopwatch in good working order and I told my wife to breathe. "Don't forget to breathe," I'd say, or, "you should breathe, you know." She, on the other hand, was unusually cranky. For example, she didn't want me to use my stopwatch. Can you imagine? All that practice, all that squatting on the natural-childbirth classroom floor, and she suddenly gets into this big snit about stopwatches. Also, she almost completely lost her sense of humor. At one point, I made an especialy amusing remark, and she tried to hit me. She usually has an excellent sense of humor.

Nonetheless, the baby came out all right, or at least all right for newborn babies, which is actually pretty awful unless you're a fan of slime. I thought I had held up well when the

423

doctor, who up to then had behaved like a perfectly rational person, said, "Would you like to see the placenta?" Now let's face it: That is like asking, "Would you like me to pour hot tar into your nostrils?" *Nobody* would *like* to see a placenta. If anything, it would be a form of punishment:

**Jury:** We find the defendant guilty of stealing from the old and crippled.

**Judge:** I sentence the defendant to look at three placentas.

But without waiting for an answer, the doctor held up the placenta, not unlike the way you might hold up a bowling trophy. I bet he wouldn't have tried that with people who have matching pillowcases.

The placenta aside, everything worked out fine. We ended up with an extremely healthy, organic, natural baby, who immediately demanded to be put back into the uterus.

All in all, I'd say it's not a bad way to reproduce, although I understand that some members of the flatworm family simply divide into two.

This article is reprinted with permission of Feature Associates. It originally appeared in the *Philadelphia Inquirer* and later under a different title in the *Miami Herald Sunday* magazine "Tropic," July 19, 1981.

# A Meditation
# on
# Being Useless

*by Leslie Todd Pitre*

I am lying on my back in bed. My husband is cleaning the bathroom, my mother-in-law is putting our baby to bed, and my father-in-law is cooking supper. Because I am recovering from surgery, I am not allowed to help anyone do anything. But I am a doer, and I feel useless.

Five days ago, my emergency surgery elicited an astounding outpouring of love from family, friends, and acquaintances. Blood was donated readily; people offered to take over my classes and to take care of our baby. My gratitude was swift and deep — but already I find my ego is agitating me. I am a burden.

Obviously, there has to be a lesson somewhere in this — one I had not mastered last year when I was forced to spend a total of four months in bed during a high-risk pregnancy.

> God, what is thy will for me?
> *Why are you so quick to turn down these love offerings, child?*
> Because they shame me, God.
> *Why are you ashamed?*
> Well, because it's better to give than to receive, and I'm only receiving.
> *No, to give and to receive are one and the same.*
> What am I giving?

As I ruminate on this, a vision of my beloved friend Peace Pilgrim comes to mind. Peace walked all over the country for 28 years, speaking of our need to achieve outer world peace by cultivating inner peace. She owned nothing but the clothes she wore and had no home and no family. Or rather, everywhere was her home, and everyone was her family.

If anyone was ever "useless" in worldly terms, it was she. But Peace was, in my estimation, a saint, for she offered grace to everyone who met her: she offered them the chance to see the Christ in her and therefore in themselves. Anyone who offered her food or shelter was richly blessed because they had recognized this stranger as a sister. Peace Pilgrim's earthly function, I realized, was to receive graciously.

> So, God, to receive graciously is to give. Then I would not deny anyone the gift of giving to me. But why do I feel ashamed?
> *Can a child of God be unworthy?*

425

Never, God. I guess I'm guilty of pride — of trying to be "independent"; I've tried to separate myself from my sisters and brothers. And if I judge myself as unworthy, surely I cannot see them truly, either.

Memories flooded my mind of instances when my husband and I had given help to people in need, telling them not to "repay" us, but to "pass it on" to someone else when the opportunity arose. I had understood that to give truly one must not desire to "even up" the relationship with the giver.

Then I recalled the conversation I'd had last night with a new but already cherished friend who asked what practical help he could provide — money? child chare?

I had hastened to refuse his further aid: "You've already given your very blood! Besides, ever since we've met, I've always been on the receiving end of this relationship. The scales are already too unbalanced!" I protested.

"Ah," he sighed sadly. "So you are only measuring tangibles. . ."

My friend had lovingly reminded me of what my threatened ego wouldn't allow me to remember: my gifts to him were not quantifiable but were nonetheless real and precious.

I have intrinsic worth, God, because I am your child. If for two weeks I am to receive aid from others, I am doubly blessed: because my needs are being provided for by divine order, and because I am offering these dear ones a chance to bless themselves by blessing me.

And so I offer these words of thanks:

O Creator, in my weakness lies my strength. As you help me give up my illusion of self-sufficiency, I will learn to relax in the waiting arms of Love. As my body heals, you will help me heal my mind, to recognize my atonement. God, thank you for keeping me still long enough to understand what is to be "useless."

Leslie Todd Pitre is an instructor of English at Louisiana State University, Baton Rouge. A member of Columbia (S.C.) Meeting, she is working to reestablish the currently inactive meeting in Baton Rouge.

Reprinted by permission of the *Friends Journal*, Volume 23, Number 20, © 1977.

426

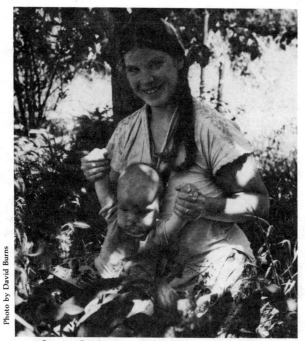

Photo by David Burns

*Lorin Graham and Jediah (see page 127)*

"You must teach your children that the ground beneath their feet is the ashes of our grandfathers. So that they will respect the land, tell your children that the earth is rich with the lives of our kin. Teach your children what we have taught our children — that the earth is our mother. Whatever befalls the earth befalls the sons of the earth. If men spit upon the ground, they spit upon themselves.

"This we know. The earth does not belong to man: man belongs to the earth. This we know. All things are connected like the blood which unites one family. All things are connected.

"Whatever befalls the earth befalls the sons of the earth. Man did not weave the web of life; he is merely a strand in it. Whatever he does to the web, he does to himself."

— Chief Seattle

427

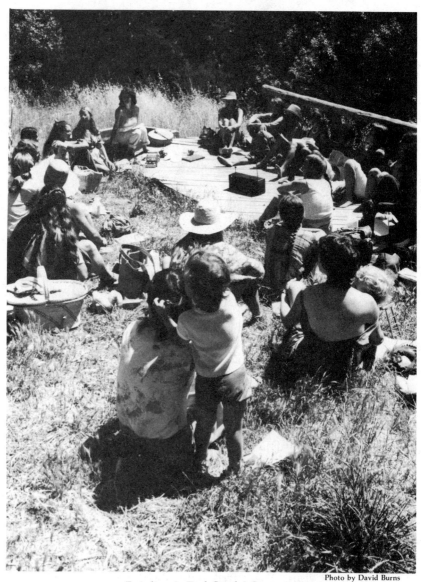

Photo by David Burns

*Rainbow's End Study Group*

428

# PART VI

# Taking Care of the Baby, Husband and Yourself

# *Caring for Your Baby*

I just finished reading a book which puts into words many of my beliefs and observations. Since many of you are seeking help with a natural birth I am hoping you will all become "natural" parents as well! The following are some quotes from the *Continuum Concept* by Jean Liedloff which summarize her message.

"A very widely held view is that giving a baby or child too much attention will prevent him from becoming independent and that carrying him about full time will weaken his self-reliance. We have already seen that self-reliance itself comes from a completed in-arms phase, but it is one in which the infant is always present, but rarely the center of attention. He is simply there, in the midst of his caretaker's life, constantly experiencing things, safely being held. When he leaves his mother's knee and begins to crawl, creep, and walk about in the world beyond her body, he does so without interference ("protection"). His mother's role then is to be available when he comes to or calls for her. It is not for her to direct his activities, nor to protect him from dangers from which he would be fully capable of protecting himself if given the chance. This is perhaps the most difficult part of switching to continuum ways. Each mother will have to trust her baby's capability for self-preservation as far as she is able. Few could manage to allow the free playing with sharp knives and fire and the freedom of waterslides that the Yequana do without a thought, knowing the enormous self-protective talents of babies as they do; but the less the civilized mother takes over responsibility for her baby's safety, the sooner and better he will become independent. He will know when he needs help or comfort. He should never be kept from his mother, but she ought to offer the absolute minimum of guidance to him. . . ."

"Once a mother realizes that seeing that her baby is carried about for the first six or eight months will insure his self-reliance and lay the foundations for his becoming social, undemanding, and positively helpful for the next fifteen or twenty years he will be at home, even her self-interest will tell her not to spare herself the "trouble" of carrying him while she is doing her housework or shopping.

I believe that the vast majority of mothers truly love their children, and deprive them of the experiences so essential to their happiness only because they have no idea what they are causing them to suffer. If they understood the agony of the baby left to weep in his crib, his terrible longing and the consequences of the suffering, the effects of the deprivation upon his personality development and potential for making a satisfactory life, I do not doubt that they would fight to prevent his being left alone for a minute." (pp. 160-161)

"It would help immeasurably if we could see baby care as a nonactivity. We should learn to regard it as nothing to do. Working, shopping, cooking, cleaning, walking and talking with friends are things to do, to make time for, to think of as activities. The baby (with other children) is simply brought along as a matter of course; no special time need be set aside for him, apart from the minutes devoted to changing diapers. His bath can be part of his mother's. Breastfeeding need not stop all other activity either. It is only a matter of changing one's baby-centered thought patterns to those more suitable for a capable, intelligent being whose nature it is to enjoy work and the companionship of other adults." (The authoress is talking about an older infant and after you've recovered from childbirth. The first two to three months are best spent as quietly as possible.) p. 163, Jean Liedloff, *The Continuum Concept*, Alfred A Kopf, Inc., 1977.

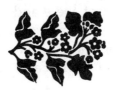

# Childbearing

*by Michael Tierra, N.D.*

The physical and emotional health of a child depends in large part upon the condition of its parents before conception. Not only the diet and lifestyle, but the thoughts and emotions of the mother and father immediately before and during conception have a permanent effect upon the resultant progeny.

If we think thoughts of peace, love and bliss, which should be associated with the act of love, this will give rise to peaceful, loving and blissful children. If, on the other hand, our thoughts are negatively based on lust, violence and power, this will produce children who are prone to violence, disrespect of others and a damaging competitive attitude.

Since the physical constitution of an individual can be no better than the physical constitution of its parents, a separate branch of therapy was denoted in ancient China and in East Indian ayurvedic medicine in preparing the parents for child conception. Herbal tonics classified as aphrodisiacs were primarily used to strengthen the reproductive power of both the man and woman. Thus, a balanced, healthy sex life was based upon inspiration, rather than a superficial need to satisfy a sexual "itch." Regularity and moderation in rest, diet and exercise will make the body strong, and that strength will automatically be imparted to the coming progeny. Meditation is also very beneficial, as it will help normalize the nervous system and therefore regulate the hormonal secretions.

Failure to conceive can be due to the condition of either the man or the woman. If men have an insufficient sperm count or weakness, herbs such as ginseng, sarsaparilla, don Quai, lycii berries, and Shou Wu can be very helpful to restore sexual potency. Special medicines are sold in Chinese herb stores made of a combination of these and other herbs along with powdered extracts of the sexual organs of various animals, including those of the dog and deer. Women can use herbs such as False Unicorn root (aletris Farinosa), Sarsaparilla, Don

432

Quai (Angelica Polymorpha), Rehmania Glutinosa and Comfrey Root. Extract of human placenta is one of the most effective female fertility treatments. A Chinese patented medicine that is very beneficial is called Unborn Fawn pills. Ayurvedic medicine uses a combination of gold and mercury, which has been detoxified through a very elaborate method of preparation. The special "pitch" of certain kinds of Himalayan granite rocks is also a good treatment (Shilajit) for infertility.

## Diet

The very purest and most wholesome diet possible should be adhered to before, during and after pregnancy. It should consist of whole grains as a primary food, supplemented with steamed vegetables, seasonal fruits and very little meat or dairy products. During pregnancy, the energy of a woman goes through a radical change which may create an increased desire for sour and sweet foods. It is appropriate for a woman to eat a little more fruit to help satisfy those desires. However, the primary food should still be whole grains and cooked vegetables.

Pressed salad is a good yin food for the pregnant mother (and for everyone else as well). It will not have any of the disadvantages of being totally raw and therefore difficult to assimilate (which can lower one's physical immunity), and yet it will have the much appreciated cool qualities of a raw salad.

Directions: Finely chop greens and wrap in a layer of cheesecloth. Dip the cheesecloth with the greens into a pot of boiling salted water for 10 or 15 seconds. Remove from the water and set in a bowl with a weight over it for one to two hours. This will help extract some of the water and aid in breaking down the hard cellulose which surrounds the various nutrients found in vegetable greens. A dressing such as lemon and olive oil, or a sauce of miso, tahini, lemon juice and water is delicious with this salad. If one eats a wholesome balanced diet, one should experience a sense of satisfaction which will be reflected in all areas of one's life. This is the ideal mood which the expectant mother should strive for and maintain. On the other hand, an unbalanced diet will create anxiety and dissatisfaction, which definitely are not good attitudes for a mother to experience during pregnancy. Therefore, a balanced diet is essential to the health and future personality of the child.

# Morning Sickness

The period of transition to a more yang condition by a mother during the early stages of pregnancy is often accompanied by feelings of nausea and distress, commonly known as morning sickness. This is actually a detoxification of the body which prepares the mother for growing a healthy fetus and a healthy labor. Some natural remedies which have been found to be effective for this condition include a combination of 1/8 tsp. of golden seal, 1/8 tsp. of powdered rhubarb root, and 1/4 tsp. of powdered cloves taken with a cup of raspberry and spearmint leaf tea twice a day. Other excellent remedies are umeboshi plum extract, false unicorn root, raspberry leaf tea and homeopathic nux vomica 6X. A tea of raspberry leaf and oat straw is good to take throughout pregnancy to help maintain the blood, facilitate delivery during labor, and prevent hemorrhage after the birth.

The best food for the newborn infant up to the time it cuts its first eye teeth is mother's milk. This places the responsibility of nutrition of the growing infant on the mother's diet. Any problems an infant might have in the form of disease or imbalance are either due to fate (karma) or the mother's diet. Whatever the symptoms the child may have, the herbs should be taken by the mother and the proper dosage will be transmitted through her milk. Recently a mother noticed some small red spots on her newborn son's face. She was eating a fairly balanced diet, except she was in the habit of drinking too much mint tea. Oftentimes the volatile oils of peppermint or spearmint will be excreted through the pores of the skin, which, in this case, was on the baby's face. After stopping the mint for a few days, all the red spots disappeared. This demonstrates how directly the herbs and foods are taken into the milk of the mother and passed on to the child.

One mother wrote and asked whether her child should be immunized. I and many other naturopaths are of the opinion that children who are raised in New Age families with a good wholesome diet are best not subjected to immunizations, whose effects are often stored in the body at a very deep cellular level. Immunizations can have negative effects later in the child's development and furthermore, much of the evidence of the effectiveness of immunizations is highly controversial, anyway. (If the reader is interested in learning more about the questionable effects of immunizations I would direct them to read *The Poison Needle* and/or *Confessions of a Medical Heretic* by Robert Mendelsohn.) I wrote back that if the child eats a healthy, wholesome diet it need never worry about contracting any of the diseases for which it is being immunized. And if the child did become diseased, it would be a mild occurrence at most, best treated naturally with whole foods, herbs and naturopathic treatments such as homeopathy and acupuncture, for instance.

I have found that for most of the common childhood illnesses, such as colic, fever, colds and flu, teas of lemon balm and calendula flowers are most effective. Lemon balm is one of the best anti-fever teas, not only because of its tremendous effectiveness as a sweating herb, but also because it has a pleasant taste and is soothing to the nerves. Calendula can be applied externally as a salve to minor cuts and burns or taken internally for various eruptive diseases which young children are prone to get.

In conclusion, I feel that we are in a time when many people, including parents and their children, are making a radical change in their lifestyle. This change, for most of us, puts us into a new way of thinking with a lot of habits, fears and approaches suggestive of the culture from which we are departing. The old culture is based upon fear, alienation, and lack of trust, and its foods and customs have degenerated into the use of T.V. dinners, McDonald's hamburgers, fast foods, with a diminishing sense of nurturing family. Its medicines reflect this degenerate lifestyle, including aspirin, high potency antibiotics, and immunizations. The new Aquarian age culture is centered around the ideals of trust, sharing wholesome foods, and a lively interest in practical ways to achieve and maintain health. Mild foods and herbs are the best medicines for the Aquarian age and there is no need to resort to the use of debilitating, harmful, strong drugs. We must all dedicate ourselves to inspiring each other with the fundamental truth of Holistic Health; that the body heals itself.

Michael Tierra, N.D. is a natural healer and expert on herbs. He is the author of *The Way of Herbs*, a teacher at Heartwood, and in private practice. He has also created the **East West Master Course in Herbology**, 3254B Mission Drive, Santa Cruz, CA.

# *Fathering and Career: A Healthy Balance*

## *by David Stewart*

*The following is excerpted from a pamphlet written by David Stewart of NAPSAC (International Association of Parents and Professionals for Safe Alternatives in Childbirth). Reprinted by kind permission of the author. Although this article is about fathers and careers, we think that it applies equally well to mothers and their careers.*

Few people do anything in their entire lives more far-reaching than raising their families. It is a rare professional accomplishment to be so significant as to make any great difference fifty years later, but the way you raise your children

436

will make a difference fifty, and even one hundred years hence.

Although you may not realize it, the effect that you have on a society today is influenced for good or ill by the things that your great-grandparents did a century ago. A well-raised child is a happy child. Happy people make others happy and make good parents themselves. The product of good parenting is a well-adjusted adult who can get down to the business of producing without having to spend his/her energies on a treadmill overcoming difficulties created in childhood. Generation after generation benefits. The results of the secure family go on and on like an atomic chain reaction.

But so also do the results of a neglected family. The root of most social problems — crime, violence, drug abuse, prostitution, neurosis, divorce, delinquency, and general unhappiness — may very well be poor family life. Deficiencies at home are manifested as deficiencies in society. Considering the amount of misery that can be brought into the world by a parent who puts career before family to the extent of breaking the home, one wonders if the good wrought by the professional achievement can be enough to offset the harm done. But the greatest loser is the father himself, who, driven by career to forsake his rightful family role, may finally realize in his old age that he has sold his birthright of parental fulfillment for recognition and "success." Then it is too late. Old folks' homes are full of such people — filled with regret, their opportunity to parent irrevocably lost.

This can wait, but the growth of your child does not wait. To enjoy a two-year-old, you must do it when he or she is two.

Family freindships afford one of the greatest sources of happiness on earth. Acquaintances come and acquaintances go. We have our business friends, our fellow-worker friends and our neighborhood friends, but among the only friends we can truly count on are those in our families. Children relate to you as you, not as career-successful, moneymaker, publicly famous, or whatever. Your children may feel proud of your

437

accomplishments, they may even brag about them, but what they care about most is simply that you are their daddy and care about them.

You must be willing to give up the desire to work at other peoples' pace. By their extra effort, they will receive extra rewards and they deserve it. But look at what they may be giving up, too. Material efforts reap material rewards, but to reap the heartfilling rewards of parenthood, your efforts must be there. It is much more difficult to achieve that goal than to throw oneself single-mindedly into one's work.

Making career and parenting compatible boils down to this: first, you must determine (and this is a completely personal choice) the minimum level of achievement in your job that you can accept and still maintain your self-respect. Then after you have decided what you can accept, then you see if this minimum level still leaves enough time for your family. Now, realistically, for some people that won't be possible. Their acceptable achievement level may be so high that they will have to spend weekends and evenings working to attain it. Ambitious young people should seriously consider a single life before committing themselves to family responsibility which they may later regret, and perhaps, even abandon.

On the other hand, you can choose a minimum level of acceptable achievement that does leave adequate free time for your home. By investing your spare time in your family, you can be happy both in your career and in your home life. Although you may not achieve the outstanding professional status of those who can dedicate a larger portion of their time to their work, you are still to be counted as a success, because success is measured by setting a goal and achieving it.

Although you may sometimes feel that society or other people set the goals which you should achieve, this is not so. You alone set your goals. You may be influenced by society and your friends if you choose to be influenced. But it is your free choice to do so or not. If you want to be a good parent, you cannot let society be a dominant influence on your goals. You and your family must be the dominant influence.

438

Put in your time at work as productively as possible and when the time is up, quit and go home. By applying your energies wisely and efficiently, you may find it possible to excel in your career and have time at home, too. The secret of career success lies not in long hours, but in properly ordering priorities and always attending to the top ones first.

I only do so much and no more. I do not compare myself with others. They have set their goals and I have set mine. While much of my mind, time and energy goes into my work, beneath it all my heart rests at home.

Happy are they who can achieve and maintain such a balance. They will have achieved the ultimate worldly accomplishment whose true reward is itself. Careers are fickle, but parenthood is forever.

# 10 Tips for Happier Fathering

## 1. RESPECT YOUR CHILDREN AS EQUALS.

It is easy in our culture to think of children as something less than adults, but souls are equal and without age. It is to your advantage as a parent to begin thinking of this equality at your baby's birth. Treat your children with respect when they are young and they will treat you with respect when you are old. Generation gaps may manifest themselves during adolescence, but they begin at birth.

## 2. BE AT HOME AS MUCH AS POSSIBLE.

Ninety percent of being a good father is being at home. All problems between people can be resolved by rapport. But rapport cannot be developed in absence. The greatest obstacle to good fathering is absence, and absence has only one cure — presence.

## 3. TUNE IN WITH YOUR FAMILY.

It is not enough to be home in body. You must also be present in mind and spirit. The absence of your genuine attention when at home can adversely affect your children almost the same way as the absence of you physically. If at home your mind is full of work worries or you feel compelled by duty to spend time at home, your family will sense that and they won't like it. To be a good father, your time at home must never be considered a burden or a sacrifice. You must choose it because you enjoy it. So concentrate on your family when you're home. You cannot enjoy that upon which you have not placed your attention.

## 4. FONDLE YOUR CHILDREN A LOT.

Learning to be a good father is learning to enjoy it. And one of the sweetest pleasures of parenthood is to love and fondle one's children. Everyone benefits. Children and babies feel more secure and such tactile skin sensations can even stimulate brain development in infants. An evening of television can be relaxing, but it usually leaves one empty. Taking pleasure in your children leaves you full.

## 5. DON'T PRETEND TO KNOW IT ALL.

If you want your words to be respected, they must always be respectable. If you want your children to believe you when they are teenagers, you must be honest with them when they are young. Without credibility, there can be no communication. So maintain credibility with your children at all costs. This means never extending your statements beyond your knowledge. It means readily admitting, "I don't know." Some people think that to admit ignorance is to destroy confidence. But nothing destroys confidence more quickly than a pretense exposed.

## 6. DON'T BE AFRAID TO SHOW SHORTCOMINGS.

Your children see your strengths and your weaknesses and accept you with both. So you might as well be open and

440

honest about your shortcomings. They probably know already and they don't care. To pretend otherwise is to paralyze your own progress and to confuse your own children who see one thing with their eyes and hear another from your mouth. Parents are the yardstick by which children measure the world. In order that the yardstick be a true measure, it is not necessary that it be perfect. It is only necessary that it be accurately represented to the child for whatever it is — perfect or not.

## 7. DON'T BE OVERLY CONCERNED ABOUT CONSISTENCY.

Sometimes parents hesitate to change before their children even when the change would be for the better. They are afraid to appear inconsistent. They fear that if they give in their child will no longer respect them. But what's wrong with giving in to a better way? You expect such changes from your children. By showing flexibility in your own example, you are helping your children to be flexible too. Nobody is perfect. To remain consistent throughout life is to make no progress. It would be simple if raising children were possible by a rigid set of rules by which parents needn't deviate. But inconsistency and unpredictability are intrinsic to human nature. Be consistent in your ideals such as truthfulness, kindness, and respect. But do not be afraid to be inconsistent with your family, if by such inconsistency you are progressing in your parenthood. Consistency properly applies to principles, not to particulars.

## 8. DON'T INSIST ON AN IMMACULATE HOUSE.

Show me a home sprinkled with the objects of child's play, and I'll show you a home scattered with the evidence of happiness. To have a neat room and house all the time is not a natural state of affairs for children. They have more important things to do. A house is to live in, not to look at. The less time spent on housecleaning, the more time you can spend with your spouse and the children. To demand a neat house of a mother with children, is to demand the impossible and create a frustrated, uncooperative wife. And don't demand too much of the children either. If neatness is important to them, they will do it voluntarily. If it is a triviality in their minds, they won't respond. If you demand trivia of them, they may be exacting in their demands of you. Order is transient and all natural processes tend toward disorder. To fret over misplaced furniture or dirty dishes is to fret forever. These things you will always have. But your children are only here for a short time as children. Enjoy them now. You will have plenty of time to enjoy a neat house when they are gone.

## 9. DON'T PRETEND THAT YOU AND YOUR WIFE AGREE ON EVERYTHING

Parents are people and people are different. For people to disagree on one thing or another is a natural state of affairs. For any two people to agree on everything is to be false to themselves. Why then, should parents pretend to their children that they always agree on family matters? Don't underestimate the understanding of a child. You don't have to water down life for them. They can handle it better than many adults. They will not be upset to learn that their father has a point of view that differs from their mother's. This is not to suggest that parents should fight and bicker in front of their children. That would be harmful. Speak frankly and openly in front of your children. That is beneficial. It is not an act of disloyalty for a mother to contradict a father or vice versa, if done in mutual respect. It is an act of recognition of human individuality, as it is, and should not be hidden from children who are in the process of growing into an understanding of their own individuality and of what human nature is truly like.

## 10. LISTEN TO YOUR WIFE.

Listen to your wife. She can be your greatest potential helper in being a good father, tuning in with your children and

442

developing the feelings so essential to good fathers. Who knows the children better than their mother? Realize that feelings and maternal inclinations are pretty reliable guides to follow in caring for children, while logic and step-by-step reasoning often fall short. If you and your wife discuss each other's feelings frequently and openly, not only will the children benefit, so will you. I only know that had I not had my wife's guidance all these years, I could easily have set different priorities that would have led me to a considerably less happy and satisfied existence today. Most of what I know about fathering I have learned from my wife.

The 14-page pamphlet entitled *Fathering and Career: A Healthy Balance,* from which this was excerpted is available for $1.00 from NAPSAC International, Box 267, Marble Hill, MO 63764.

# *Feeding Your Baby*

*Notes from lectures by Bill Gray and Jim Greene, August 1976, with additions by Nan Koehler, August 1977.*

Many physicians find that Adele Davis' dietary advice doesn't work. We recommend following Paavo Airola. Read his book *Are You Confused?.* Airola has several other good books. (I'd also recommend a book from the Rodale Press called *Confessions of a Sneaky Organic Cook.*) More good information comes from Rudolf Hauschka's book *Nutrition,* published by Steward & Watkins, 45 Lower Belgrave St., London, 5W1, 1967.

First point to keep in mind is that *food isn't just food.* We don't live in an exclusively material world: everything is unbalanced if the child doesn't get love — attention.

Second point is to observe your child carefully. Everyone is different and what might keep one child healthy will make another child sick.

443

1. Good nutrition for the child starts in pregnancy and before. Major points are below.
   A. PROTEIN (60-80 grams a day)
      a. Too much; the symptoms of too much protein are sluggishness, trouble getting out of bed, headaches, rashes, and intestinal problems.
      b. Too little; toxemia can be considered a disease of poor nutrition — specifically lack of protein, fatigue and dehydration.

   B. LIQUIDS
      a. Urinate at least every 4 hours and drink 3 quarts of water a day.
      b. Vascular expansion is normal in pregnancy, slightly swollen ankles especially in first pregnancies are normal in the summer.
      c. Toxemia: kidney failure — drink water.

   C. CRAVINGS
      a. Follow cravings, but *no sugar* (need B Vitamins), *no smoking,* and *no alcohol.*

   D. VITAMINS
      a. Folic acid — 1-2 mg/day
      b. Iron — anemia is natural in pregnancy because of the increased blood volume. 70 mg/day.
      c. Vitamin E — 800 IU/day prevents stretch marks and miscarriages.
      d. Vitamin C — with Bioflavanoids — prevents tearing and trauma. 1st trimester 1000/3x's day; 2nd trimester 2000/3x's day; 3rd trimester 3000/3x's day.
      e. Vitamin A — 25,000 Units/day — helps liver detoxify poisons.
      f. Vitamin D — Sun yourself daily.
      g. Vitamin B Complex — get Super B's with at least 50 mg in each tablet. Take 2-4 a day.
      h. Calcium-Magnesium — take as Dr. Bronner's

Calcium food, or volcanic clay tablets 2,000 mg/day.

    i. Take your vitamins 2 or 3 times a day with your meals. They are a food supplement, not a medicine!

2. BREASTFEEDING

The longer you totally breastfeed your baby, the healthier your child will be. Introduce other foods (see below) when your child shows a desire to eat them—usually at 5-6 months. (When they can sit in a high-chair and grab for stuff!) The best time for weaning (unless you want to breastfeed until the child is about 3) is around 18 months when they have all the milk teeth in and their gastric juices flow better. Their main source of nutrition until three is milk; and, by then, they will be very interested in all kinds of foods, so don't worry too much about *what* you give them.

    a. Marshmallow root strengthens the milk.

      b. Holy Thistle or Blessed Thistle increases flow.

      c. Keep up the liquids, keep taking vitamins and build up your blood again from the birth with Cherry Juice, Nettle and Comfrey tea, and eat organ meats.

3. INTRODUCING FOOD

    A. The kind of food you give the baby helps shape their consciousness. For example, it's very frightening for a heavy thinker to space out too badly—give them grounding foods. You will observe them craving them anyway.

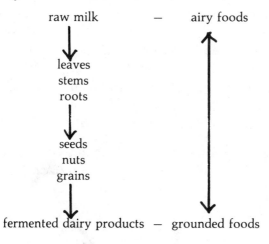

raw milk     —     airy foods

leaves
stems
roots

seeds
nuts
grains

fermented dairy products   —   grounded foods     445

B. Feed your child according to his/her growth and age.
   a. Introduce them first to: goat's milk and oat straw, blended in a 1:1 ratio; or plain goat's milk, or goat's milk with a little molasses added. Then fruits—non-citrus fruits; then goat's milk yogurt.
   b. Introduce foods slowly every 3-4 days so you observe the effect on your child.
   c. When the teeth come in, give steamed vegetables.
   d. When they can stand, introduce strong vegies like potatoes.
   e. When they can talk, give them nuts and seeds. Introduce benign grains such as millet, buckwheat, oats and rice.
   f. Avoid: wheat, citrus fruits, cow's milk, egg whites. All can be allergy-forming if introduced too early in the child's diet.
   g. Mucous formation comes from over-eating! Sugar or dairy.
   h. Keep the child away from meat, honey and/or sugar, and salt until 3-4 years old.

C. An even easier way to feed your little one is to hold them on your lap while eating and let them taste what's on your plate. They can't really *eat*, they just explore the food. It's a mess, but this introduction to food will pay off when they are older and happily eat what is set before them. If your child really wants food, then chew a morsel and feed him/her from your mouth. This mixes the food with amylase and grinds it on nature's babyfood grinder—your teeth! If the food isn't good for the baby it's not good for you either. The babies digestive track is built for milk until their 2nd year molars come in (between the 2nd and 3rd year of age), so don't worry about food until they are weaned from milk at 3-4 years of age.

4. Additional thoughts about keeping your baby healthy:
   a. Fire turns clay into porcelain, or "maturity comes

446

with experience."

b. Trust your inner program — do what feels good.

c. Health isn't just eating. Child needs sleep; Child needs to be in water alot; Child needs space to grow.

d. Don't use any synthetic clothes for your child. The skin can't breathe.

e. Use regular diapers. Synthetic, disposable diapers feed the psychosis that child-rearing is easy. *It's Not Easy! Don't think it will be!*

f. Do gardening. Give your children herbs.

g. Spagnum moss and mullein leaves in the diaper are good for diaper rash. Corn starch is good also. Remove rubber pants. Make sure all the soap is rinsed out of the diapers (4 rinses).

h. For fevers — use lemons as juice in tea and garlic oil in the ears. Keep your child warm and put down for a nap. Help them sweat it out.

i. For diarrhea — suck on lemons, eat blackberries, or drink blackberry leaf tea. Give liquid acidophilis pure culture in whey.

j. For screaming — dill tea or the seeds to chew on.

## READINGS:

Retundi — *Your Vegetarian Baby*
Juliet De Baircali Levy — *Nature's Children*
Ann Wigmore — *Healthy Children Nature's Way*
Joseph Chilton Pierce — *The Magic Child*
Arthur Janov — *The Feeling Child*
Hazrat Inayat Khan, Teachings of, Vol. 3 — *Education and Marriage*
Polly Berrien Berends — *Whole Parent, Whole Child*
Fredrick LeBoyer — *Loving Hands*
Sheila Kippley — *Breastfeeding and Natural Child-Spacing*
Shivalila (Children's Liberation Front) — *The Book of the Mother*
Jean Liedloff, *The Continuum Concept*

447

# Using Herbs with Children

## Gardening — Eating — Smelling
## Drinking — Bathing
## Rubbing — Seeing!

### by Nan Koehler

*Gardening* is first because all other uses of herbs follow from that activity. I love having herbs right at my door. Instead of ornamental flowers and shrubs—or maybe along with them—it's nice to have mint, thyme and lavender within easy reach. The hummingbirds come close to my door where I have a big pineapple sage. Along with parsley, dill and basil, my children love to plant and then help themselves to carrots (great for a teething baby), radishes and beans. My kids are very proud of the garden and love to work in it and talk about it. The lessons are numberless; life and death, patience and timing, cycles and recycling, garden pests and garden helpers, proper methods and harmful ones. I could go on and on. Having herbs as neighbors is the best way to learn about them and their uses. What better way is there to be grounded and connected with life than knowing where our food comes from and being part of that process?

*Eating* herbs right from the start brings health to the child and educates the palate to fresh, raw, strong tasting food. For those who rely on milk for the child's source of minerals, it's nice to know that herbs are just as useful. A leaf of comfrey, dock, and kale minced into a salad are a terrific source of minerals. Topped with delicious homemade mayonnaise, my children will eat anything! They like to dip their greens in salad dressing or some sort of dip. If your kids complain alot about salads or herbs in their food, a guess would be that they aren't really hungry. When we went camping this summer and

448

came upon watercress my children ate it with as much relish as we did. If your children don't like greens, it's a good idea to begin meals with the salad when their appetite is the strongest.

*Smelling* is the most primitive sense we have, and the one that influences us the most profoundly. Because that sense operates on a very unconscious level, it influences our whole being very powerfully. Besides making our food taste delicious, smells can help us feel good, help us sleep or help us rid ourselves of colds, bugs, headaches and imbalances of all sorts. I love to make sleep pillows; little herb-filled-sacks to be placed by someone sleeping. For my children I have little pillows stuffed with hops (to put them to sleep) and camomile. For my oldest, I made a pillow of rosemary when he had bad dreams. Bay, sage and mint are nice to clear the nose and sinuses. Pennyroyal (and Bay) keep fleas and mosquitoes away. To make these powerful smells delightful, add dried roses and dried orange peels. All these materials are free and easy to obtain! Another nice thing to do with sleep pillows is to collect wonderful smelling plant material while on a holiday, dry it and then stuff small pillows with it to inhale later to remind you of the time away in the woods and fields. Incense cedar from Yosemite. Sage from the desert.

*Drinking* herbal teas is the gateway to health and harmony. When any ailment or irregularity pops up, I give my children teas. For cuts, comfrey; for stomach aches, dill, peppermint or fennel; for colds I usually make the child his own tonic out of mugwort, dock, honeysuckle, mint and sage. For excess mucus, white pine bark, sow thistle or dock work very well. Whatever is handy beckens. Often chewing the leaves fresh is easier for a child than drinking a tea. For sore throat or canker sores have them chew thyme; for a fever, basil. Whenever we have tea, they always want some. Needless to say, it's definitely better than soda-pop!

*Bathing* with herbs is pleasing to everyone and nice to do as a family all together. It can be restful and cleansing, as well as therapeutic. If the child's circulation seems sluggish a very hot rosemary bath for several days in a row will make a new person appear in your life. It's especially effective with babies. Jeanne Rose has many recipes for herbal baths in her book that are wonderful. Children often drink their bathwater which makes that a virtue when you are trying to administer some herbal cure. Hot followed by cold bath water — especially saunas — are good for everyone, young and old! When my children have a fever, I take them in the sweat with us. They perspire alot, sleep alot afterwards and wake up OK.

*Rubbing* herbal oils, salves or just plain herbs on the skin is one of life's greatest pleasures. It's especially fun to rub someone else or to be rubbed. Children thrive by it. Massage oils made with comfrey, sage or mint are soothing to the muscles. Add some rosemary or lavender and your child's skin tone will perk up. Old fashioned liniments are very easy to make. One with golden seal, myrrh and cayenne pepper is very cleansing and soothing. We all know how our kids love to plaster iodine on themselves when they have a cut or scratch. Next time, try cutting an aloe leaf or crushing some sow thistle for them rub with. Another bonus is the milkweeds (and relatives, the spurges) and wild lettuces with their milky juice. When applied regularly, they will rid your child of worts.

*Seeing* flowers and greenery all around is a true delight. Children and flowers go together. The bees and children have a continual parade of flowers all year round. My three year old loves to gather small bunches of radish flowers with as much enthusiasm as the crysanthamums and calendulas. The children can easily speak with the plants and be reverent toward them. I tell them that the snap or squash a plant makes when it breaks or is tred on, is it's cry. We all belong together.

*Nature's Children*, Juliette de Bairacli Levy, Warner Paperback Library, $1.25. *Herbs and Things*, Jeanne Rose, Grosset and Dunlap, 1973, $2.95. *Healthy Children and Nature's Way*, Ann Wigmore, Hippocrates Health Inst., Boston. *The Herb Book*, John Lust, Bantam Book, 1974, $2.50.

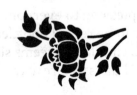

450

# Children and Herbs

*by Bhavani Worden, Metalink #8, 1979*

I wish we were talking face-to-face, so that there would be real contact and interaction. This is a subject close to my heart, and I'm sorry it's so impersonally written down. Herbs at their best are very personal and intuitive, used with a lot of feeling.

Herbs and children are basic and honest; to be successful with either, you must be relaxed and open to pure energy. Herbs do not work mechanically on the body, but rather through the spirit, through the earth as Mother. The nourishment, comfort and healing one receives from a well-chosen and prepared cup of tea is total, like a mother's feeding. Children are more open than anyone to this healing, and when used properly, herbs are especially effective with them. Children's bodies are clean, and assimilate elements readily: the minerals and healing factors in the herbs are almost instantly absorbed, and the effects soon manifested.

There are several herbs that have been found through the ages and verified by my experience to be especially useful for infants and children:

*Peppermint* is a safe and powerful stimulant, warming the body, aiding the digestion, and improving the state of mind through its high mineral content. As a stimulant, increasing circulation, it also acts to enhance the effect of other herbs combined with it.

*Raspberry* leaf is a stimulant and tonic very high in healing vitamins and minerals, including iron. It draws toxins and serves as a relaxant. Dr. Christopher recommends it specifically for a sick child who doesn't feel like eating: serve raspberry tea all day to nourish, soothe, rebalance and heal.

*Catnip* is one of the safest and most widely acclaimed remedies for babies and children. It is effective for any kind of pain, gas, cramps, spasms (e.g. hiccups), fevers, and to induce sleep.

451

*Sweet* or *lemon balm* is a mild, tasty herb useful as a general tonic as well as for digestive upsets, and trouble in any internal organ. It expels poisons, as for insect bites, dog bites, boils, etc. For this purpose, it should be taken internally as tea, as well as applied externally as a poultice (see below).

*Marshmallow* root is a demulcent, soothing and lubricating to tissues and inflammed membranes. It is invaluable for lung or throat troubles and diarrhea; it also serves as a demulcent for any mixture of herbs.

*Licorice root* is high in potassium and other minerals, soothing to throat and chest, useful for coughs and thirst, serves as a mild laxative, strengthens the muscles, and sweetens an herb mixture to make it taste good to a child.

*Ginger* is a safe and potent stimulant, promoting perspiration and good for sore throat, coughs, diarrhea, gas, nausea, and colds, especially when combined with other herbs for the specific problem.

*Honey* is not really an herb, but is too important to exclude from any discussion of treatment, particularly of children. It is absorbed into the bloodstream without digestive distraction or strain. It must be raw (not "uncooked") and organic (not "natural"). Taken by the teaspoonful, it will stop intestinal cramping, or vomiting; combined with crude safflower oil (½ teaspoon of each), it has produced a normal bowel movement within an hour from a constipated child. In addition to soothing and healing the intestines, it does the same for the kidneys and heart. Its calcium content is good for building strong bones, and its high vitamin and mineral content nourishes the entire body.

Honey can also be used externally: rubbed on gums, it has a soothing effect during teething; applied to scrapes, cuts, or other wounds, it serves as an antiseptic (preventing infection), soothes pain, and promotes rapid healing. If combined with chewed-up plantain or comfrey leaf (the saliva is part of it), honey can cause even the deepest cut to close without stitches and without scarring. (I have had remarkable experiences with each of the above uses — they are real awe-inspiring.)*

*There is some evidence pointing to a connection between a few cases of botulism in infants and raw food. So it is advised not to feed babies under 15 months raw honey.

452

All the herbs mentioned above can be combined in pleasing proportions to make a children's tonic, to be given in a spirit of love after any upset, during an illness, before sleep, or at a tea party. This tea can be served iced as punch at a birthday party, with hibiscus flowers and orange slices floating in it, or frozen as popsicles (put the honey in when the tea is still hot). For illness, select the herbs from this group that seem most relevant to the child's state and add one or two from below that apply specifically to his or her condition (include a stimulant and a demulcent in each blend).

To make tea, place the herbs in a cup (since you want between 1 and 2 teaspoons, it works best for me to make a blend in a jar, mix well, then take a teaspoon or two of blend); add pure water brought to a boil, and steep covered about 5 minutes. If too strong, dilute with water. If the child doesn't like the tea without honey, I put honey in—the healing experience is a positive one.

For a poultice, first serve a cleansing tea, then boil chopped or pounded herbs to a jelly, spread on a cloth and bandage on. Keep it warm. Change often, using new herbs, until desired effect is achieved. Slippery elm powder can be combined with prepared herbs to make a paste.

You can also make a syrup, especially for a cold or cough, by making the cup of tea with a tablespoon of herbs (instead of a teaspoon) and adding an equal amount of honey to the strained tea. We put it in a small jar (as from vitamins) and give to the child to carry to school, or just around.

Here are some herbs for specific conditions in children:

*Teething:* angelica root, pimpinella, mullein, lemon balm. To chew: whole licorice root, marshmallow or orris root, stalk from fennel plant, peeled.

*Fever:* chamomile, catnip, lemon balm, echinacea, elder flowers. (Seek medical advice if fever does not subside in a few hours.)

*Diarrhea:* blackberry leaf; carob powder mixed with water and honey.

*Gas:* peppermint, valerian (can be nausea-producing if given without a stimulant).

*Intestinal cramps:* ginger, licorice, honey; chew fennel seeds.

For any digestive, stomach or intestinal upset, there is no equal to slippery elm gruel: put 1-2 tablespoons slippery elm powder in a cup with a tablespoon of honey. Slowly add boiling water, stirring to a paste and one step beyond to a porridge consistency. It should be eaten immediately, as it hardens when cool.

*Cough:* wild cherry bark, chamomile, thyme, raspberry, slippery elm bark.

*Mucous congestion:* sage, licorice, peppermint, lemon balm.

*Rashes and insect bites:* to apply externally — aloe vera, chamomile tea, opened dandelion stem, chewed-up mugwort or plantain leaf. For bee stings: honey. For swellings: slippery elm/lobelia poultice.

Herbs are one part of what we can do to bring out the best in our children: the best of spirit, health, self-healing powers and happiness. Our whole way of life and attitude can be consistent with our approach to healing with herbs; thus diet and communication skills loom even larger than healing skills in serving to prevent illness and encourage rapid self-recovery.

Some useful books about herbs and children:

Dr. Christopher, *Childhood Diseases*

Juliette de Bairchi Levy, *Nature's Children*

Jethro Kloss, *Back to Eden*

Nicholas Culpeper, *Culpeper's Complete Herbal*

Bhavani Worden has studied nutrition and worked with herbs for the past ten years. She formulates the recipes for Red Dust Tea Co. and has been giving Health Workshops around Sonoma County for years. She has two children.

Reprinted with permission from Bhavani Worden, P.O. Box 234, Cazadero, CA 95421.

454

## Poisonous Plants

Many common house and garden plants are dangerous and can cause various injuries. The numbers that follow plants names are keyed to the four different reactions listed below.

1. skin irritation,
2. mouth-and throat-lining irritation
3. stomach and intestinal irritation, and
4. poisoning of the system.

| Houseplants | |
|---|---|
| Angel's Trumpet | 4 |
| Caladium | 2,3 |
| Castor Bean | 3,4 |
| Dieffenbachia | 1,2 |
| Elephant's ear | 1,2 |
| Mistletoe | 3,4 |
| Philodendron | 1,2 |
| Poinsettia | 1 |

| Ornamental | |
|---|---|
| Bleeding Heart | 1,4 |
| Daphne | 1,2,3 |
| English Ivy | 3 |
| Mountain Laurel | 4 |
| Oleander | 4 |
| Rhododendron | 4 |
| Wisteria | 3 |
| Yew | 3 |

| Forest Growth | |
|---|---|
| Baneberry | 3,4 |
| Bittersweet | 3,4 |
| Bloodroot | 3,4 |

| | |
|---|---|
| Deadly Amanita | 4 |
| Fly Agaric Mushroom | 4 |
| Jack-in-the-Pulpit | 2,3 |
| Mayapple | 3 |
| Moonseed | 4 |
| Poison Ivy | 1 |
| Poison Oak | 1 |
| Rosary Pea | 4 |
| Snakeroot | 3,4 |
| Yellow Jessamine | 4 |

| Flower Garden | |
|---|---|
| Autumn Crocus | 4 |
| Belladonna Lily | 3,4 |
| Christmas Rose | 1,3 |
| Daffodil | 3 |
| Four O'Clock | 3 |
| Foxglove | 4 |
| Hyacinth | 3 |
| Hydrangea | 3,4 |
| Iris | 3 |
| Larkspur | 4 |
| Lily of the Valley | 4 |
| Monkshood | 4 |
| Morning Glory | 4 |
| Narcissus | 3 |

| | |
|---|---|
| Snowdrop | 3 |
| Sweet Pea | 3 |

| Vegetable Garden | |
|---|---|
| Asparagus (unripe shoots) | 4 |
| Flax | 4 |
| Potato (eyes, stems, spoiled parts) | 4 |
| Rhubarb | 4 |
| Tomato (leaves) | 3,4 |

| Field Plants | |
|---|---|
| Buttercup | 2,3 |
| Death Camas | 4 |
| False Hellebore | 4 |
| Lupine | 4 |
| Milkweed | 4 |
| Nettle | 1 |
| Nightshade | 4 |
| Poison Hemlock | 4 |
| Poison Ivy | 1 |
| Pokeweed (Inkberry) | 3,4 |
| Snow on the Mountain | 4 |
| Sour Dock | 4 |
| Tobacco | 3 |

| Trees | |
|---|---|
| Apple | 4 |
| Black Locust | 3,4 |
| Box | 3,4 |
| Cherry | 4 |
| Chinaberry | 3 |
| Elderberry | 4 |
| English Holly | 3 |
| Fig | 1,2 |
| Golden Chain | 3,4 |
| Horse Chestnut | 3,4 |
| Lantana | 3,4 |
| Oak | 3,4 |
| Osage Orange | 1 |
| Peach | 4 |
| Privet | 3 |

| Marsh | |
|---|---|
| Cowslip | 3 |
| Lady's Slipper | 1 |
| Skunk Cabbage | 2,3 |
| Sneezeweed | 4 |
| Water Hemlock | 4 |

Distributed by the Marin County Department of Public Health, 1976.

455

# Childhood Illnesses

*by Nan Koehler, March 30, 1979*

Usually the first illness a baby gets is a mucous discharge from the nose, eyes, and/or throat (commonly known as a cold) or a rash on the face, chest or buttocks. These, in turn, may lead to something worse; an earache, cough, severe rash, or more frightening, a fever. Don't panic. Remember that to do home remedies you must catch everything early—before it gets out of hand—and you must be willing to follow the principles of natural healing. These principles can be found in a multitude of books. Basically they are fasting, rest, and dietary changes which allow the body to heal itself.

It's very important for speedy results to understand that illness is the outward manifestation of some internal imbalance. The idea of a germ invader is nice, but that concept doesn't help when you are doing home remedies. The internal imbalances (which we all experience as we "grow up") can be developmental in origin, that is—the child is ready for a growth spurt, but is disoriented; or external in origin, diet or disharmony in the environment. If the sickness is developmental, then it's best to devote an entire day to the child. Treat them as though they were younger, as though they were an infant—catering to their every need. Feed them the same way, have them take frequent naps (preferably on you) and give them a nice herbal tea. The next day they should be dramatically changed. If the diagnosis was correct, they should be well and doing whatever it was that seemed so hard for them; walking, talking, whatever.

If the sickness is environmental (you'll know if you tried the above and it didn't work), there are two basic areas to bear in mind which might need altering. First, the child's diet, or yours, if you are nursing. Second, the child's sleep patterns, the amount of rest they are getting or, in other words, the amount of stress they have to deal with. Usually simply altering the diet, changing your attitude toward your partner and loving yourself more will heal the child. The child is your mirror. They are you. Painful as that seems sometimes, it is

456

the truth. The child is your mate's and yours. The child is the physical manifestation of your combined energies. If that energy is off, then the child will have a hard time. As long as the mother and father keep their hearts open to each other, no matter if they are together or apart, the child will thrive. The more sexual energy you can flow to your child, the juicier they will look. I mean rubbing them, stroking them, hugging and kissing them, looking at them, just giving them attention. SEXUAL-ENERGY-IS-LIFE-FORCE-IS-ATTENTION!

In summary, here are some "rules-of-thumb" that help keep kids healthy. Bath them every day. Not only for cleanliness (avoids impetigo, scabies, lice, ringworm, etc.), but to also cleanse their aura. Water washes other peoples' (and places) energy off the body. It's good to do before bed for the soothing effect. Don't give them any foods with white flour or anything refined in it. This eliminates alot of junk foods. Don't give them sugar or honey.* It's acid forming in the body, throws their metabolism out of balance, and inhibits learning to taste and appreciate foods.

When they do have a runny nose, put them on an alkaline diet — mainly vegetables, no fruits, no citrus, no dairy, no meat, no grains. Soybeans are okay, almonds are okay, as well as bananas (but not too much). Just lighten up on food in general. Let them fast; most kids do that on their own anyway. Last but not least, learn some good herbal teas (trial and error) that your child really responds to. A cup of *that* tea and a nap are the best remedies I know. You might have to experiment to find which herbs your child needs (if you are nursing *you* take the tea or do the alkaline diet *and* rest more). Using astrology can be really helpful. For example, basil works well on Scorpio energy, comfrey on Capricorns, and kelp for Pisces — this is common knowledge found in the back of many herbals. You might need a combination. Usually if you use what attracts you (don't consciously think about it), that will be the right plant. If all else fails, then give your child as many cups of apple cider vinegar "tea" as they will drink. It's made by adding $\frac{1}{4}$ teaspoon of apple cider vinegar to a glass of warm water.

*A note on honey. Most honey available in the stores has been treated in some way or another. Even those that say natural untreated have been filtered and cooked. Raw honey with all the bee junk in it is a good food, but very hard to get. Therefore I'd recommend eliminating it altogether. Bhavani recommends it but I know she assumes that you will be buying the best available. Don't give honey to a little baby!

# Look Your Child Over Every·Day!
## Love is Attention: Attention is Love!

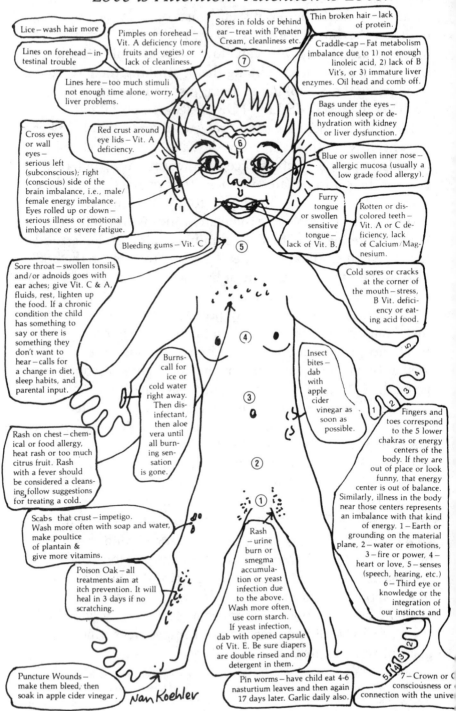

Lice – wash hair more

Lines on forehead – intestinal trouble

Pimples on forehead – Vit. A deficiency (more fruits and vegies) or lack of cleanliness.

Sores in folds or behind ear – treat with Penaten Cream, cleanliness etc.

Thin broken hair – lack of protein.

Craddle-cap – Fat metabolism imbalance due to 1) not enough linoleic acid, 2) lack of B Vit's, or 3) immature liver enzymes. Oil head and comb off.

Lines here – too much stimuli not enough time alone, worry, liver problems.

Cross eyes or wall eyes – serious left (subconscious); right (conscious) side of the brain imbalance, i.e., male/female energy imbalance. Eyes rolled up or down – serious illness or emotional imbalance or severe fatigue.

Red crust around eye lids – Vit. A deficiency.

Bags under the eyes – not enough sleep or de-hydration with kidney or liver dysfunction.

Blue or swollen inner nose – allergic mucosa (usually a low grade food allergy).

Furry tongue or swollen sensitive tongue – lack of Vit. B.

Rotten or discolored teeth – Vit. A or C deficiency, lack of Calcium/Magnesium.

Bleeding gums – Vit. C

Sore throat – swollen tonsils and/or adnoids goes with ear aches; give Vit. C & A, fluids, rest, lighten up the food. If a chronic condition the child has something to say or there is something they don't want to hear – calls for a change in diet, sleep habits, and parental input.

Cold sores or cracks at the corner of the mouth – stress, B Vit. deficiency or eating acid food.

Insect bites – dab with apple cider vinegar as soon as possible.

Burns – call for ice or cold water right away. Then disinfectant, then aloe vera until all burning sensation is gone.

Rash on chest – chemical or food allergy, heat rash or too much citrus fruit. Rash with a fever should be considered a cleansing, follow suggestions for treating a cold.

Fingers and toes correspond to the 5 lower chakras or energy centers of the body. If they are out of place or look funny, that energy center is out of balance. Similarly, illness in the body near those centers represents an imbalance with that kind of energy. 1 – Earth or grounding on the material plane, 2 – water or emotions, 3 – fire or power, 4 – heart or love, 5 – senses (speech, hearing, etc.) 6 – Third eye or knowledge or the integration of our instincts and

Scabs that crust – impetigo. Wash more often with soap and water, make poultice of plantain & give more vitamins.

Poison Oak – all treatments aim at itch prevention. It will heal in 3 days if no scratching.

Rash – urine burn or smegma accumulation or yeast infection due to the above. Wash more often, use corn starch. If yeast infection, dab with opened capsule of Vit. E. Be sure diapers are double rinsed and no detergent in them.

Puncture Wounds – make them bleed, then soak in apple cider vinegar.

Nan Koehler

Pin worms – have child eat 4-6 nasturtium leaves and then again 17 days later. Garlic daily also.

7 – Crown or consciousness or connection with the unive

458

# Special Books for Parenting

*by Jeannine Parvati Baker*

*The Kin of Ata Are Waiting for You* by Dorothy Bryant, 1976. From Ata Books, 1920 Stuart Street, Berkeley, CA 94703. $5.00 pap. (plus $1 shipping).

*The Mermaid and the Minotaur, Sexual Arrangements and Human Malaise* by Dorothy Dinnerstein, 1977. From Harper and Row, 10 East 53rd Street, New York, NY 10022. $4.95 pap.

*The Continuum Concept* by Jean Liedloff, 1977, 248 pages. From Warner Books, 75 Rockefeller Plaza, New York, NY 10019. $2.50 pap.

There are certain books which merit the status of milestones in our journeys in parenting. In my own, they often come grouped together, with each building upon the body of knowledge of the others. This body of knowledge helps to carry me forth, comfort me, and provide the context of meaning for mothering. In other words, books are like a mother to me.

A dozen or so years ago, when I was in college and preparing for my first pregnancy, a vision of the ideal mothering found me. This ideal has served me well through the deliverance of four beautiful children. The image, which I still hold as ideal (by definition implying that I am in process of realizing it in my own experience), shows mother and children together with a peaceful glow, becoming more and more conscious of who they really are. There is a mutual respect and acceptance of the archetypal positions — mother and child — and agreement that these are *equal yet different*. The seeming paradox provides the opportunity, ultimately, for spiritual unity. Lastly, the mothering process is a healing one which affects all whom we may meet along the way. Healing one mother is healing our Earth. When I came upon these three books (actually several hundred others as well, but for the purposes of this short review I've had to limit the discussion to mainly three titles) it was like meeting dear friends. Here was the support for my vision; the careful and logical information for my intuition. I am moved to share them because they are loyal friends and have made mothering a joy.

It wasn't until pregnant with the fourth baby, that the first of these three books came. *The Kin of Ata* by Dorothy Bryant had been in the periphery of my friendship circle for quite a while but I hadn't time for "novels." Well, in this pregnancy, I indulged in many imaginal treats and when Bryant's book was given to me, I read it in one sitting. Here was the portrayal of a culture in which my ideal of parenting could live. The values were very similar. There was only one disparity; birth was presented as an excruciating ordeal and that didn't match my experience at all. (I found this same portrayal in Bryant's *The Garden of Eros*, wherein pain during labor is emphasized, perhaps without the important context of "initiation ritual.") My favorite line in *The Kin of Ata* is in response to the protagonist's question, "How do you know when you are fertile?" She answers, in true maiutic* style, "How do you know when you are thirsty?" In the culture Bryant describes, it is given that mothers are in tune with themselves and their babies, both present and forthcoming. Here is a community which acknowledges that babies come for one another, their peers, and not just for their parents. This book gives us a less threatening look at community than *The Book of the Mother* by the Shivalila Children's Liberation Front. Both of these titles address a core issue of spirituality and mothering which has confused us all for millenia; i.e., that *attachment is pain.* This is the precept of yoga or union. It is the primary dogma of what I term patriarchal spirituality. The following two titles (which I'd like to suggest each and every parent read) lend support to another view, which is that *attachment is bliss.*

460

If it is true that we haven't ever fully experienced a complete attachment and that it is the lack of and thwarting of attachment which is painful, then *The Mermaid and the Minotaur* and *The Continuum Concept* bring us the tools to remedy this. Both are books of the feminist renaissance in spirituality. Dorothy Dinnerstein's brilliant book is rough going for those of us who have avoided developing the "upward mobility of the mind" (M. Daly). I have completed graduate work in archetypal psychology and so the book read easily, but some of my students who aren't facile with this language couldn't read it. There is great depth and richness in these pages and so I encourage the reader to "hang in there." *The Mermaid and the Minotaur* brought to light all the "whys" behind my ideal of *mothering as a shared process for both the parents.* Briefly, the idea is this; our planet needs a mother's guidance now. Fathers could share early childcaring duties (to their great benefit) and thus free the mothers for work in the world with the men leaders. When we've let men run the show, as we know, it tends to be horror movies. Our attitude of "boys will be boys" boomeranges as "the boys" have us on the edge of an apocalypse. If mothers had help with young children, we would also be less frazzled and kinder, and children would grow up imprinting on the feminine as less of an ambivalent image. The "negative mother" would less often rear her ugly head and there would be greater respect for all mothers, including our great mother, the Earth. Pollution, rape, and other forms of male chauvinism would decline. (And while I'm on the subject; there is a movement to transform this world into a peaceful one. The slogan is, "People are not for hitting — and children are people too." Write to Humanethic 3629 Mossman, Wichita, KS 67208 for further information, bumper stickers, etc.) My only disagreement with *The Mermaid and the Minotaur* is the suggestion of bottle-feeding and contraceptives, both decidedly unfeminist tools. Total mothering and fertility awareness do not preclude sharing of our babies with the papas, as our experience has shown. In fact, I have found that these practices increase my creative

461

energy to fully give myself to our babies and to know when we might possibly conceive another. I've been able to write and publish a couple of good books, found a college, practice lay midwifery, astrology, and herbalism, take a Master's degree, and enjoy being a mother *all at the same time.* How? By bringing my babies with me. Which brings us to the last title I'd like to share with you — *The Continuum Concept* by Jean Liedloff.

Here, at last, is the support needed to attach deeply to our babies! When birth is a healing, that unity between mother and babe is honored. No separation. No taking away of the baby to be "assessed" or rated or cleaned. The mother delivers her own baby and s/he's allowed to stay in her arms until s/he is ready to crawl or creep away. I've done this with all my babies, including twins, and have found that when they do walk away from our bodies, it is with full confidence that their mother supports them and they are loved. This translates into a knowing that mother Earth as well is a friendly body. I know that it is easy to say and harder to do, that I surrender my body (soul and spirit) in service to my baby. Especially since we do not have a primal imprint or active present day model of how to do it. JoAnn Groham's book *Born to Love,* Arthur Janov's *The Feeling Child,* and my own *Prenatal Yoga* are suggested supplementary reading on *how* to do it.

My favorite part in *The Continuum Concept* is on meditation. Often I have felt that "surrendered mothering" is meditation. Being a yogini for 23 years, I've had phases of disenchantment with the yoga practices being seemingly at odds with my mothering. A Guatemalan story about weaving comes to mind that is germane here. When weavers in that culture become pregnant with their first baby, they go away from the loom. It is not until they have weaned their last babe that they resume their work. At that point they are masters. Even though they have not practiced for all those years, they are still expected to have kept up with their barren sisters in the art of weaving. And they do. When I apply this metaphor to spiritual practice, I am heartened. When my husband awakes at 4 a.m. to do the spiritual practices we both used to do together before the birth of our latest baby, I don't feel left out. By truly giving myself to our littlest one, I am doing the Goddess' work. And I therefore have the fantasy that when our last babe is weaned and I am free to change the form of my daily worship from breast-feeding to pranyamam, there won't be any lost time. In fact, perhaps we both will become masters.

In summation, *The Kin of Ata, The Mermaid and the Minotaur,* and *The Continuum Concept* provide us mothers with the knowledge base we need to bring a healing to our best spiritual practices — the caring of and for our babies and the means to share this with their fathers. If healing one mother is healing our Earth, then healing one father is bringing heaven here and now.

Jeannine Parvati Baker, M.A. (née Jeannine O'Brien Medvin) is the founder of Hygieia College offering programs in Lay Midwifery and Gyn/Ecology-Feminist Holistic Health Care. She is the author of *Hygieia: A Woman's Herbal* (1978), *Prenatal Yoga and Natural Birth* (1974), *Conscious Conception* (1982) and numerous articles on mothering, feminism, rituals, etc. Her current projects include a book order service for her own and other books, and a Home Study Correspondence Course in healing birth and non-medical ritual for lay midwives and families. The full tuition is $200 for ten lessons. Sample lesson #1 is available for $15. For more information write to Jeannine Parvati Baker, Freestone Innerprizes, Hygieia College and Home Study, P.O. Box 398, Monroe, UT 84754.

Reprinted from *Childbirth Alternatives Quarterly*, Winter 1983, Vol. IV, No. 2.

*"In the manner of a midwife."

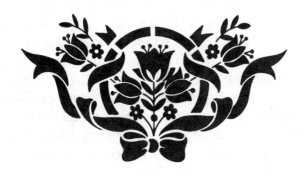

463

# Circumcision: My Own Story

*by Rosemary Romberg Wiener*

When children are born and people grow up in this world, we expect each individual to keep all parts of his or her body. All people have hands and feet, fingers and toes, noses and ears. People are unquestionably accorded that basic right. Most people would be aghast at the idea that any individual should be unwittingly deprived of any part of his or her body. People without their expected body parts are usually regarded as unusual.

Our feelings toward tiny babies inspire emotions of tenderness and protection. Babies are to cuddle and hold, to be kept secure in their parents' arms. Babies should nurse (preferably) at their mother's breast and sleep peacefully, safe and secure from any harm. Parents want to protect their infants from any unnecessary pain, discomfort, or unhappiness. The idea of cutting, pinching, or tearing the baby's skin, of injuring that baby, causing him to experience pain, crying, or bleeding, is totally against what most parents want for their infants.

In the United States, people make one glaring exception to these "rules" in that the foreskin of the penis of most newborn baby boys is routinely amputated shortly after birth. Most American baby boys undergo the following procedure: The infant is placed on his back in a plastic "Circumstraint" tray where his arms and legs are strapped down. Paper drapes are then placed over him with a hole where his penis is exposed. A hemostat is applied to the tip of the foreskin to crush it and then a slit is made to enlarge it. The operator then takes a small instrument and goes inside to free the foreskin from the glans of the penis—essentially tearing one layer of skin away from another since at birth the foreskin is noramlly adhered to the glans. A small protective "bell" is placed over the glans and under the foreskin. By one method a metal clamp is placed

464

over the foreskin and left in place for 5 minutes. Then the foreskin is cut off and the clamp removed. By another method, a string is tied tightly over the foreskin and the plastic bell. Then some of the foreskin in front of the string is trimmed away. The handle of the bell is removed and the ring of plastic remains in place around the end of the penis. The remaining foreskin atrophies (dries up) within approximately one week and the plastic ring then falls off.

In most cases this is done to the infant without anesthesia, although when the same operation is performed on an older child or an adult it is considered painful enough to warrant an anesthesia.

As an American middle class woman, I had always thought penises were supposed to look a certain way with the exposed, rounded head at the end. It never occurred to me that anything had been changed or cut off to make it appear that way. As far as I knew, males were born with penises that looked like that. I had heard of the term "circumcision" and knew vaguely that it had something to do with the penis and that the Bible said some things about it. However, this was something that I never questioned, thought about, or really understood.

I am a person who seeks to educate myself and prepare myself for every experience in whatever way possible. Therefore in 1972, when my husband and I were expecting our first child, I read books, asked questions, watched films, and attended classes in natural childbirth. I believed that I knew everything that I needed to know about pregnancy, birth, and care of the new baby.

I gave birth to our first child, a son, by the Lamaze method, and successfully nursed him. However, I gave birth in a "traditional" hospital in which the baby was separated from me, kept in a central nursery, and brought to me on a four hour feeding schedule. Therefore I had little knowledge or control over what was being done to my baby.

When the baby and I came home and I first began changing his diapers, I found that he too had a penis in the style and

465

shape to which I was culturally accustomed, with the rounded glans exposed. The end of the baby's penis was bright red for the first few days, but soon healed. The baby screamed every time his diaper was changed. Being a naive new mother, I had no idea why diaper changing upset him so much — perhaps all babies did that. I never gave the appearance of my baby's penis any concern.

Shortly after our baby's birth I became a childbirth instructor and soon enjoyed challenges and rewards of educating other expectant parents about pregnancy, birth, infant care.

Two and a half years later, in 1974, our second son was born in another hospital, again by the Lamaze method. This birth experience included several "progressive" practices such as "rooming in." I was also more aware of the baby undergoing circumcision. The morning following his birth the doctor came by, took the baby to another room where he cut off his foreskin, and brought him back to me about 15 minutes later. Although I expected that the procedure would be painful for the baby, it never occurred to me not to have it done. Again this baby had a penis in the style which seemed "normal" to me. The new baby's penis healed within a few days and I forgot about it.

Two years later after our second son's birth I again became pregnant. During this time I underwent a tremendous amount of change in my thinking about what I wanted for this birth and baby. We made the unconventional and daring (for that time and place) decision to go outside the traditional medical system, seek the services of a lay midwife, and give birth at home. I was intrigued with Dr. Frederick Leboyer's philosophy of *Birth Without Violence* and wanted to use some of these practices for our baby's birth. I read that the baby who is welcomed into the world in this manner is calmer and more peaceful than the baby who is born to conventional bright lights, loud noises and rough handling. Our first two sons were fussy and cried a great deal as new babies, so I was very much interested in trying a different approach for our new baby's birth.

466

We made plans to use only dim lighting when our baby was born. We would hold, massage, and speak softly to our new baby and welcome him into the world with gentleness and love. We would delay the clamping of the umbilical cord. No silver nitrate or other chemicals would be placed in the baby's eyes.

During this time I also took additional training as a childbirth instructor in preparation for teaching more technical classes for people planning home births. I did extensive studying in many areas of obstetrics and newborn care. I considered myself more educated and knowledgeable about all aspects of pregnancy, birth, and baby care than most new parents.

The idea occurred to me that if our new baby was a boy, perhaps he should not be circumcised. However, I knew practically nothing about it. None of our doctors ever gave us any information about the operation—pros, cons, why or how it was done. Although mothers regularly discuss at length all aspects of pregnancy, birth, and infant care, I had never heard anyone else talk about circumcision. While I regularly discussed in detail such things as nutrition, breastfeeding, exercises, breathing techniques, and postpartum care in my Lamaze classes, it never occurred to me to discuss circumcision.

Despite my extensive knowledge in many other areas, and my wholehearted desire to do the very best for my children, my awareness of circumcision consisted of nothing more than a basic concept that that was the way that penises were "supposed" to look and a vague idea that it was somehow supposed to be cleaner.

Early one morning in April of 1977, our third little son came into the world in the peace and comfort of our home. He coughed, sputtered, then breathed quietly as he emerged into dim light and was placed on my tummy to be massaged, comforted, and held close to me. Babies do not have to do a lot of screaming to announce their arrival in the world. There is a profound difference in the experience of birth and the nature

467

of the baby when he is welcomed into the world in this manner.

During the next few days our new son nursed contentedly, slept peacefully, and rarely cried. He had a peacefulness and serenity that I had never known with my first two babies — something very special and rare.

Another thing that was different about this baby was that he had a penis that was straight and long, coming to a point at the end. While I had always thought that intact penises looked "strange," this baby's penis seemed normal and natural the way it was. The first few days of our new baby's life were peaceful and joyous and our new little son was whole and perfect.

What incomprehensible force brought me from this beautiful, untraumatized birth at home to a strange doctor's office one week later — sitting their frightened and reluctant, holding my sleeping, peaceful, trusting newborn infant? "He shouldn't be different from his brothers or father." "I'm afraid he'll have problems." "Our relatives would object if we didn't have it done." All these thoughts went through my head, while all the while I wanted so much to protect my baby from any harm.

My husband and I found ourselves relinquishing our baby and leaving the building. When we returned about 15 minutes later the office was filled with our baby's screams! I found our precious baby on the doctor's operating table with a penis that was cut, raw, and bright red! I remembered his brothers' penises looking that way, but while they, to me, seemed to have been "born that way," this baby had definitely been injured, damaged, and traumatized! My maternal protective instincts had been violated! I immediately held and nursed him, trying to relieve his pitiful screams. Soon he mercifully fell asleep and I took him home. I felt like I had brought home a different baby. His tense, agonized little body reminded me of the way his brothers had been as newborns. Within a few days the redness around the end of his penis healed. But this time I was not about to forget! The trauma and torture that

468

was inflicted upon this tiny, helpless little being was to come back and haunt me again and again. From this sprang my quest to do extensive research for a book which will be entitled *Circumcision: The Painful Dilemma.*

As emotionally difficult as my own baby's circumcision was, I still began my research with a neutral stand on the subject. My sole concern was that the operation was so painful for a baby. My American middle class upbringing had led me to believe that circumcision conferred a number of health benefits on the individual. As a *result* of my research I have become opposed to neonatal circumcision. None of the popular myths about circumcision are valid. The startling facts that I have unearthed all stack up overwhelmingly against the operation.

The practice of male genital mutilation—drawing blood from, causing pain to, and changing the appearance of the penis finds it origins in prehistoric times. It is not known where, how, why, or with what group of people the practice began. Several possible explanations have been offered as reasons for circumcision. Among these are blood sacrifice, an initiation rite in which it was a test of torture and pain by which young boys "became men," a fertility ritual, a means of subjection to torture and humiliation on conquered enemies and slaves, a means of "purification" that accompanied shaving of all body hair, a means of diminishing sexual desires, and an expression of envy of the female menstrual process. For some peoples what has been labeled as "circumcision" actually consisted of a gashing of the foreskin rather than a complete amputation as we know it today. It is clear that explanations such as "cleanliness" or "cosmetic value" had nothing to do with the operation's primitive origins. Female circumcision, which is repugnant to the Western mind, but is still practiced in other parts of the world, originated in much the same manner as did male genital mutilation. Rarely has circumcision been the personal choice of the individual. However, with the exception of the Jewish culture and the present day American medical profession, extremely few peoples have ever performed circumcisions on babies. (1, 2, 3)

In Western society, since the time of early Christianity when St. Paul declared circumcision unnecessary to conversion to the Christian religion, it was rare for non-Jewish people to be circumcised, until the late 1800's. The practice, as an American medical fad, arose out of the antimasturbation hysteria of the Victorian era. (4, 5, 6) People feared that if a boy had his foreskin he would learn to masturbate while washing his penis. At that time it was believed that masturbation led to insanity. Today, most people accept the fact that masturbation is harmless, and that circumcised individuals certainly do masturbate. Yet American parents continue to accept the operation as appropriate for their infant sons, knowing little or nothing as to why or how the practice originated.

During the 1920's and 30's many articles appeared in American medical publications advocating infant circumcision on the grounds that lack of foreskin would somehow prevent cancer of the penis and the female uterine cervix. Since the rates of these diseases are low among Jewish and Moslem people, both of whom practice male circumcision, many authorities concluded that circumcision must prevent these diseases. *However,* upon comparing the rates of penile cancer among America's (mostly circumcised) and Europe's (intact) males, one finds that the rates of this disease in Europe are as low or lower than in the United States. (7) Among American non-Jewish women, when comparing those married to circumcised and those married to intact husbands, studies have found no differences in the rates of cancer of the cervix. (8, 9) Clearly other significant factors are related to both of these diseases and circumcision is not justified as a cancer preventative.

There have been many astonishing and tragic complications of the operation. Infants have both hemorrhaged and developed severe infections of the circumcision wound. Plastic surgery has been required when too much skin was removed or the glans or penile shaft was accidentally damaged. Occasionally troublesome cysts, fistulas, and keloid

470

formations have developed at the site of the circumcision wound. (10, 11, 12, 13, 14) There are documented cases of infants who were born male who have had to be raised as females as a result of total loss of the penis due to complications of circumcision. (15)

The most common complication of circumcision is called meatal ulceration. The exposed glans, without protective foreskin, develops painful urine burns from contact with wet diapers. (16, 17, 18) My own sons had this problem. Our doctor never advised us that this was a complication of circumcision. Probably they did not know this.

Many people choose not to believe that the newborn infant feels any pain when his foreskin is smashed, slit, torn back from the glans, clamped and cut off. Circumcision, in its primitive origins, was often deliberately intended to be a means of torture and a test of endurance in adolescent initiation rites. We think of that as barbaric, yet regularly do the same thing to babies. There have been NO documented studies to support the popular assumption that babies have little or no feelings. Curiously, the earliest modern writings on infant circumcision, those that appeared in medical publications around the turn of the century, were full of concern for the feelings of the helpless infant. (19, 20) The belief that infants feel no pain came about years later, during the 1920's, 30's, and 40's, during an era that advocated bottlefeeding instead of nursing, rigid schedules, separation from mother and baby following birth, and rigid toilet training. Parents were warned not to rock, hold, or cuddle their babies for fear that they would "spoil" them. Popular attitudes and practices during that time totally ignored the baby's feelings and needs in many different areas.

Recent, scientifically controlled studies on the reactions of newborns to being circumcised have revealed that the infant characteristically lapses into a deep, "semi-coma," non-rapid-eye-movement type of sleep which is an abnormal sleep pattern for newborn infants. This is clearly a stress-withdrawal reaction. (21) Because some babies do not cry out in response

471

to being circumcised, but instead lapse into this deep sleep, some observers have falsely believed that the operation is not painful for infants.

Another study, attempting to evaluate gender differences among newborn infants, found that boy babies were generally fussier and more restless than baby girls. However, it was found that the greater fussiness on the part of the baby boys was due to recent circumcision—not gender. When the study was repeated, using only non-circumcised newborn boys, no behavioral differences between girl and boy babies were found. (22)

Today, many American parents and doctors are becoming aware of these facts. There is a growing trend *against* choosing infant circumcision, which is following the recent trend towards natural childbirth and breastfeeding. Many parents do not wish to have their infants experience such a painful ordeal as circumcision. Also there is a growing acceptance of the fact that the body is designed correctly as it normally comes into the world and does not need to be surgically made different. Another facet of the issue is that of individual human rights. Many are questioning the ethics of altering another person's body in this manner without his permission, in the absence of medical or perhaps religious indications. Many parents are realizing that their child's foreskin is rightfully his, and by consenting to circumcision they are causing the destruction of a valuable and useful part of his body. Parents should be aware that there are a substantial number of men who DO resent the fact that a part of their body was cut off and that they had no say in the matter.

Some parents still do choose circumcision for their infant sons. Usually these reasons are vague and uninformed. Many have accepted it as an automatic medical procedure when giving birth in a hospital or have believed that they had to have it done. Some believe that circumcision is important for cleanliness, just as people in other countries believe that female circumcision somehow makes women cleaner. Some people are turned off when they hear that smegma collects under the foreskin and must be washed away. However, smegma is the same substance that collects on the genitals of women and girls and must be washed away regularly. In our society we have running water and bathing facilities unparalleled to any other time or place in history. Like all other body parts, cleanliness of the intact penis is not difficult or complicated. In contrast to the myriad of dirty diapers, runny noses, and spit up that all parents must attend to regularly, smegma is an extremely minor concern.

Some parents worry that their son will be "different" from other boys if he is not circumcised, or feel that he should "match" his already circumcised father or older brother(s). However, with the growing trend to choose against circumcision, the intact boy born today should have plenty of peers who also have foreskins. Many intact males have enjoyed their "individuality." There are many families in which the father and son or different brothers "don't match." This does not appear to cause problems within the family.

Some parents fear that if their infant son is not circumcised he will have to have it done at a later age. Many people believe that the operation is more painful for someone who is older than it is for an infant. This belief is unfounded, and the likelihood that he will have to undergo circumcision for a medical reason is slim. Undoubtedly some doctors prescribe circumcision for problems that can and should be corrected by less drastic means. Newborn babies do heal rapidly and do not normally require stitches for circumcision. However, older children and adults are given anesthesia for the operation, and most importantly are able to understand what is being done to their bodies. If a boy or man chooses circumcision because he would simply rather be that way, then it is his body and he has made that decision for himself, therefore the operation should not be traumatic.

Certainly people's religious beliefs must be respected. Some devout Jewish people believe that circumcision of their infant

473

sons is an expression of their "covenant with God." Yet today even many Jewish people question this aspect of their faith, considering it merely a tradition, or like the other American parents, merely accept it as a medical procedure. There are Jewish parents who have chosen to leave their sons intact.

Many people, doctors included, do not understand the normal development and correct care of the infant's foreskin. We have been led to believe that circumcision is "cleaner" and therefore believe that the care of the intact child's penis is very difficult and complicated. Frequently doctors forcefully retract the infant's foreskin during the hospital stay or at one of the baby's office visits. Parents are sometimes instructed to retract and clean under the baby's foreskin every day. This practice is more traumatic to the baby than circumcision (since circumcision happens only once) and is what causes such problems as infections, phimosis (foreskin attached to the glans of the penis) and paraphimosis (foreskin retracted and cannot be replaced). We are having to be educated to leave the normally tight and non-retractible foreskin of the infant alone until it gradually loosens of its own accord which can take up to three or four years. (23, 24)

In 1980 I became pregnant with our fourth child. This time, based on my learning through all of my research, there was absolutely no question that if the child were a boy, he would keep his foreskin. In January of 1981 our daughter was born. Today as I care for my baby girl who is so sweet, pretty, and perfect, the idea of anyone cutting up her genitals, making her bleed, or hurting her in any way is totally repugnant to me! I am thankful that our society has not developed any medical fads that cause pain and anguish to baby girls! Perhaps some day soon American people will accord that same protection and respect to our boy babies as well!

REFERENCES:

1. Bryk, Felix. *Sex and Circumcision: A Study of Phallic Worship and Mutilation in Men and Women.* Brandon House, North Hollywood, CA. c. 1967.

474

2. Loeb, E.M. "The Blood Sacrifice Complex." American Anthropological Association Memoirs, 30, p. 3-40.

3. Bettelheim, Bruno. "Symbolic Wounds" p. 230-240, from *Reader in Comparative Religion*. Lessa, William A., & Vogt, Evon Z. Harper & Row, Publishers, New York, 2nd Ed., c. 1965.

4. Remondino, P.C. *History of Circumcision from Earliest Times to the Present*. Arms Press, New York, c. 1974 (original ed., F.A. Davis Co. 1891).

5. Marcus, Irwin M., M.D., & Francis, John J., M.D. *Masturbation: From Infancy to Senescence*. National Universities Press, Inc., N. Y. c. 1975, ch. 16, "Authority and Masturbation," p. 381-409 by Spitz, Rene A., M.D.

6. Baker-Benfield, G.J. *The Horrors of the Half-Known Life*. Harper Colophon Books, New York, c. 1976.

7. Persky, Lester, M.D. "Epidemiology of Cancer of the Penis." Recent Results of Cancer Research, Berlin, 1977, p. 97-109.

8. Aitken-Swan, Jean, & Baird, D. "Circumcision and Cancer of the Cervix." British Journal of Cancer, Vol. 19, No. 2, June 1965, p. 217-227.

9. Terris, Milton, M.D.: Wilson, Fitzpatrick, M.D.: & Nelson, James H., Jr., M.D. "Relation of Circumcision to Cancer of the Cervix." American Journal of Obstetrics and Gynecology, Vol. 117, No. 8, Dec. 15, 1973, p. 1056-1066.

10. Gee, William F., M.D. & Ansell, Julian S., M.D. "Neonatal Circumcision: A Ten-Year Overview: With Comparison of the Gomco Clamp and the Plastibell Device." Pediatrics, Vol. 58, 1976, p. 824-827.

11. Grimes, David A., M.D. "Routine Circumcision of the Newborn Infant; A Reappraisal." American Journal of Obstetrics and Gynecology, Vol. 130, No. 2, Jan. 15, 1978, p. 125-129.

12. Kaplan, George W., M.D. "Circumcision — An Overview." Current Problems in Pediatrics, Year Book Medical Publishers, Inc., Chicago, IL., Vol. 7, No. 5, March 1977.

13. Limaye, Ramesh D., M.D. & Hancock, Reginald, A., M.D. "Penile Urethral Fistula as a Complication of Circumcision." The Journal of Pediatrics, Vol. 72, No. 1, Jan. 1968, p. 105-106.

14. Shulman, J., M.D.: Ben-Hur, N., M.D.: & NEUMAN, Z., M.D. (Israel) "Surgical Complications of Circumcision." American Journal of Diseases of Children, Vol. 107, Feb. 1961, p. 149-154.

15. Money, John Ph.D. "Ablatio Penis, Normal Male Infant Sex-Reassigned as a Girl." Archives of Sexual Behavior, Vol. 4, No. 1, 1975, p. 65-71.

16. Mackenzie, A. Ranald, M.D. "Meatal Ulceration Following Neonatal Circumcision." Obstetrics and Gynecology, Vol. 28, No. 2, August 1966, p. 221-223.

17. Freud, Paul, M.D. "The Ulcerated Urethral Meatus in Male Children." The Journal of Pediatrics, Vol. 31, No. 2, August 1947, p. 131-141.

18. Brennemann, Joseph, M.D. "The Ulcerated Meatus in the Circumcised Child." American Journal of Diseases of Children, Vol. 21, 1920, p. 38-47.

19. DeLee, Joseph B., A.M., M.D. Obstetrics for Nurses. W.B. Saunders Co., Philadelphia, PA, 7th ed. 1924 (1st ed. 1901), p. 436-440.

20. Valentine, Fred C., M.D. "Surgical Circumcision." Journal A.M.A, March 16, 1901, p. 712-713.

21. Emde, Robert N. M.D.; Harmon, Robert J., M.D.; Metcalf, David, M.D.: Koenig, Kenneth L., M.D.: & Wagonfield, Samuel, M.D. "Stress and Neonatal Sleep." Psychosomatic Medicine, Vol. 33, No. 6, Nov.-Dec. 1971, p. 491-497.

22. Richards, M.P.M.; Bernal, J.F.; & Brackbill, Yvonne. "Early Behavioral Differences: Gender or Circumcision?" Developmental Psychobiology, Vol. 9, No. 1, 1976, p. 89-95.

23. Gairdner, Douglas, M.D. "The Fate of the Foreskin — A study of Circumcision." British Medical Journal, Dec. 24, 1949, p. 1433-1437.

24. Reichelderfer, Thomas E., M.D. & Fraga, Juan R., M.D. Reprint from Care of the Well Baby, by Shepard, Kenneth S., M.D. (ed.). J.B. Lippencott Co., 1968, p. 10.

© Rosemary Romberg Wiener, 1981.

Reprinted from Mothering Magazine, No. 22, Winter 1982. P.O. Box 2208, Alburquerque, NM 87103.

This article is a publication of INTACT Educational Foundation. INTACT stands for Infants Need To Avoid Circumcision Trauma. Copies of this article are aviailable at the following rates: Single copy — 45¢ plus business sized self-addressed, stamped envelope. 12 copies — $4.50 plus $1.00 postage & handling. 50 copies — $8.00 plus $2.00 postage & handling. 100 copies — $15.00 plus $3.00 postage & handling.

Order from: Rosemary Romberg Wiener, Prepared Natural Childbirth/INTACT Educational Foundation, 4521 Fremont St., Bellingham, WA 98226; or Jeffrey R. Wood, Box 5, Wilbraham, MA 01095.

Other information sheets, technical articles, books, slide sets and teaching aids also available.

476

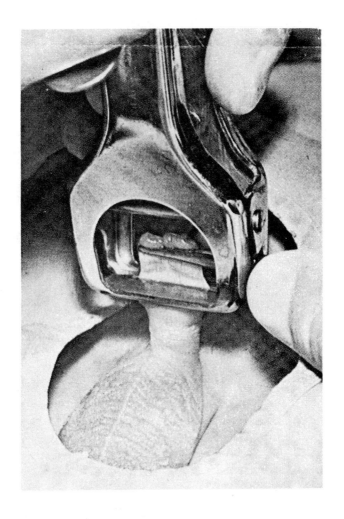

*Sheldon Circumcision Clamp — manufactured by Olympic Medical Supplies, Seattle, WA.*

*Handout available —*

# *When Your Baby Boy is Not Circumcised*

*by Edward Wallerstein,*
*author of "Circumcision: An American Health Fallacy"*

The United States is the only country to practice nonreligious circumcision almost routinely. Since about 80% of male newborns are circumcised, it has not seemed important to pay attention to the care of the uncircumcised penis. There were so few of them. The result is widespread misunderstanding of its proper care and hygiene.

Within the past five years, however, we have witnessed a trend away from routine newborn circumcision, led by the American Academy of Pediatrics and the American College of Obstetricians and Gynecologists. Dozens of articles in both professional and popular magazines have urged prospective parents to question this newborn surgery. It is, therefore, important for those who are or will be responsible for infant care to learn the essentials of caring for the uncircumcised penis — a simple task indeed.

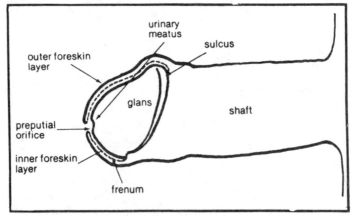

Diagramatic Representation of the Inner and Outer Foreskin Layers. (Reproduced with permission of Edward Wallerstein.)

478

# Summmary: Care of the Uncircumcised Penis

BEFORE RETRACTION TAKES PLACE

1. Frequent bathing or sponge bathing of your baby is necessary.

2. Make sure all the folds and wrinkles of the genitals are cleansed after bowel movements and with diaper changes. The uncircumcised penis requires no extra cleaning—just wash, rinse, and dry it, along with the rest of the baby's bottom.

3. Wash away any smegma appearing on the outside of the penis, but don't try to wash or clean under the foreskin.

4. DO NOT retract (pull back) the foreskin over the glans of the penis. In a newborn, the foreskin is almost always attached to the glans. Forcing the foreskin back may harm the penis, causing pain, bleeding, possible scarring and adhesions.

5. DO NOT Let your pediatrician or anyone else forcibly retract the foreskin of your newborn. Some pediatricians today remain uninformed on this matter, and believe that at birth the foreskin must be retractable. If it is not, they force it. As familiarity with the normal uncircumcised penis increases, there will be less of this improper care and improper advice.

6. Separation of the foreskin from the glans may take years.

7. To test whether or how much the foreskin has separated, either:
   a. Observe an erection (most baby boys have them). If full erection occurs, full retraction may also occur; or
   b. Hold the penile shaft with one hand and with the other hand, GENTLY push the foreskin back, only as far as it goes easily. STOP if the baby seems to be uncomfortable or if you feel resistance.

8. You may test for retraction every few months.

479

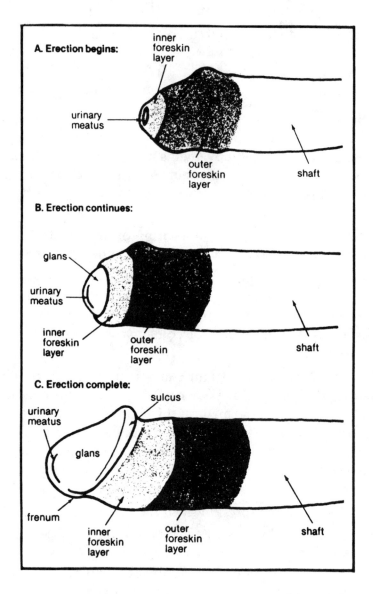

Diagrammatic Representation of the Erection Process in the Uncircumcised Penis. (Reproduced with permission of Edward Wallerstein.)

## AFTER FORESKIN IS FULLY RETRACTABLE

1. Until the child can bathe himself, an adult bathes him.
2. When washing the penis, retract the foreskin gently, wash the glans, rinse, and replace the foreskin, teaching the child that this is how the penis should be washed.
3. Sometimes, after the child takes over his own bathing, he may be careless and the glans may become red and sore. Washing the penis and applying a protective ointment will quickly clear up the problem.

## A FINAL WORD

Remember, soap and water work wonders; they are all that is necessary for foreskin hygiene. As Dr. Alex Comfort wrote: "Wash, don't amputate."

Excerpts reprinted by permission of Pennypress, Inc.

*Circumcision: An American Health Fallacy,* by Edward Wallerstein, is published by Springer Publishing Co., 200 Park Avenue South, New York, NY 10003. $14.95 plus $1.10 postage.

Copyright © 1982 by Edward Wallerstein. All rights reserved. No part of this pamphlet may be reproduced by any means without written permission of the author.

*When Your Baby Boy is Not Circumcised* is published by and available from Pennypress, Inc. 1100 23rd Avenue East, Seattle, WA 98112. Price: 1 to 5 – $0.50 each (including postage). For quantity prices, write for our flyer.

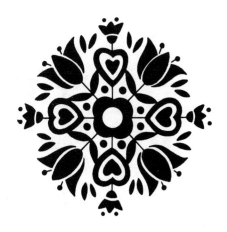

# Discipline

## Age 1–7
### Vital – Physical Adaptation

1. Discipline is physically based

   *Non-verbal communication is what they get, lectures are wasted.*

2. Create child's reality moment to moment.

3. *Bodily intimacy is the Key.*

4. Don't talk and rationalize – act!

5. Use loving force to move them bodily into a different disposition.

*Discipline over and over and over. They won't remember.*

(Praise should be generalized, not specific – then self-love doesn't develop.)

## Age 7–14
### Emotional – Sexual

1. Discipline is emotionally based

   *Don't punish, no spankings, redirect negative emotions.*

2. Encourage self-generated responsibility (learn consequences).

3. *Service is the Key.*

4. Establish agreements, rights and privileges.

5. Encourage emotions. Only true emotion is *Love.* Other emotions are perversion of love.

*Then they practice and remember.*

## Age 14–21
### Mental – Intentional

1. Discipline appeals to the understanding

   *Don't keep telling what to do. Become sympathetic friend. Don't be in opposition.*

2. Child becomes responsible as the will develops through understanding.

3. *Understanding is the Key.*

4. Teach natural consequences of their actions.

5. Expanding intimacy to the total culture via compassionate friendship.

*Relax concern that the child respond immediately.*

Notes from a seminar given by the Laughing Man Institute, Feb. 20, 1982, *Discipline Is An Act of Love.* Nan Koehler

482

# The Hormonal Cycle

The hormonal cycle is one of many parts that fit together to form the menstrual cycle, beginning at puberty when the ovary develops, and ending with menopause when the ovaries stop functioning.

It is important for us to understand how our bodies function and how each of its parts are related. With this information we will feel closer to ourselves and to each other as women. We will draw our own conclusions about our bodies. We will give up some of the erroneous myths that have developed and that we, through ignorance about ourselves, have helped to perpetuate. We are making connections in regard to our psychological state and our emotional beings. When we finally put physiology and psychology together, it will not be surprising to find that they are the same.

The following is an outline of hormonal, ovarian, and cervical cycles that we experience each month. I have tried to tie this information together with the *basic self-exam* as I have experienced it on myself, as well as with many other women. It is meant to be a practical guide, leaving room for the fact that each of us is unique, respecting each other's physical differences.

Normal Menstrual Cycle: Day one of the cycle begins with the day that you begin to menstruate. The level of *estrogen* (a hormone secreted by the ovary) is low enough to send a message to the *Pituitary Gland*, which in turn secretes *Follicle Stimulating Hormone* (FSH). The FSH causes a follicle in one of the ovaries to begin to mature into what is called a *Graafian Follicle*. An egg is maturing inside of the Graffian Follicle.

Self Exam: You will see that the os (cervical opening) is somewhat open and the menstrual blood is oozing out of it. There usually is no other discharge during this time.

*Menstrual Cycle: Day 5-14:* The Graafian Follicle produces estrogens. The level of estrogens will increase as you progress towards the day of ovulation. Estrogens cause: 1) the uterine walls to grow thicker. Glands form which will secrete nourish-

483

ment if the egg is fertilized; and 2) the fallopian tubes to contract to help propel the egg into the uterus.

*Self Exam:* During much of this time there will be very little discharge. The os is closed; it appears as a slit. The cervix may be light pink in color. The walls of the vagina usually have a somewhat textured surface and will also be a light color. Because each of us is different from the other, it is important to keep in mind that these are very loose guidelines, helpful only in that they will make you more aware of what to look for.

As the time of ovulation nears, the os will become more open. As the estrogen level rises the discharge from the cervix will become profuse; it will be clear and wet.

*Menstrual Cycle: Day of Ovulation:* The day of ovulation is usually fourteen days before you begin to menstruate. Estrogens are at a high enough level to send a message to the pituitary gland to cut off FSH, and to release *Lutenising Hormone* (LH), which will stimulate the ovarian hormone, *progesterone.* This will trigger the release of the egg. It will break out of the ovary and begin to travel down the fallopian tube, into the uterus. This takes about six and one half days. If the egg is fertilized it will be during the first 24 hours, when the egg is in the outer one-third of the fallopian tube.

*Self-Exam:* The os is open, the cervical mucous is greatly increased, and a clear mucous is commonly found in the open os, called the *Mucous Plug.* This transparent mucous plug is a sign of ovulation. It helps the sperm to get through the cervical opening into the uterus. If you touch it with a sterile Q-tip, you will find that it is stringy and thin. In a few days, if fertilization has not occurred, the mucous plug will disappear. If fertilization occurs the plug thickens and acts as a barrier to keep bacteria from entering the uterus.

Ovulation may be felt by some women as an abdominal pain called *Mittleschmertz.* Some women have a small amount of midcycle vaginal bleeding during this time.

There is a rise in temperature of about 1°F after ovulation,

484

due to a sudden rise in progesterone. This rise occurs abruptly and will remain until the menstrual flow is near or until it begins, when the temperature drops. This temperature shift is useful in determining ovulation. A basal thermometer is recommended in order to give an accurate reading. However, readings with a basal thermometer should be taken over a period of several months in order to be accurate.

*Menstrual Cycle: Days following ovulation. 14-26:* The burst follicle is now called the *Corpus Luteum,* which produces progesterone under the influence of the pituitary hormone *LTH* (leteotropic hormone), as well as estrogens. The corpus luteum continues to secrete progesterone for about eight days.

The uterine walls become thicker and the glands secrete a sugary substance which is used as nourishment if the egg is fertilized. Movement in the fallopian tubes and uterus decreases.

*Self Exam:* The cervical mucous becomes thick and dry; it resembles white paste. This thick dry mucous acts as a barrier to sperm. The os is closed.

*Menstrual Cycle: Days 26-28 or more:* If no fertilization occurs, the estrogens and progesterones production slows to a low level. The corpus luteum is reabsorbed into your body. The lining of the uterus, no longer supported by hormones, starts to disintegrate, and will be sloughed off, coming out of the os as menstrual flow.

*Self Exam:* Many women perceive no visable changes in the vagina, cervix or os during this time. Some women may notice a deepened hue, or the cervix may look larger, the os may be somewhat opened prior to menstruation. It is common to notice a vein or veins on the surface of the cervix immediately before menstruating as well as puffiness in the walls of the vagina. This is usually a sign of water retention. It will disappear after you have menstruated.

*Menstrual Cycle: Days 1-5:* The low level of estrogen will begin sending a message to the pituitary gland. The pituitary

485

will release FSH, which will increase the level of estrogen from the ovary, and the cycle continues.

*Self Exam:* By keeping a log of what you have observed, each time that you examine yourself, you will have a basis for comparison. After several months, you will be able to draw your own conclusions about what is normal for you and when your body deviates from this norm. This information is important for you, in order to have a better understanding of your body. It will also be helpful when you decide to visit a doctor. You will feel more confident about what is happening to you and you will be better equipped to make decisions concerning the type of medical care you want and need.

One of the main focuses of self-help is the cervical self exam. Cervical self-exams are a powerful tool both personally and politically. The knowledge we gain through self-exam enables each of us to reclaim our bodies and gives us the power to decide how they are treated. Becoming familiar with our bodies enables each of us to know what is normal for us. Each woman's body is unique. She will have her own distinct coloring, smell, size, shape, etc. We have found that by doing a cervical exam every other day we have been able to determine what is normal for us and the changes we can expect from one part of our monthly cycle to another.

## *The Basic Self-Exam*

Have a mirror and a flashlight within reach. You will be more comfortable if you urinate before starting the exam.

Start the exam by looking at the outer genitals with a mirror. The most obvious features will be the outer lips (the labia majora) which are covered with pubic hair and the inner lips (labia minora). The labia minora extend toward the pubic bone to form a hood over the shaft of the clitoris. The tip of the clitoris can be seen as a small smooth pink bump. When you spread the lips, the vaginal and urinary openings come into view. During your first examinations you will become

486

familiar with what is normal for you. Later on you will be looking for unusual color changes, irritations, bumps and swellings, breaks in the skin or parasites (such as crabs) which would appear at the base of the pubic hair as small light or dark specks. You should also feel for swellings in both the Skeenes glands and Bartholins glands. The Skeenes glands are located on the sides of the urinary opening. If there is nothing wrong with these glands, you won't be able to see or feel them. The Bartholins glands are located just inside the vaginal opening on both sides of the vagina, just back toward the anus. These glands also will be undetectable if there is nothing wrong.

Next is the examination of the interior genitals with a speculum (an instrument used to spread the walls of the vagina open for easier viewing). Before inserting the speculum, spend some time opening and closing it. Don't insert it until you can open, close and lock it into place easily. The speculum can be inserted in various positions, whichever is most comfortable for you. You can lie down with your knees bent, squat or stand with one leg on a chair or bed. Insert it in whatever position is comfortable for you and stop if it is painful. Relax, take your time. If you need a lubricant you can use water or a water soluable jelly such as KY jelly. Don't use vaseline as it disturbs the natural balance of the vagina. Lubricate your speculum with the paddles closed and the handle in an upright position. Grasping it by the paddles, gently insert it with the paddles closed into the vagina, as you would insert a tampon, until the handle touches the pubic area. Many women prefer to insert the speculum sideways and then turn the handle up. After the handle is in an upright position, pull the two handles together; this will lock the speculum open. When you remove the speculum, pull on the short handle to release it. If you have trouble, have someone help you. Hold the mirror so that you can see your vagina and shine the light into the mirror so that it is reflected into the vagina.

Once the vagina is open, the hymen can be seen just inside the opening. It is different in each woman. It varies from a slight ridge to a flap of skin projecting into the opening. The walls of the vagina will be some shade of pink and textured. The texture and color will vary during the menstrual cycle and from one woman to another. If you're breast-feeding, the walls may be lighter in color and less firm, this also occurs during and after menopause. Water retention may cause puffiness.

At the end of the vagina, you will see the cervix, a smooth round protrusion 1 to 1½ inches in diameter if you have not had children, and larger if you have. The cervix is the tip of your uterus. If you cannot see it, relax, massage your abdomen and it may pop into view. You may have to move the speculum around inside the vagina a bit to find the cervix; sometimes the speculum goes in underneath it. Take your time; if you still can't find it have someone help you. The color as well as the size of the cervix varies from woman to woman and from one part of the menstrual cycle to another. Just before menstruation, the cervix may deepen and become bluish in color. This is due to the build-up of blood and hormonal changes.

In the center of the cervix is the os, the opening to the uterus. The os is usually round in women who have no children and slit-shaped and larger in women who have children. The size and shape of the os will vary from one part of the menstrual cycle to another. There will be a secretion of mucus from the cervix. This is normal. The quantity of mucus varies with each woman. The consistency and color of the mucus change during the menstrual cycle, see the paper on the hormonal cycle for a description of these changes.

After examining yourself, don't unfasten the handles of the speculum, but pull it straight out of the vagina. The paddles of the speculum can pinch the walls of the vagina if they are closed while the speculum is inside the vagina. However, some women find it more comfortable to unfasten the handles before removing the speculum. Do whatever is comfortable for you. After you have removed the speculum, smell the mucus and check the consistency.

The smell will be helpful in detecting infections. A trichamonas infection usually has a strong unpleasant odor and a yeast infection a definite yeasty smell. When you are finished, the speculum should be washed in hot soapy water and kept in a clean place. During the class, it is a good idea to put your name on the handles with masking tape so it won't get mixed up with someone else's.

It's a good idea to record your observations each time you self-exam in a diary or on a calendar. It's valuable to be able to look back and see your natural patterns. Over a period of time, you will be able to tell which changes are normal and recur and which are unusual and may require treatment. Basically, keep track of the day of your cycle, the color and any discolorations of your cervix, the size and shape of your os, the texture and color of your vaginal walls and the amount, kind and smell of secretions.

Following is a guideline for observation:

*Vulva:* color of outer lips; color of inner lips; clitoris, size and position; bartholin and skeenes glands—not normally noticeable unless infected.

*Vaginal Walls:* hymen—shape, color, position; color of walls; texture—puffy, firm, ridged, smooth; surface—clean, patchy, tender.

*Cervix:* color—pink, red, bluish; any spots or discoloration; position.

*Os:* shape—round, slit, smiling, frowning; size—open, closed; IUD string.

*Mucus secretion from os:* color—clear, milky, yellow, brownish, greenish; consistency—thick, thin, stringy, foamy; amount—a lot, little, moderate; smell—bland, acidic, yeasty, fishy; menstrual blood—color, amount.

*General Health Information:* ease of speculum insertion; went off pill, IUD removed; painful intercourse, cauterized; any medication; whatever else you think pertains.

San Francisco Women's Health Center.

# How to Avoid Menstrual Problems

*by Nan Koehler and Donald A. Solomon, M.D.*

First of all, every woman has trouble at one time or another. Our bodies are constantly changing and just when we feel at an equilibrium, we are ushered through another door of life's mysteries. Second, learn as much as you can about the menstrual cycle. Read *Our Bodies, Ourselves; Hygiea* by Jeannine Parvati; *Everywoman's Book* by Paavo Airola; *The Curse: A Cultural History of Menstruation* by Delaney, Lupton & Toth; *Menstruation* by Maddux; *Woman's Body, An Owners Manual,* by the Diagram Group.

Usually, trouble during the period has several origins. I've listed below all the variables I know which effect menstruation (and there must be others). Scan the list and follow the advice that speaks to your condition . . .

1. Follow your cycle carefully so your period doesn't catch you by surprise. One week before it's due, lighten your diet. Eat alkaline foods which means no animal protein, no starches, no acid fruits; just vegetables and whole grains. During this time, eat alot of parsley or drink parsley tea.

2. Keep your fluid intake high — drink at least two quarts of water or tea per day. Starting one week before your period, drink a female toner tea blend such as Blessed (Holy) Thistle, Red Raspberry leaves, Skullcap leaves, and Licorice root.

   It's very important that you prepare and ingest the teas properly. Mix the herbs in equal parts and store them in an air tight container (not metal). Place a tsp. of herb mixture in a one quart jar with a lid. Boil the water in a separate pot and pour a quart of boiling water into the jar containing the herbs. Let it steep for several minutes, then sip the tea all day as though you were taking medicine. This is to

490

maintain the level of the herbal alkaloids in your body. The most important thing is to keep all metal; spoons, tea balls, pots, etc.; away from the herbs. Metal deactivates the alkaloids, the plant chemicals which alter or affect your body chemistry.

Teas you can try:

*Irregular cycles*—Sarsaparilla, Holy Thistle, Squaw Vine (Mitchella repens), Black Haw and Licorice Root. Drink 3-4 cups daily for at least 3 cycles.

*Menstrual cramps*—Calcium and Magnesium and herbs high in Calcium and Magnesium such as Parsley, Sage, Comfrey, Borage, Horsetail, Oat Straw, Nettles. Camomile tea helps you to relax which relieves cramps, as well as Catnip, Ginger Root, Lemon Balm, Peppermint or Alfalfa. Use what you have.

*To increase the flow*—Squaw Vine; make a tea of the berries and sip all day.

*To decrease the flow*—Shepherd's Purse, White Oak Bark, the root of Rushes or Blackberries. For severe bleeding, press the inside of the leg about 5" below the knee on both legs at the same time.

*To bring on your period*—Pennyroyal, Rue, Ginger, Tansy, Sweet Basil, Birthwort, Rosemary, Black Cohosh, Mugwort, or Cotton Root. There are many emmenagoges. Use them singly or in a combination and use what you have.

3. Take vitamins on a regular basis and you'll be amazed how terrific they make you feel.

   A—25,000 IU/day to prevent infections, especially herpes.

   B Complex—50 mgm/day for edema and irritability.

   C Complex—2,000 mgm/day (at least) for fighting infections and increasing cell wall strength to prevent excess bleeding. (Recent research shows that along with Ascorbic Acid, 2,000 mgm, you need at least 100 mgm of Bioflavinoids, 50 mgm of rutin and 25 mgm of hesperidin.)

Iron and Folic Acid — 20 mgm/day elemental iron and 1 mgm/day of folic acid to prevent anemia.

E — 800 IU/day to improve circulation, control excess bleeding and regulate hormones.

Minerals — especially Calcium and Magnesium. 2,000 mgm/day Ca and at least 40 mgm/day Mg for cramps relaxation.

4. Many of the other symptoms of menstruation are due to a faulty diet which results in low blood sugar and/or anemia. In summary, these are the changes which will strengthen your body and eliminate the uncomfortable symptoms of our monthly changes. Eliminate meat (or eat meat sparingly), eat Brewer's yeast, cold pressed oils (at least 1 Tsp,/day), kelp, lecithin, Calcium, Magnesium, iron rich foods such as eggs, apricots, whole grains, seeds, legumes, nuts, grapes, raisins, beets, spinach, prunes, bananas, liver and high quality proteins. High quality proteins are buckwheat, millet, sunflower seeds, pumpkin seeds, sesame seeds, soybeans, peanuts, almonds, cheese, eggs, fish, green leafy vegetables, avocados, and potatoes. See pp. 345-355, *Everywoman's Book* by Paavo Airola.

5. Take hot baths, several times a day if needed, especially submerging your legs and hips.

6. When your period is due, try to make love. It's a relatively infertile time of your cycle so you can relax about pregnancy worries and let the sexual stimulation give relief from the lower pelvic engorgement. If you don't have a sexual partner, masturbate to relieve the engorgement.

7. Many "primitive" people consider the time of menstruation a time of taboo for the woman. She can't cook, work in the fields, eat certain foods or participate in many of the normal tribal activities. In short, it's a rest period when her normal duties are suspended and she can totally relax. Wouldn't it be wonderful if we had such an institution today. At least we can give ourselves some space to retreat during that time of the month.

February, 1980.

This handout is intended for women who have had a Gynecological evaluation to rule out organic disease and then choose biological remedies rather than chemical treatment.

# To Help Your Flow

*by Laura Burns*

## To Aid Elimination During Menstruation

Menstruation is the eliminative cycle in a woman's body. It is a natural form of detoxification. Often, right before the period starts, there are lymphatic swellings, maybe a slight sore throat, mucous discharge, etc. As soon as the period begins, these symptoms are gone. Take advantage of this time and help your body out! Eat lightly or fast a couple of days before menstruation is to begin. Drink a good tea that will help build the blood and facilitate the eliminative process: 1 part Yellow Dock Root; 1 part Red Clover Blossoms; 1 part Burdock Root; 1 part Nettles; 1 part Cassia Bark (Chinese Cinnamon).

If your blood is strong, it is easier to eliminate toxins through it without any debilitating effects on your system.

## Strengthening Your System

Next, work with the building and strengthening cycle. It is best to do this right around ovulation (both physical and lunar) as this is the height of this flow. Drink a food uterine tonic: 1 part Holy Thistle; 1 part Sarsaparilla; 1 part Cramp Bark; 1 part Licorice Root; 1 part Squaw Vine.

Remember as you strengthen and build your system, you also increase your fertility. Your cycle should become more regular and your flow healthier.

## Normalizing Your System

If you are relating to your menstrual cycle with herbs that

493

are being used for their abortive effect (see *Well-Being* issue #4), please be aware of what they do to your system. You are depending upon their irritating quality on the uterine lining and muscles to be effective. The constant use of irritants can tend to weaken the organ and create imbalances within your entire uterine system. If you do take any of those herbs (pennyroyal, tansy, etc.) regularly during your menstrual cycle, a good tonic at some point each month should be drunk to help normalize and tone up your glandular system: 1 part Holy Thistle; 1 part Raspberry Leaves; 1 part Blue Vervain; 1 part Nettle Leaves; 1 part Siberian Ginseng. This tea will *not* increase fertility.

To prepare these teas use 5 cups of water and 1 Tbs. of each herb. Simmer roots and bark for 20 minutes, add leaves and blossoms and steep 10 more minutes.

In Chinese medicine, the female system is related to the bladder meridian. The time of elimination of this flow is about 3:00-5:00 in the afternoon. Try drinking tea at this time! By working with our natural flows in this way, a balance begins to be created within us. Relating to our body with such a harmonious attitude not only strengthens us physically, but also has a positive effect on our emotions as well.

Laura Burns is Vice President of the Christos School of Natural Healing, Taos, New Mexico.

Reprinted from Well-Being Magazine, Feb. 1978.

# *Treating Mild Vaginitis*

## *by Nan Koehler, June 1980*

It's important to understand that the yeast, trichomonas, or bacteria that are bothering you now have overgrown the bacteria that normally reside in your vagina. The organisms that are causing symptoms multiply on the vaginal secretions when your body chemistry is out of balance. Their waste products irritate the tissues of your vagina, which in turn causes itching, which when indulged, irritates the area even more.

The usual medical remedies will give you prompt relief, but won't solve the underlying problem which set off the chain of events resulting in the vaginal infection. Treating it with home remedies and some change in your basic diet and lifestyle will permanently solve your problem. (If the condition is advanced pharmaceutical remedies may be required, however lasting resolution will come only with additional basic change.)

The first rule for using home remedies is to catch whatever condition you are treating early! So at the first hint of vaginal disturbance—odd smell, increased discharge, itching, raw sensation, burning (especially with urination or coitus), check where you are in your cycle. Then take the appropriate steps enumerated below.

1. Stop eating sugar or honey.

2. Go to bed early; get more rest.

3. Drink more fluids. Aim for 2-3 quarts of water or, even better, 2-3 pots of a blood purifying tea a day.

4. Do an alkaline diet—lightly steamed or raw vegetables, nuts, and alkaline grains—until the condition clears.

5. Take extra vitamins. 2-4 grams C, 100 mg B complex, 50,000 IU A, 1000 IU E; and Minerals with at least 1000 mg Ca and 500 mg Mg.

6. Wash more often. You might enjoy a water spash after urination or a baking soda or apple cider vinegar sitz bath 3-4 times a day. 1-2 tsp. baking soda or 1/8 cup apple cider vinegar per quart warm water.

7. Fast for fast results. Liquids and vitamins only for 24 hours. During the fast, drink apple cider vinegar tea (2 tsp. per cup of warm water) every 4 hours.

# Herbal Abortion

November 10, 1981                    Nan Ullrike Koehler

What follows is a how-to guide for doing an herbal abortion. I and several of my friends have used this method and know it to be *safe* and effective.

*Prerequisites* for using this method:

1. Keep a chart of your monthly cycle in some reliable way (ovulation method, mucus, basal temperature, etc.). You need to be aware of your rhythm so that you can accurately predict your fertile and menstrual times each month.

2. Procedures for an herbal abortion must be started before you expect to bleed. *If you wait until you have missed your period, it will be too late to use this method effectively.*

If you made love with a man during your fertile time (for example, on days 10-16 in a 28 day cycle), and you do not wish to be pregnant, here is what you do:

1. After unprotected intercourse on a potentially fertile day, begin eating 5-10 apricot kernels 3 times a day. Continue this until your period comes. This prevents implantation. (The same effect can be achieved with high levels of Vit C. But I personally haven't used Vit. C in this way. Use more than 10 grams per day.)

2. Three to five days before you expect your period, do a fast or a semi-fast (eat lightly, aiming for an alkaline diet, and eliminate all animal proteins). Also make an effort to be extra physically active during this time. This will give your body the direct message that this is not a time to foster the growth of a baby.

3. Do herbal teas. Choose from the emmenagogues: bay, black cohosh, cotton root, pennyroyal, rue, squaw vine,

496

tansy, yarrow, etc. To make the tea: Pour one quart of boiling water over one teaspoon of the herb or herbs in a glass quart jar. Do not let the tea come into contact wth metal. Sip this tea throughout the day. The idea is not to poison yourself, but rather to keep the level of the herb constant in your body. Again, you are giving your body the message that this is not an appropriate time for growing a baby. Continue with the teas until your period comes.

4. Insert fresh parsley into your vagina. Wash the parsley, cut off the stems and place the parsley high up in your vagina. The herb is irritating to the uterus and it will help encourage your period to come.

An additional method may be used in conjunction with the above steps. I have not tried this method, but my friend Jeanine Rose has reported success with it: Take one capsule of evening primrose oil (prostaglandins) 3-4 times a day. Theoretically, this will help soften the cervix, which opens to release the menstrual flow. The oil may also be applied directly to your cervix.

In summary, this regime is simple, easy and safe. Chart your cycle, chew apricot kernels, sip teas, work hard and take positive action to achieve your goal of total self mastery.

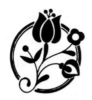

# Reading List on Birth Control, Abortion, and Related Subjects

*compiled by Nan Koehler, February 1984*

## BIRTH CONTROL

1. Billings, John, *The Ovulation Method.* American Edition, Borromeo Guild, 1530 W. 9th St. Los Angeles, CA 90015.
2. Garfink, Christine and Piper, Hank, *The New Birth Control Program.* Bolder Books, Hampstead Hall Press, 10 East 40th St., New York, NY 10016. $4.95.
3. Guay, Terrie, *Creation of Life, Your Choice* (Expansion of *Avoid or Achieve Pregnancy Naturally*). Emergence Publication, 185 Beacon Hill, Ashland, OR 97520. (503) 482-0666. $6.95.
4. Jackson, Mildred, *Mental Birth Control.* Lawton-Teague Publication, P.O. Box 656, Oakland, CA 94606. $3.00.
5. Kass, Barbara-Annese, et. al., *Fertility Awareness.* Telesis Corporation, P.O. Box 681, San Francisco, CA. $10.00.
6. Kippley, John and Shelia, *The Art of Natural Family Planning.* Couple to Couple League International Inc., P.O. Box 11084, Cincinnati, Ohio 45211. $4.95.
7. Kippley, Shelia, *Breastfeeding and Natural Child Spacing.* Penguin Press.
8. Lacey, Louise, *Lunaception.*
9. Nofziger, Margaret, *A Cooperative Method of Natural Birth Control.* The Book Publishing Company, Summertown, Tenn. 38483. $3.95.
10. Nofziger, Margaret, *The Fertility Question.* The Book Publishing Company, Summertown, Tenn. 38483. $4.95.
11. Rosenblum, Art, *The Natural Birth Control Book.* Aquarian Research Foundation, Box P-4120, 5128 Morton St., Philadelphia, Penn. 19144. $3.00.
12. Shivananda, Mary, *Natural Sex.* Berkeley Books, Berkeley Publishing Corp., 200 Madison Ave., New York, NY 10016. $2.75.
13. Tucker, Tarvez, *Birth Control.* Women's Library Tobey Publication Company Inc., Box 428, New Canaan, Conn. 06840. $2.95.
14. Emergence Publication, *Avoid or Achieve Pregnancy Naturally.* 185 Beacon Hill, Ashland, OR 97502. $3.00
15. Baker, Jeannine Parvati and Rico, *Conscious Conception; Elemental Journey Through the Labyrinth of Sexuality.*

## RELATED SUBJECTS (Herbs, Health, Spirituality)

1. Adsen, Coral and Horowitz, Deena, *Taking Control: A Guide to Self Healing for Women.* C/O P.O. Box 2324, Santa Cruz, CA 95063.
2. Airola, Paavo, *Everywomen's Book.* Health Press Publication, P.O. Box 22001, Phoenix, Arizona 85028.
3. Inayat, Taj, *The Crystal Chalice, Spiritual Themes for Women.* Sufi Order Publication, P.O. Box 396, New Lebanon, New York, $4.75.
4. Morgan, Robin, *Sisterhood is Powerful.* Vintage Book, V-539 Random House. $2.45.
5. Parvati, Jeannine, *Hygieia, A Woman's Herbal.* Freestone Collective Books. Bookpeople, 2940 7th St., Berkeley, CA 94710. $10.00.
6. Hamilton, Richard, *The Herpes Book.* J. P. Tacher Inc., 911 Summit Blvd., Los Angeles, CA 90069. $9.95.
7. Shafrey, Mary Jane, *The Nature and Evolution of Female Sexuality.* Penguin Press.
8. Washborn, Penelope, *Seasons of Woman.* Harper and Row Publication, 10 E. 53rd St., New York, NY 10022. $7.95.
9. Lichtendorf, Susan S., *Eve's Journey: The Physical Experience of Being Female.* A Berkeley Book, 200 Madison Ave., New York, NY 18016. $2.95.
10. Padus, Emrika, *The Woman's Encyclopedia of Health and Natural Healing.* Rodale Press, Emmaus, PA. $19.95.
11. Britton, Bryce, *The Love Muscle.* A Plume Book, New American Library, Inc., 1633 Broadway, New York, NY 10019. $7.95.

## ABORTIONS

1. *The Right to Abortion.* A Psychiatric View by Group for the Advancement of Psychiatry Committee on Psychiatry and Law. Charles Scribner's Sons. New York, NY $1.95.
2. Gage, Suzanne, *When Birth Control Fails.* Speculum Press, P.O. Box 1063, Hollywood, CA 90028. $5.95.
3. Lett, Alexsandra, *Herbal Abortion: Using Plants to Induce Miscarriage.* P.O. Box 430, Yellow Springs, Ohio 45387. $3.50.
4. Wilke, Dr. and Mrs., *Handbook on Abortion.* Hiltz and Huges Publication Co., Inc., Cincinnati, Ohio 45224. (513) 681-7559. $1.50.

P.S. There are two new books soon to appear to watch for: one on *Conscious Conception* by Jeannine Parvati, and *A Woman's Herbal* by Jeanne Rose.

# Herpes Handout

*from Common Women's Health Project, Santa Rosa, CA*

Since 50% of the population has had cold sores/fever blisters (type 1), they will have an elevated antibody level whether or not their present sore is herpes. The titer *is* useful in confirming the diagnosis of an *initial* outbreak of herpes when there has been no previous exposure to either Type 1 or Type 2.

## TREATMENT

While there is no "cure" for herpes, many remedies, prescription and non-prescription, are available to minimize the length of time of an outbreak as well as some to possibly prevent recurrences.

*Acyclovir*, a synthetic substance sold under the brand name Zovirax, is the newest treatment for genital herpes infections. Zovirax is a prescription cream, which is applied to the sores six times a day for a week. It costs about $20 a tube. Studies show that the ointment speeds healing in initial outbreaks, but is less effective in recurrent infections. Acyclovir does not prevent new lesions from appearing during an outbreak and does not prevent recurrences. As a new drug, the long term safety is not known.

*Lysine* is an essential amino acid derived from food sources and also available in capsule supplements. It has been found effective in suppressing recurrences and speeding healing time. Recommended doses during an outbreak range from 1500 mg to 3000 mg daily (500-1000 mg taken 3x/day). Maintenance doses of 500 mg/day may prevent recurrences. When obtaining supplements, *L-Lysine* is preferable to Lysine. Lysine in combination with arginine should not be used because arginine, another amino acid, may support the growth of herpes. It is thought that a diet deficient in lysine and high in arginine can trigger an attack. (See food chart for lysine and arginine amounts in certain foods.

500

*Ice* has been found to be effective by some people. It can shorten an attack, relieve its discomfort, and can even prevent an outbreak. When the "prodrome" is felt or a sore appears, apply ice (in a plastic bag) directly to the sensitive area for 90 minutes.

One basic rule is to keep the genital area clean and dry with normal bathing. Besides this, there are dozens of methods that have been tried by people with recurring herpes. These methods are not standard treatments nor have they been proven effective by medical scientists, but they are methods devised and used successfully by those who have Herpes. Keep in mind that each remedy may not work for everyone. Remember that mucous membranes (urethra, vagina, cervix, inner labia, anus) are more sensitive than your skin so try remedies a little at a time.

## EXTERNAL REMEDIES TO RELIEVE SYMPTOMS OF ITCHING AND PAIN:

1. *Baths:* Hot baths, cold baths and baking soda baths.

2. *Local Anesthetics:* Apply to the affected area; Compress soaked in a tea made with cloves (boil 1 Tbsp. cloves for 10 mins.). Black tea bags which have been soaked in hot water. The tannic acid is the anesthetic. Pepperment oil, Clove oil.

3. Baking soda, corn starch, hone, witch hazel, wheat germ oil, vitamin E oil, aloe vera gel, have all been recommended to be applied to the sores or infected areas.

4. *Poultices:* Make a paste using any of the following with warm water; spread between layers of sterile gauze or apply paste directly to sores; keep moistened with warm water. Pulverized calcium tablets; powdered slippery elm, myrrh, comfrey root; volcanic ash (moisten frequently with water, as it's hard to remove when dry); cold milk compresses applied locally for 5-10 minutes 5-6 times a day.

5. *Clendula Tincture:* Applied directly to active sores.

6. *ViraHelp:* Is a new topical ointment that is an herbal/homeopathic combination of the following ingredients: comfrey, zinc, lysine, lithium, thymus, copper, manganese, ranunculus and BHT as a preservative, in natural gels. Applied in the "prodrome" this gel has for some people relieved itching and burning symptoms almost immediately and many times the outbreak did not occur.

7. *G-Jo Acupressure Point:* Pressure by fingertips if used just as symptoms begin to appear, may prevent an attack. Also relieves pain and discomfort. The point is located the width of 3 thumbs forward of the crown of the outer ankle bulge, along a line between the ankle bulge and the little toe. To stimulate the point, probe the area with the tip of your finger or thumb, until you feel a distinct twinge of sensitivity. Stimulate both feet as deeply as you can tolerate.

8. *Acupuncture:* A treatment may be effective, if you can locate someone who performs this service.

9. *Topical Xylocaine:* May help soothe and numb the area of outbreak.

## THESE REMEDIES MAY HELP SHORTEN AN ATTACK:

1. To dry up sores: Aloe vera, rubbing alcohol (may be quite stinging—but works for some people), calendula tincture, eucalyptus oil. Sunlight may help dry up sores, but it has also been shown to trigger an outbreak.

2. It's helpful to wear cotton underwear or no underwear at all during the prodrome or outbreak. Nylon underwear, pantyhose, and tight pants create a very moist and irritating environment.

3. Some use mind visualization and/or meditation of healthy genitals, to help shorten or lessen your attack.

4. The healing philosophy of color therapy maintains that the visualization of certain colors can affect your health. Visualizing blue is good for inflammations; reds and oranges bring up inflammations; gold is a strengthening color and green is a balance.

*Remember:* Everyone's body is different and different remedies will affect us differently. In managing herpes, it is important to have a test *first* to confirm the presence of this particular virus as opposed to your rash/outbreak being caused by something other than herpes. Talking with a practitioner, friends/partners with herpes will help in deciding which path to take in using different remedies.

## VITAMINS AND NUTRITION

Maintenance of good physical condition will be very helpful in preventing recurrent outbreaks, length of outbreaks, and susceptibility to contracting herpes in the first place.

*Nutrition:* As mentioned under "treatment," the ratio of amino acids lysine and arginine should be balanced in our diets to help prevent recurrences of herpes outbreaks. A 1:1 ratio is advised during latent stages and a balance favoring lysine is recommended during active outbreaks. L-lysine capsules can help with this maintenance also. See the chart "Diet for Herpes Control" for a list of foods high in lysine and arginine. One helpful hint is to avoid those foods highest in arginine or at least balance them immediately with foods equivalently high in lysine or with L-lysine capsules. When you are in a lowered state of resistance, (Fatigue, emotional stress, fever, menstruation, etc.) you may even want to avoid the foods which are at the middle or low end of the scale in amounts of arginine.

*Vitamins:* Vitamins A and C, in combination with L-lysine are believed to interfere directly with the spread of herpes virus in the infected tissue. Vitamin E and B are thought to improve circulation and allow greater amounts of the L-lysine to

503

## Diet for Herpes Control

### High-Lysine Foods
(Foods to Eat)

| mg excess lysine | food | portion |
|---|---|---|
| +930 | fresh fish | 4 oz |
| +880 | shark | 4 oz |
| +810 | canned fish | 4 oz |
| +740 | chicken | 4 oz |
| +720 | beef | 4 oz |
| +520 | goat's milk | 1 cu |
| +420 | cow's milk | 1 cu |
| +420 | lamb | 4 oz |
| +410 | mung beans, cooked | 1/2 cu |
| +380 | pork | 4 oz |
| +280 | cheese, all types | 1 oz |
| +270 | beans, cooked | 1/2 cu |
| +240 | lima beans | 1/2 cu |

### High-Arginine Foods
(Foods to Avoid)

| portion | food | mg lysine deficency |
|---|---|---|
| 1/2 cu | hazel nuts | −2250 |
| 1/2 cu | brazil nuts | −2110 |
| 1/2 cu | peanuts | −2060 |
| 1/2 cu | walnuts | −810 |
| 1/2 cu | almonds | −710 |
| 1/2 cu | cocoa powder | −650 |
| 2 tb | peanut butter | −510 |
| 1/2 cu | sesame seeds | −450 |
| 1/2 cu | cashews | −420 |
| 1/2 cu | carob powder | −310 |
| 1/2 cu | coconut | −290 |
| 1/2 cu | pastachio nuts | −240 |
| 1/2 cu | whole wheat flour | −230 |

| | | | | |
|---|---|---|---|---|
| +220 | cottage cheese, dry | ½ cu | ½ cu chickpeas (garbanzos) | −210 |
| +210 | mung bean sprouts | ½ cu | ½ cu brown rice | −190 |
| +190 | yeast, brewer's | 1 tb | ½ cu pecans | −180 |
| +170 | crustaceans | 4 oz | 4 sl whole wheat bread | −160 |
| +130 | soybeans, cooked | ½ cu | ½ cu oatmeal, cooked | −130 |
| +120 | egg | 1 | ½ cu raisins | −130 |
| +100 | human milk | 1 cu | ½ cu sunflower seeds | −120 |

These foods contain more lysine than arginine. For example, a 4 oz. serving of fish contains 930 mg of excess lysine. This is about equal to two 500 mg L-lysine tablets.

These foods contain more arginine than lysine, so there is a deficiency in lysine. For example, if you eat ½ cup of peanuts, you have about a 2,000 mg lysine deficiency. You need to balance this with four 500 mg. tablets of L-lysine, or by eating 2,000 mg of high-lysine foods.

Used by permission © 1981 Crittenden-North Concepts.

reach remote skin tissues. B complex also helps with stress. A very good source of B vitamins is Brewer's Yeast. Increasing your intake of Zinc and Calcium supplements may also be helpful.

NOTE: Large doses of some vitamins and minerals can sometimes be harmful. Check with health food store personnel, health practitioners, and resource books on vitamins. HERBS can also be helpful topically in poultices and taken in capsule forms or teas. Like vitamins/minerals, some are very potent and should be taken with full information/research in regards to dosages.

HERPES AND PREGNANCY

If you have recurrent genital herpes, your major concern is that the baby may pick up the virus by contact during passage through the birth canal at the time of delivery. Infections of the fetus in the womb have been reported. These are very rare and only occur from primary infections acquired during pregnancy. The virus manages to be transported by the bloodstream across the placental barrier to infect the fetus. This does not occur with recurrent herpes, since it is highly localized. The important thing to remember is to work closely with your physician or midwife during the last few months of your pregnancy to determine if there is an outbreak on your cervix. If everything is clear, a caeserean will not be necessary. Close monitoring of the state of the birth canal all the way through the pregnancy and especially near the time of delivery is what's important. You can nurse your baby, just don't let her/him come in contact with the sores in any way. Exercise the same precautions for cleansing as discussed above and be careful not to transfer the virus from your sores-fingers-to the baby. This is very important since herpes presents a great risk to newborns and infants up to six months, as they have a 50% fatality rate if infected.

We encourage you to call us here at Commonwoman's Health Project with any questions, experiences, or information about herpes. **578-1700.**

## REFERENCES USED IN THIS SHEET:

*Herpes: What To Do When You Have It,* by Oscar Gillespie, Ph.D., co-founder of New York Help. Grosset & Dunlap, 1982. $4.95.

*Santa Cruz Women's Health Center Newsletter,* March 1983 and *Herpes* pamphlet and supplement.

Advances in Preventive Health Series; *HERPES! Something Can Be Done About It!* Third printing. $1.50.

## OTHER RESOURCES:

The Herpes Resource Center; 260 Sheridan Avenue, Palo Alto, CA 94306, (415) 328-7710. This group has a lot of up-to-date information about research on herpes.

National VD Hotline: 800-982-5883.

Reprinted by permission of Commonwoman's Health Project, Suite H, 2200 County Center Drive, Santa Rosa, CA 95401.

# *Herbal Directory*

*pages 14-15 from the 1984
Calendar of Herb School Events*

A partial listing of herbalists and organizations that, through their services, are creating a better Planet. Most of the following are friends we have worked with over the years and each comes highly recommended as a resource for well being. If we have forgotten a name, please forgive us (hold it not personally) — just send us names and addresses and we'll include in next years directory.

**Hygeia College.** c/o Jeannine Parvati Baker. Author, herbalist, midwife, correspondence course. Hygeia College will happen in Hawaii, May 13-20, 1984. To register: Box 953, Captain Cook, Hawaii; Box 398, Monroe, Utah 84754.

**Emerald Valley Herb Nursery.** c/o Tim Blakley. Teacher and staff of CSHS. Specialize in medicinal and culinary herbs and native plants. 9309 Hwy. 116, Forestville, CA 95436.

507

**Trinity Herb Co.** Wholesaler of organic and wildcrafted herbs. 874-3418, P.O. Box 199, Bodega, CA 94922.

**Rob Madrone Menzies.** Naturalist, botanist, herbalist, author and teacher. Box 915, Cecilville, CA 96018.

**Breitenbush Hot Springs.** Retreat Center, mineral waters, healing community. P.O. Box 578, Detroit, Oregon 97342.

**Optimal Health Institute.** c/o Svevo Brooks. Full service health clinic, Bach flower remedies, bee products and hydrotherapy. Classes and seminars. 81900 Mahr Lane, Creswell, Oregon 97426.

**Heartwood Health Institute.** Certified Massage Program and wholistic Health Program—beautiful country campus and heartfelt staff. 220 Harmony Lane, Garberville, CA 95440.

**Jane Bothwell.** Staff member CSHS. Private counselling, herb classes, Bach flower remedies. Box 155, Camp Meeker, CA.

**Bear Tribe Society.** c/o Wabun and Sunbear. Authors and hosts of the Medicine Wheel Gatherings—a tribal gathering for all on Native American healing ways and walking in balance. Seminars. Box 9167, Spokane, WA 99209.

**Atlantis Rising.** c/o Joseph Montagne. Educational Center, Botanical Research Center, Herbal pharmaceutical company. 15 volume Universal Pharmacopoeia, People's Desk Reference Correspondence course. 7909 S.E. Stark, Portland, Oregon 97215.

**Nalini Chilkov.** Herb classes and walks, private practice. (415) 388-0421.

**Herbalist & Alchemist Inc.** c/o David Winston. Teacher and wildcrafter. Wholesale/retail Chinese herbs, herbal products, correspondence courses. 63 Franklin Park, NJ 08823.

**National Institute of Medical Herbalists.** c/o Silena Heron. One year correspondence course, classes, herb walks and leader of ceremony/ritual. 115 Oak Drive, San Rafael, CA 94901.

**Dance of the Deer Foundation.** c/o Brant Secunda. Ceremony and ritual of the heart. Classes, retreats, apprenticeship program, teaches the art of prayer. Box 699, Soquel, CA 95073.

**Self Heal Herbal Center.** c/o James and Mindy Green. Herb store, school. Classes, apprenticeship program. 4725 Eales Rd. RR6, Victoria, B.C., Canada.

**The Herbal Gazette Newsletter.** Box 491, Mt. Kisco, NY 10549.

**The Business of Herbs Magazine.** P.O. Box 559, Madison, Virginia 22727.

508

**Association for the Promotion of Herbal Healing.** Prints a quarterly newsletter update of herbs. 2000 Center St., Suite 1475, Berkeley, CA 94709.

**Earth Star Botanicals.** c/o Garbriele Howearth. Seed Catalogue. All bio-organically homegrown.

**Rosemary's Garden.** Old fashion herbal apothecary. Mail catalogue. Box 350, Guerneville, CA 95446.

**Healing Yourself.** c/o Jay Gardner. Books on herbs. 45 Linden St., Victoria, B.C., Canada V8V.4C9.

**Steven Foster.** Herbalist, author. Box 454, Mt. View, AR 72560.

**Independent Chemistry Consulting.** For the advanced use of natural substances. P.O. Box 606, San Rafael, CA 94915.

**Peter Holmes.** Herbalist, teacher. 314 West Gomez, Santa Fe, New Mexico 87501.

**Jade Easter.** Herbalist, teacher, author. c/o Heartwood College, 200 Harmony Lane, Garberville, CA.

**Norma Meyers.** Native Indian herbalist, teacher and healer. Box 46506, Station G. Vancouver, B.C. V6R.4G7. Norma moves around a lot, so this address may have changed.

**Orr Hot Springs.** Healing waters, Retreat center and community. 13201 Orr Springs Rd., Ukiah, CA 95482.

**School of Clinical Herbology.** c/o Michael Moore. Teacher, author, counsellor. An excellent school and clinic with wildcrafted herbs and herbal products. 319 Aztec, Sante Fe, New Mexico 87501.

**New Age Creations.** c/o Jeanne Rose. Herb classes, books, products. 219 Carl St., San Francisco, CA 91342.

**Herb Pharms.** c/o Ed Smith. Excellent wildcrafted herbal products, apprenticeship program. P.O. Box 116, Williams, Oregon 97544.

**Nan Koehler.** Excellent botanist, herbalist and midwife. Classes, herb walks. 13140 Frati Lane, Sebastopol, CA 95472.

**Marina Bokelman.** Teacher, herbalist and researcher. Wildcrafted herbal products. Medicine Flower. 14670 Blind Shady Rd., Nevada City, CA 95959.

**Dr. Paul Lee.** (408) 423-7923. 129 Spring, Santa Cruz, CA.

**Oak Valley Herb Farm.** c/o Kathie Keville. Herbalist. Classes, retreats, products, garden. Star. Camptonville, CA 95922.

509

**Trout Lake Herb Farm.** A beautiful herb farm located near Mt. Adams. Wholesale organic medicinal and culinary herbs. Rt. 1, Box 355, Trout Lake, Washington 98650.

**Ethen Nebelkopf.** Author, teacher and herb counsellor. Clinic classes. 1614A Harman, Berkeley, CA 94703.

**Ojai Foundation.** Wholistic programs. P.O. Box 1620, Ojai, CA.

**Subhudti Dharmananda.** c/o Institute of Traditional Medicine School Newsletter. 215 John Street, Santa Cruz, CA 95060.

**East West Master Course in Herbology.** c/o Michael Tierra. Teacher, author, acupuncturist and clinic, 36 lesson correspondence course, classes, treatments and private counselling. 3254B Mission Drive, Santa Cruz, CA

**Wishing Well Distributing Co.** New Age health products and aids. P.O. Box 819, Sebastopol, CA 95472.

**Well Being Community Center.** A non-profit educational organization dedicated to spreading information on health and well being. Offers a free monthly publication called Well Being Community Calendar. 6270 Carlotta Ct., Sebastopol, CA 95472.

**Cascade Anderson.** Classes, counselling, herb walks, seminars. 1934 S.E. 56th Ave., Portland, OR 97215.

**Christopher Hobbs.** Herbal botanist. Classes, wildcrafter. c/o Platonic Academy, Box 409, Santa Cruz, CA 95061.

**Christopher Nyerges.** Author. Classes, herb walks. 5830 Burwood Ave., Los Angeles, CA 90042.

**Nam Singh.** Chinese herbalist and Taoist minister. Private counselling. Chinese herbal medicine classes, Tai Chi classes, acupuncture treatments. 654 Cole St., San Francisco, CA 94117.

**Gabriell Howearth.** Master gardener and seed man. 10417 Highway 238, Jacksonville, Oregon 97530.

**Granpa "Hugs" Roberts.** 90 year old Elder and Medicine Pipe Man. Classes and counselling. 9309 Hwy. 116, Forestville, CA 95436.

**Flower Essence Society.** P.O. Box 459, Nevada City, CA 95959.

**Bea Meyers.** Teacher and saint. Gardens, herbs and plants. 9710 River Road, Forestville, CA 95436.

**Taylors Herb Garden.** A huge variety of beautiful herb plants and gardens. Classes, herb walks. 1535 Lone Oak Drive, Vista, CA 92083.

**Chela Bear.** Herbalist and teacher. c/o Heartwood College. 200 Harmony Lane, Garberville, CA.

510

**Marylee Bytherwin.** Herbalist, botanist, plant identification walks. Box 1655, Redway, CA 95560.

**Christine Devai.** President of Ontario Herbalists Association. General delivery, Macksons Point, Ontario, Canada LOE ILO.

**Herb News.** Newsletter. P.O. Box 12602, Austin, TX 78711.

**School of Natural Healing.** c/o David Christopher. Herbal training, seminars, products, books. P.O. Box 412, Springville, Utah 84663.

**Turtle Island Herbs.** Mail order catalogue specializing in tinctures. (303) 442-2215, Salina Star Route, Boulder, Colorado 80302.

**North American Herbs.** Herbal products catalogue. Organic and wildcrafted products. (503) 863-6115, 309 N. Myrtle Road., Myrtle Creek, OR 97457.

**Platonic Academy.** c/o Dr. Paul Lee. Herb School. Box 409, Santa Cruz, CA 95061.

**Peace Seeds.** Planetary gene pool service—a seed collection. 1130 Tetherow Rd., Williams, OR 97544.

**Old Mill Farm.** School of country living. Box 463, Mendocino, CA 95460.

**Herb Research Foundation.** c/o Rob McCaleb. Newsletter and research program. 1780 55th St., Boulder, CO 80301.

**Rosemary House.** Herb catalogue of delightful items. 120 S. Market St., Mechanicsburg, PA 17055.

**River City Herb Society.** c/o Harvest McCampbell. Newsletter of local events for Sacramento area. Box 30, Carmichael, CA 95609.

**Mother Earth Works.** c/o Cindy Parker. Herb shop and wholistic learning center. 373 Mt. Vernon Rd., Newark, Ohio 43055.

**Talisman.** c/o Gwendolyn Raush. Newsletter of Seattle wholistic events. 2970 30th Ave. S., Seattle, WA 98144.

**Medicine Ways.** c/o Adelle Getty and Sunwater. Teachers of Native American healing ways. Classes, seminars, apprentice programs. 6000 Gericke Rd., Petaluma, CA 94952.

**New Age School of Massage.** c/o Catherine Osterbye. Certified massage program, special herbs and massage program. Box 958, Sebastopol, CA 95472.

**David Cavagnaro.** Extraordinary gardener, author, botanist and nationally published photographer. Photography workshops. 2665 Leslie Rd., Santa Rosa, CA 95404.

**Denise Diamond.** Author, maker of flower essences, gardener and teacher. Box 1101, Bolinas, CA 94924.

**Abundant Life Seed Foundation.** c/o Forest Shomer. Dedicated to perpetuating the seed life-force. Experimental gardens, research foundation, store and mail order company. Lectures. Box 772, Port Townsend, WA 98368.

**Kim Blair, herbalist.** c/o Windflower Herbals. Herbal products, classes, walks. 21697 Montgomery Rd., Sonora, CA 95370.

**Jessie Longacre.** Botanist, herbalist, naturalist and author, mushroom and seaweed expert. Weekly herb walks, camping trips. 9309 Hwy. 116, Forestville, CA 95436.

**Marcia Stark.** Medical herbalist, author and lecturer. P.O. Box 893, San Rafael, CA 94915.

**Robyn Klein.** Wildcrafter, plant walks. P.O. Box 836, Big Sky, MT 59716.

**Rainbow Oils.** c/o Robert Seidel. P.O. Box 88, Sandy, OR 97055.

**Don Ollsin.** Herbal consultant. 1221 Whart St., Victoria, B.C., Canada.

**Vj Keating.** Veterinarian specialising in wholistic animal care. 37820 Hwy. 26, Sandy, OR 97055.

**Mara Levin.** Tinctures, wildcrafter. 7867 SE 9th, Portland, OR 97202.

**Ron Spector.** Wildcrafter. 2292 Grant St., Vancouver, B.C., Canada.

**Peter and Nancy Bigfoot.** Plant identification. Director of Reerts Mt. School, school of survival education. Box 543, Payson Star Route, Globe, A 85501.

**Ryan Drum.** Lecturer, Dominion Herbal College. Walden Island, WA 98297.

**Judy Nelson, DC.** Dean and Vice President of Dominion Herbal College. 7527 Kingsway, Burnaby, B.C., Canada.

**Marleen Mulder.** Herbal trance work. 4640 Sonoma Hwy., Santa Rosa, CA 95405.

**Wish Garden Herbs.** Herb catalogue. P.O. Box 1304, Boulder, CA 80306.

**Bill Roley.** Gardner, herbalist, teacher. 1027 Summit Way, Laguna Beach, CA 92651.

# Herbal Bibliography

## compiled by CSHS and Bill Roley

*Medicinal Plants of the Mountain West.* Michael Moore. Museum of New Mexico Press, Santa Fe, 1979.

*The Herbal Body Book; Kitchen Cosmetics; Herbs & Things;* and other books. Jeanne Rose. Grossett & Dunlop, NY, 1976.

*A Modern Herbal,* Vol. I and II. M. Grieve. Dover Publ., NY, 1971.

*School of Natural Healing.* Dr. John R. Christopher. Biworld, Orem, Utah, 1979.

*Science of Herbal Medicine.* J. Heinerman. Biworld, Orem, Utah, 1979.

*Medicines from the Earth.* W. Thomson. McGraw-Hill, NY, 1978.

*Natures Healing Arts.* Lonnelle Aikman. National Geographic Society, 1977.

*Rodale Herb Book.* ed. William Hylton. Rodale Press, Emmaeus, PA, 1974.

*Green Medicine.* Margaret Kreig. Rand McNally, Chicago, IL, 1961.

*A Guide to Medicinal Plants of U.S.* Arnold and Connie Krochmal. Quadrangle Books, New York Times Book Co., NY, 1973.

*A Field Guide to Wildflowers.* Roger Tory Peterson and M. McKenny. Houghton Mifflin, Boston, 1968.

*Herbs: A Concise Guide in Color.* F. Story and V. Jirasek. Hamlyn Publ., Prague, 1973.

*Old English Herbals.* E.S. Rohde. Dover, NY, 1971.

*Culpepper's Compleat Herbal.* N. Culpeper. W. Foulsham & Co., Great Britian.

*The Herbal.* J. Gerard. Complete 1633 edition revised. ed. T. Johnson. Dover, 1975.

*Of Men & Plants.* Maurice Messegue. MacMillan Co., NY, 1973.

*The Herbalist.* Joseph Meyer. Indiana Botanic Gardens, Hammond, Indiana, 1939.

*Planet Medicine.* R. Grossinger. Anchor Press, NY, 1980.

*Back to Eden.* J. Kloss. Lifeline Books, Santa Barbara, CA, 1975.

*Earth Medicine – Earth Foods.* M. A. Weiner, MacMillan, NY, 1972.

*The Medicine Wheel.* Sunbear and Wabun. Prentice Hall, Englewood Cliffs, NJ, 1980.

# Artemis Speaks, Part VI: Creating A Family

*A Barefoot Doctor's Manual.* Running Press, Philadelphia, 1977.

*Profitable Herb Growing at Home.* Betty Jacobs. Garden Way Publ., Charlotte, VT.

*Herb Gardening in the 5 Seasons.* Adelma Simmons. Hawthorn, NY, 1971.

*Herbal Handbook for Farm & Stable.* J. de Baircli Levy. Farber & Farber, London, 1963.

*Compleat Herbal Handbook for the Dog.* J. de Baircli Levy. Transatlantic Arts, Levittown, NY, 1971.'

*The Herbal Connection.* Ethan Nebelkopf. Biworld, Orem, Utah, 1981.

*Hygieia: A Woman's Herbal.* Jeannine Parvati. Freestone Collective, Cotati, CA, 1978.

*Organic Garden Medicine.* Jean Valnet. Erbonia Books, New Paltz, NY, 1975.

*Natures Children.* J. de Baircli Levy. Schoeken, NY, 1971.

*Natures Healing Agents.* R. S. Clymer. Humanitarian Society Press, Quakertown, 1973.

*Staying Healthy with the Seasons.* Elson Haas. Celestral Arts. Milbrae, CA, 1981.

*Star Botanicals.* Rob Menzies.

*Living with the Flowers.* Denise Diamond.

*Herbal Bounty.* Seven Foster. Gibbs Smith, Layton, VT, 1984.

*The Way of Herbs.* M. Tierra.

*Herbal Pathfinders.* R. Conrow and A. Hecksel. Woodbridge Press, Santa Barbara, CA.

*The Web That Has No Weaver.* T. Kaptchuk. Gongdom & Weed, New York, NY, 1983.

*Pharmacognosy.* Tyler, Brady and Robbers. Lee & Febiger, publ., Philadelphia, PA, 1976.

*A Manual of Material — Medica and Pharmacology.* D. Culbreith. Eclectic Med. Publ., Portland, OR, 1983.

*The Eclectic Material-Medica.* H. W. Felter. Eclectic Med. Publ., Portland, OR, 1983.

*American Material-Medica, Therapeutics and Pharmacognosy.* Eclectic Med. Publ., Portland, OR, 1983.

Reprinted by permission of CSHS, Box 350, Guerneville, CA 95446.

514

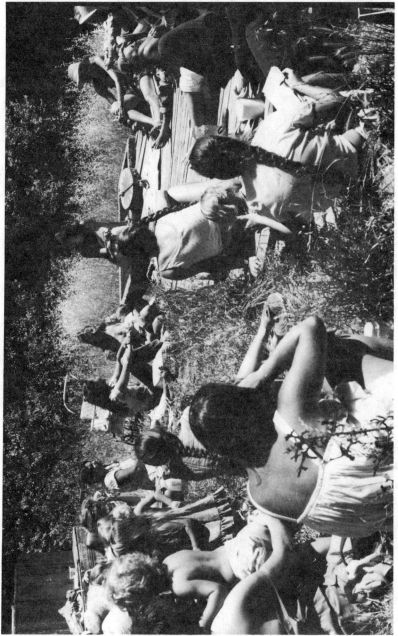

*Rainbow's End Study Group*    Photo by David Burns

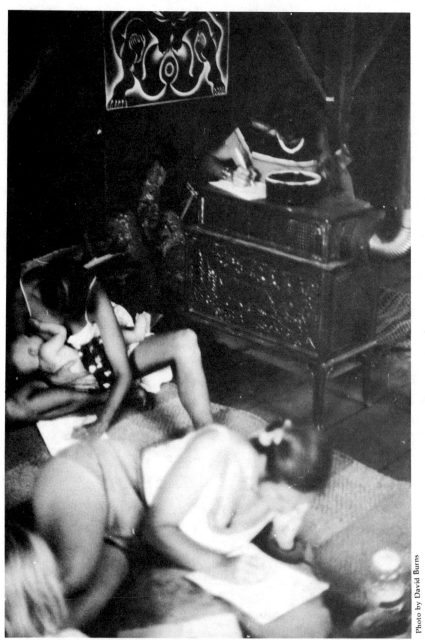

Photo by David Burns

*Rainbow's End Study Group*

516

# Part VII

# Conclusion: What You _Really_ Need to Know!

# Transcript of First and Last Class Talks

*by Nan Koehler*

There are a couple of things that I like to tell everybody in this first class. Had someone told these things to me the first time I was having a baby, it would have made my experience unimaginably more pleasurable, and this little bit of knowledge that I'm going to tell you is something that I've painfully learned. I know that what I'm telling you is the truth. It's what everybody experiences at some level or another. We're all the same. We're all different in detail, but we're all the same in the fundamentals and the basic process; the biological experience of pregnancy and birth are pretty much the same for everyone. The way we do the dance, of course, is unique for each of us.

The first thing I want to tell you is especially for those of you who are having their first pregnancy. Being pregnant forces you, whether you want to or not, to go through some changes—to go through some doors. It takes energy from your body to make a baby, and if you're not eating exactly right for you, resting properly and being around the right kind of people who really support you and what's happening to you, you're going to be sick in one way or another. You have to do some homework on one of those three aspects of your life for you to feel okay. The more spiritual work you do now, the more you can figure out what it takes to feel good while you're pregnant (especially as your pregnancy advances and you get closer to giving birth), the better you'll feel. If you don't take care of yourself, in one way or another, you will feel worse and worse. You'll feel really crabby, nauseated off and on, immobilized, unable to do anything; you'll feel vic-

518

timized and at the mercy of the process that is happening to you.

Hopefully, you will pay meticulous attention to your body and the signals that you get about what's going on: take the vitamins, drink the teas, eat good food, avoid junk food. Do whatever it takes for you to feel really good. Then when you're not pregnant, if you continue on whatever regime you've worked out, you'll feel like a million dollars. You'll be able to take care of your baby, your husband, everybody around, and you'll be able to work harder. And, of course, the truth is that in this process we're all learning how to work, how to really take care of someone else, nurture a being who's completely dependent on us and bring them life. You're bringing life to another person by your willingness to surrender yourself to the process.

When we're having babies is a really nice time in all our lives, because that's mother nature's intent for us. When you finally make love with your partner for the purpose of having a baby, it feels so good, and then it's so good to feel the life forming within you. You'll feel a lot of energy coming towards you, a lot of people taking interest in you. People whom you haven't heard from in ages will call you up; your family will flock around. Babies draw attention to themselves. The closer you get to giving birth and the actual arrival of your child, the more intensely that energy is focused on you. And, of course, mother nature has your best interest in mind by making it be that way, because you do need a lot of support and you need the protection of your family and your close circle of friends in many ways, and on many levels, when you're having a baby.

One of the main things I want to tell you about pregnancy, though this may sound strange, is that I want to give you permission to fight with your partner. It feels funny saying that, but please don't be afraid to confront each other. Be willing to acknowledge that you're feeling bad about something or other or you feel like crying or you're hurt or things aren't going the

519

way you want. Let it out, open yourself up to your negativity, work it out together. "Well, maybe this needs to change, that needs to change, or I can do this or you should do that," and so forth. You've got to change your routine with each other. The more you do that now, the easier it will be for you to take care of the baby. If you don't do it now, once your baby comes it will be a nightmare for you. Then you've got to do it in the presence of the third person (the baby) who has come to join your family. In some ways it's much easier taking care of your baby when it's inside your body than when it's outside your body. As Don always likes to say after the woman's delivered, "Now the easy part is over, and the hard part begins." That has a lot of truth in it.

The other thing that I like to talk about is the presence of the new baby in your life. They are incredible beings to be around. Once you experience a week or two with a newborn baby—their purity, their innocence, the glow that they radiate—you will experience a love energy, a love consciousness that is very difficult to attain any other way. It is the religious experience that all holy people seek. You will have that experience with your baby right after it is born. The more you can maintain that bubble, the longer you maintain it, the more bliss you will have from your birth experience. It will burst, sooner or later, and the reality of your life will crash home, when you face the nitty-gritty job of taking care of the baby, bringing home the bacon, keeping your household together, etc. Anytime you need to you can close your eyes, take some deep breaths and jump right into that space, if only momentarily. You will have experienced it, you know it, you can tap into it at any time for a source of strength and a direction or an understanding of what's happening to you. When you feel confused or negative or hostile, either towards your child or your partner, you can ground yourself by remembering what and how you felt when the baby first came into your life.

I was quite religious when I was a girl and became a really devout Christian. But the Catholic teachings particularly

520

never made much sense to me. I couldn't understand why they worshipped the Virgin Mary and the baby Jesus and what the adoration of the baby meant. It didn't hit home until I started being around births a lot and experiencing my own babies. Now, to me, every baby that's born is the Christ Child. And you will experience Christ's love through your child, through the presence of your Christ Child. He or she is your teacher. After three months the baby will give back to you everything you put into the baby. The baby is a perfect mirror. Sometimes this truth is very sweet and sometimes it is quite bitter. In summary, I want to alert you to a higher consciousness of what's happening to you. The learning about Christ love is the ultimate teaching of the baby who will open your heart, make your chest and your heart just flow with energy, and your most primal self will open up to you and each other—as though we were each other's mother and father, each other's brothers and sisters, and babies, etc. The more we can be like that to each other, the better the world will be. We all get a little taste of that when having a baby.

Another thing that I want to tell you is to prepare as diligently as you can. You cannot over-prepare for this process, this event that's going to happen to you. It is appropriate to liken it to an athletic event. *And* it isn't just a plain old athletic event; it is a monumental athletic event, like climbing Mt. Everest. The more you prepare your body, your spirit and your mind, the easier it will be. It will be like nothing if you do your homework. But if you don't put that much energy into preparing for the arrival of your child, then your birth experience can be quite confounding to you and a disturbing experience. This is because it is something that happens to you, it is not something that you do. It takes a lot of will power and control to let your body do what it needs to do: to "flow" with the process, to be "open," to be all the adjectives that you hear everyone talking about. For some of us, it comes easily. For others, it is a very painful quest, but it's definitely attainable for everybody. Everyone of you can have the perfect experience that you want.

The last point that I'd like to make, which I feel is very important, especially for the women, is thinking about the process of giving birth as a rite of passage, a passage from girlhood into womanhood, into motherhood. Whenever you have a growth experience like that, there's always pain, always pain and suffering. I first started thinking about this when I was with my second husband, who is a writer and a minister. He worked with young people, with teenagers. He was very interested in how to help young people grow into adulthood. Because of this, he became very interested in the rites of passage in our American society compared to aboriginal people. Most traditional societies have initiation ceremonies for young people to introduce them into adulthood. These ceremonies are quite elaborate and often involve bodily mutilation, severe pain and/or deprivation. The American Indians would send their young people out into the wilderness on a vision quest where they have to fast. Sometimes they were sent out without food or water to isolated places. Some tribes do it only for a few days, some do it for two weeks, and then someone will go out and get the young person. It's intended to be long enough so that a child, via a period of deprivation, hallucinates and receives some kind of message about what their life purpose is. At puberty, in many cultures all over the world, the boys are circumcized and sometimes the girls are, as well. During the circumcision rite, when the boys are in great pain, the tribal elders will whisper the survival secrets and social taboos in their ear. The little things that you need to know in order to survive properly — like how to breathe right, what women are like, how to gather the harvest and whatever it takes to survive — are whispered in the boys' ears when they're in pain. They never forget.

When you're in a crisis situation like that, and are scared, your whole reality crumbles. Everything, including your time perspective, is altered; things become crystal clear to you. Your mind works a different way. Of course, it's the hormones that do it. They change your brain pattern. So too, in labor, a

522

woman undergoes severe pain as the contractions force the baby through the bony pelvis. At that time, she will let go of her girlish selfishness, release, so that when the baby comes, she will be able to surrender her own needs for the baby's needs. You've got to when you're a mother. The baby comes first. The baby's your slave-driver. Taskmaster. You can't resent it. You have to be the selfless servant to your child in order for them to flourish and really grow into a wonderful, peaceful human being.

The pain of labor also helps you bond on the baby. The way the midwives say it is, "The more your labor hurts, the more you love the baby." The more intense the experience is, the more difficulties you have to go through in producing your baby, the more you'll love it. The better you can communicate with it. That definitely has been my experience. It seems to be true. I'm not saying that in easy labors you don't bond with the baby, but some of us need to have more intense experiences in order to become good mothers. So you see, just trust the process. Mother nature knows what she is doing.

A postscript to this talk is to remind you of what a profound political statement it is to prepare for a homebirth. In Sonoma County, there are a lot of people having their babies at home, but elsewhere in the United States it is just about unheard of. It's still a minority of us who are having our babies at home. It's quite a radical thing to do, and it is a political statement that you do not want to cooperate with the social norms and that you would like to do it differently. Hopefully, by birthing at home we will raise our children differently and we will try to create a generation of human beings who do not want to spend all their money on warheads, atomic bombs, guns and so forth; a generation who will put energy into growing good food, taking care of the earth, keeping it clean and preserving it for all living things.

# Tape Transcript from the Last Class in the Series

At this point, you are all filled with baby, on the brink of this fantastic experience, ready to greet your newborn. An experience that comes near it is Christmas, in the excitement and anticipation. (Christmas when you're a child, that is.) The adult Christmas for us is the birth of our Christ Child. There are a few points that I want to tell you that I hope will help you have an easy delivery.

One of the great hurdles that you will need to overcome is just that excitement, that feeling of Christmas, that anticipation. This over-excitement keeps you from sleeping, from eating, from being normal. With the second baby, it is easier because you have the first child to distract you. "Oh, I've got to fix breakfast. I've got to keep it together," and so on. With the first baby, it is easy to become completely engulfed with that wave of anticipation, that excitement and dread and horror and fear as well. (As many positive emotions that come forth, so too will the negative ones.) Your goal at this point is disinterest. Equilibrium. Just day to day attention to what is real. Not fantasy work. Be normal as long as you can.

The second hurdle is that it's going to be a feat for you to figure out exactly when you're in labor. It's not something that just starts, the way the books make you think. It doesn't have a beginning and an end. It's a process that you're already involved in. Your body's already starting to get ready to give birth. As soon as you get pregnant, your body starts to get ready to give birth. The hormones start circulating through your body, making you feel like you're crazy half the time . . . you're not. You're just using a different part of your brain. The hormones change your body chemistry, loosen your bones, loosen your ligaments, soften your tissues so that your cervix and your uterus are being prepared for the event that you are now on the brink of experiencing.

Usually it takes two or three days of false labor, prodromal, or early labor (whatever word you want to use for it) before

524

you're really in "active" labor. (Active labor means that the birth of the child is at hand.) This may or may not be heralded by your membranes rupturing or losing your mucous plug. Just because you've lost your mucous plug or your membranes have ruptured doesn't necessarily mean that the baby's coming within the next few hours. Usually these events are associated, but not necessarily. It depends at what point these events happen to you—early in your labor or later. Whether or not you have a three day labor or a two hour labor depends on at what point you plug into the process. Everybody's body works more or less the same, but some women notice the prodromal labor and other women don't notice it. It depends how you're carrying the baby. If the baby is really high and not squeezing out of your bones too much, you won't notice the early labor. You have contractions all the time. Even now, you are having contractions. If the baby's high, out of the bones, then you feel it as your uterus hardening or it feels like the baby's moving around. But once the head has dropped down in your pelvis, when the uterus tightens and squeezes, it will push it down in your bones even more and oooo!, you'll feel it. If the baby drops before labor or early in labor, you'll be in more pain and you'll plug into the experience earlier.

Please ignore the whole process as long as you can. Be normal, because if you act with the first pangs of labor as if "oh, this is it!" and you start laying down, not drinking, not eating, not peeing, your body will get to be in a physiologic "wacko" state. Then when you really are in labor, you won't be able to cope with it as well. You'll be too tired. It's difficult to bear the pain when you're fatigued. Your body just doesn't work right when you're dehydrated, have low blood sugar, and so forth.

No one knows exactly what sets off labor, but this is my theory, and it makes a good story. The baby grows to be a certain size, when the placenta can't nourish it as well anymore, and so the baby starts panicking and slowly secreting adrenal hormones, which are metabolized by the placenta and the membranes into a hormone called prostaglandin. The pros-

525

taglandin makes the uterus very irritable and it softens the cervical tissue. As the uterus gets irritable, you have more contractions, more Braxton-Hicks contractions, which squeezes the baby some more as well as pulling on the cervix, which ripens it some more. The contractions come closer together, and the baby starts panicking more, secreting more adrenal hormones, which are transformed into more prostaglandins, until it reaches a critical point when the cervix is mush. The cervical tissue gives way and it literally starts to pull away and open with the contractions. The process snowballs even more, because as the cervix opens and gives, the pressure of the descending forewaters and/or the baby's head pressing on the cervix stimulates you to have even more contractions. By the time you're in active labor, the contractions will be three minutes apart and a minute long, hurting you really bad. You *have* to pay attention to them. Then you lay down. At this point, if it hurts you even worse when you lay down, that's what you want to do, and then the baby will come. Usually it doesn't take very long—only a few hours. But if you lay down early, when your contractions are seven minutes apart or five minutes apart and not lasting a minute, and you act like you're in labor, then it will take you a long time. Try to ignore the early part. *I can't say it to you enough.* Easier said than done, I know—it's not that easy to ignore the coming of the baby.

The third thing that you want to remember in giving birth is *not to try to escape the pain.* Whatever you do that makes it hurt more, that's the right thing to do. If it hurts worse when you get up and walk around, then get up and walk around. If it hurts worse when you lay down, then lay down. Because the more it hurts, the more you know something is happening. Pain brings the baby. You want to make a strong association between pleasure/pain, realizing that the phenomenon of pleasure and pain in labor is one. Make yourself images and pictures of what's happening to your body so that you can visualize it, so that you don't feel overwhelmed by some

526

mysterious process. Visualize your bones opening, the baby coming through, your cervix opening up. Hang the pictures around your bed to remind yourself constantly about what's going on, so that you don't get scared.

Let's say you're starting to have contractions. You wake up one morning and you notice you're having a wave of menstrual cramp feeling which gets worse and worse, coming about every ten minutes. Just be normal throughout your day. If they start to get worse and worse as the morning progresses, then you know you'll have your baby around noon or three o'clock. You have your hormonal low point at two in the afternoon, and your hormonal peak at two in the morning. Most labors start at two in the morning. Fatigue brings false labor in the evening. So if you've had a pretty normal day and you start having labor pains after dinner, you can pretty much ignore them. Take a hot bath, drink a glass of wine or smoke some dope, whatever you do to relax. They should go away once you fall asleep. If your labor starts in the evening, it isn't always real labor, although it might seem real! But if it starts in the morning you can pretty much count on it being the real thing, because the labor pains which peak around two in the morning you can sleep through and you don't really notice them much. They might wake you up around five or six in the morning. Or again when you wake up at seven or eight in the morning they will be coming stronger and stronger. You will notice that they increase as the day goes on. Conversely, with the coming of the daylight they might peter out. But when it's nighttime and dark again, you'll have the baby. If you haven't had it during the day, you'll start having good labor after supper as it gets dark, and then by two that morning you should have had the baby. (If everything works as it should.)

Now it can be that it's the false labor that wakes you up in the morning, and you might not have the baby that night. You might not have it until the next night, depending on how ripe your cervix is and how ready you are for giving birth.

The first thing to do when you perceive yourself in labor is to eat. Eat a good meal, not just some yogurt and fruit, you want to fill your stomach with good food. If you throw up it's alright. You'll have the food in you if you need the energy. Also, the movement of the food through your intestinal tract stimulates the contractions because the nerves that innervate the uterus also innervate the lower colon. In an hour or two after eating, it will stimulate your labor as the food passes through your intestines. You can digest food while you're in labor. It's a myth that you can't eat while you're in labor. The only reason that they have people not eat is in anticipation of giving them medication or surgery. Hopefully, that will not be a reality for any of you and you will have a perfectly normal experience. You need to eat and drink. If you should need medical help your food will be long digested!

After breakfast, lunch or supper, go for a long walk. Try to walk for at least an hour. Walk about two or three miles to stimulate your labor. In early labor, the combination of eating and walking should put you in good labor. When you come home take a hot bath. Try to stay in the bath as long as you can. This should bring on the labor even more. Call the birth attendant when your contractions are three minutes apart and lasting a minute. Or call at any point when you need to have input from your birth attendant. Call when you either need feedback about whether you're in labor or not, or when you're having trouble bearing the pain, or feel confused about what's going on. Don't hesitate to call.

Once you are in labor, try to move around and be normal. When you cannot help but lay down, then lay down on your left side. Try to put everything out of your mind except paying attention to your body, except keeping your body relaxed. It will take all your will power, all you can muster, to keep from screaming, yelling, running away—"Help, I can't stand it!" It won't last long. You can always remind yourself that the sensations that you are experiencing will pass you by, and that as soon as the baby is out of your body you will feel completely normal. It is hard to believe when it's happening to

528

you, but believe me you will. You will be amazed at what a relief it is when the baby is out and how wonderful you will feel. If you take pain medication at this point ("Oh, give me something, I've got to have something!"), you might hurt the baby. Keep your sights on the fact that as soon as the baby's born you will feel okay. It's not something that goes on and on. It's not the kind of pain that's from a wound that you don't know when it's going to end. This pain is going to produce the baby for you.

I think that's why the first baby is harder. You've never experienced the pleasure of having a baby, so you can't make that association of pain = birth = baby like you can with the second or third. When you've done it before, you know how bad it's going to hurt and that it's going to bring the baby, so you don't mind as much.

When you feel like pushing (you will feel the pressure on your anus, like you have to defecate), just keep doing your transition breathing as long as you can. Then when your body tells you to push hard (follow your instincts), go ahead. Your instinct is the best advice and guide you have. Better than your birth attendant. Try to do what your body tells you to do. It will always tell you the right thing. So when you body tells you to push, you go ahead and push. You can push with all your might, until you feel a burning, and that means your baby's head is starting to stretch your vaginal opening. When you feel it burning like fire, then you pant and let the uterus push the baby out the rest of the way, so that you don't tear. Then bring the baby out, you and your partner, up on to your stomach. And give the baby some time to begin breathing. The cord will still be pulsing. The baby doesn't have to look fantastic immediately. The baby wants to live more than anyone. Clear the mucus out of the baby's mouth and rub the baby's back and feet. Usually it takes about five or ten minutes for the baby to start breathing really well. After your placenta is delivered and the cord is cut, nurse the baby. Sometimes they nurse right away, but not very often. Usually they wait until the cord's quit pulsing and their mouth is all free from mucus. Hopefully, that's how all of your births will be — easy and wonderful and natural and something that you can be proud of.

*A Postscript, something I have recently become painfully aware of, is the importance of staying home with your baby the first 3 months or so of their life. A perfect natural birth doesn't insure the bonding I had assumed it would without that time of intense isolation afterwards. Most other cultures have prescribed customs which dictate what the woman can do and who should see the baby, etc. These customs serve nature by insuring that we know our babies intimately and will support them appropriately in all situations. The difficulty for most of us lies in the fact that we don't have good support systems around us. By helping each other give birth, preparing meals for each other and looking after each others children we can become family and nurture our children in a loving way that will bring peace on earth.*

# Reevaluating Bonding — Postpartum Care

One of the driving forces of my interest in and support of home births has been the phenomenon of bonding. For over ten years, I have equated home births with good bonding. This was *my* experience, and I'd assumed it was the experience of every woman having a similar kind of gentle-home-birth. But I was puzzled by the examples of a few women I knew who had had wonderful births and biologically splendid opportunities for bonding, yet abused their children by abandoning them early to baby-sitters or using overly-harsh discipline. I had been hoping that the home birth movement would help heal families, with reverberations through

530

society — how we feed our children, where and how we send them to school, etc. It has been wonderful for me to observe the transformation of so many couples following their conscious birth experiences. But still, a few couples acted as though their children weren't connected to them.

A recent experience has led me to believe that the quality of the extended postpartum experience, and not just the bonding at birth, is a deciding factor in getting families off to a truly good start. A woman in our community birthed under general anesthesia with an emergency cesarean for a prolapsed cord. Her pediatrician overreacted to the baby's slight malformations (a cleft lip and mild hypospadias). The mother was so traumatized by the birth that she did not even want to see her baby at first. Luckily, we were there to help her over the "hump" of those first few hours postpartum. The baby nursed well, and the mother's reserves began to melt. However, two weeks after the birth, the baby was still slightly jaundiced and hadn't regained the pound he had lost since his birth. This galvanized me and the other women in my community to rally around the mother. We had been bringing her food, but now I checked her every day, with attention to every detail of how the baby was doing. We told her daily how beautiful she was and what a good job she was doing and how wonderful her baby was. They are truly a Madonna and child. The growth of their relationship and the development of the baby after this was stunning. Today, at eight weeks postpartum, both look fantastic. We have even stopped weighing the baby weekly because he so obviously is growing!

What happened with this mother? As I see it, two main factors contributed to the dramatic improvement in the child. First, the mother stayed home exclusively with the baby, in a quiet environment. Secondly, she benefited from the intense witness/support of other experienced nursing mothers. Most other cultures take care of this automatically with their taboos and so-called superstitions. In truth, they support the interests of Mother-Nature by having prescribed periods of isolation

531

and social deprivation as well as food regulations. (Only certain people can see the baby: Father, Grandmother, Aunt, etc., but *not* strangers.) In India, for example, the new mother and baby stay in a darkened room for some time, with only candle light. Of course, they take the baby outside periodically during the day, but the idea is to rest the baby's eyes and create a safe, stimulus-free environment. Most American Indian people, that I've read about, have a two week period of isolation with the baby; also often spent in a darkened room. At the end of that time, a ceremony is held introducing the baby to the world and dedicating him/her to the earth. In the Middle East and much of Asia, the isolation time is even longer. Forty days are spent in one's room with the baby. All household chores are done by someone else during this time. An anthropologist, Dana Raphel, has written a wonderful book on this subjected called, *The Tender Gift.*

By way of example, let me tell you about my birth experiences. I had no trouble giving birth to my first child; it was in a hospital setting with minimal interference of any sort. I was very proud of my 6 hour first labor! But that experience didn't bring the personal transformation that my second (home) birth did. My relationship with the two babies was also very different. As I wrote earlier, I attributed my different reactions to the setting and to the intensity of the bonding experience. In the bright hospital room the baby was caught by the Doctor, handed to a nurse who weighed, measured, dried and foot-printed the baby (while the Doctor stitched my episiotomy) and then handed back to me wrapped in a blanket. In the darkened room at home my mate caught the baby and immediately handed him to me. I nursed him right away and moved about freely because I didn't tear and felt normal in every way. In hindsight, I can see that, in fact, the more intense bonding I experienced with my second child was due not only to the more intimate birth setting, but also to the fact that I was in my mother's home! She, and several friends, nurtured me for about 8 weeks, until I moved back to California. All that time I didn't have to worry about anything except my baby and my older child. It was a blissful time for me.

In our culture, we aren't careful with our new babies. Beginning with birth, strangers touch the infant almost at will and we expose them to frightening sights and sounds. For example, one often hears young couples proclaim that their baby loved to ride in the car; s/he fell right to sleep. The reason they fell asleep was because they were experiencing sensory overload and had to shut it off. The same is true for meetings, shopping, etc., with a newborn. If you're lucky, they'll sleep the whole time you are out (or fuss so much you can't even go out)! But then upon returning home, they are hungry, wet, needing to defecate, etc., in short, screaming while you are exhausted from being out all day. This cycle results in colic. It's better just to stay home with the newborn. For how long? It's best to take your cue from the child. Some need more time than others to integrate what is going on around them, or as Joseph Chilton Pearce, in his book *The Magical Child*, puts it, they need more time to bond on the mother. This bonding on the mother can only occur as the result of days on end of mindless routine and total attention of the mother to the child. The isolation period varies from culture to culture and it varies from child to child.

In the biology books it says that sometime around ten weeks of age the fovea matures. This is the area of the retina where the rods and cones are most densely concentrated. When this happens, one definitely notices a marked change in the child. Suddenly, they are interested in what is going on around them. They aren't so preoccupied with their internal rumblings. Some children can branch out earlier, while others need more time getting used to their body. My last child (my fifth) didn't like going out at all until very recently. She is nine months old!

The biological results of this isolation is a tranquil child and an intense telepathic relationship between mother and child. The social results of adhering to a period of isolation are

533

manifold and healing to the family. With the mother home constantly, a stable base is established for the rest of the family. This source of emotional stability and comfort is underestimated by our culture. One can't create a home via interior decorating and arriving at the door at 5:00 p.m. It takes time and attention to see to all the details of creating a loving space. It takes time and attention to fill the home with loving energy and arrange it to everyone's satisfaction.

This time of sensory and social deprivation results in an intimate knowledge of the child. There are no distractions to take our attention away from the baby. In his book, Joseph Chilton Pearce describes African mothers whose babies could walk at seven months and were toilet trained very early. This can only happen when the child toilet trains the mother, and not visa versa. (No child can go on their own until they are about three or four years old.) With the mother's knowledge of the baby—their breath changes, subtle postural changes, etc.—and no other distractions, she can catch each urination before the baby fouls the living space.

Another benefit from this isolation and intense bonding is a baby who is very comfortable with its bodily functions. Alone with mom all this time, its physical needs met promptly and without haste, the child grows accustomed to eating, sleeping, urinating, defecating, burping, etc., with no trauma. The long term benefit is a child in tune with his body and able to look after themself intuitively at a later age.

Lastly, this isolation time creates a social support base for the child vis-a-vis all the women mobilized to help the new mother. In order to stay at home, we must allow other women into our home. (In a tribal setting, it would be Mom, or Sister, or Aunt who would help us. For most of us separated from our families, it will be our female friends.) It's hard to rely totally on one's mate for this support. Most men aren't that good at preparing meals and nurturing their mates. For a few days they are fine, but not for weeks on end. Other women, especially those who have been through it themselves, are

534

ideal helpers. This precious time together heightens mutual interest in each other, and in each other's children.

Here is the format that my circle of women friends and I have developed in the last few years to heal and support our families.

1. The new moon before the woman is due, give her a Blessingway. (See attached handout written by Raven Lang, midwife from Santa Cruz, California.)

2. Support the woman in whatever birth choice/place is appropriate for her, then have her stay in bed the first week after her baby's birth, except for going to the bathroom. The new mother should drink lots of comfrey tea (two pots a day at least), take her vitamins, drink a quart of carrot juice each day, etc. With a different woman friend bringing dinner each night, the husband doesn't need to worry about the evening meal. If desired, this support woman can do a few simple chores—laundry, dishwashing, etc.—but most couples like to be left alone. If someone can come stay at the home in a discreet way and serve the new mother, that's even more desirable.

3. The second week after the birth, the mother can be up, but resting and definitely at home. The suppers from friends should continue for another week.

4. At the end of two weeks, the midwife or support person, should come and give the new mother an herbal bath, review with her how to massage her baby and lead the family in a ceremony celebrating the safe passage and introducing the new child to the earth forces. Thus we dedicate the child to the healing of our earth and the strengthening of the new family. The Blessingway beforehand and this ceremony afterward serve to remind us of our higher goals.

5. Remember that six weeks after birth is the low point. If one can pass this time without getting sick, that is a feat and a real measure of how well this isolation time was handled.

In summary, the time alone with a beautiful, innocent, but crabby, up-at-night—often with inexplicable aches and pains—baby, has many benefits. The major benefit, not mentioned yet, is to the woman herself. Dealing with a being who is not interested in anything external, and who needs constant input, without anger or frustration is a feat of maturity. People pay money to go on retreats where they can't sleep, must fast, etc. to enter the state that all nursing mothers are in who really take loving care of their babies. The combination of sleep deprivation and constant selfless service, taken in stride with grace and humor, prepare the woman for any challenge in later life. And so we see that the skills gained during this period can help her become a source of strength for her whole community.

# *Blessingway*

*by Raven Lang, Midwife*

### *Notes from 1982*

It's helpful to explore myths and symbols associated with birth from different cultures to help bring to the surface your own feelings about the spirituality of birth, and to see where your perceptions echo the ones that come through in ancient cultures.

Helpful books:

*Woman's Mysteries*, Esther Harding
*The Way of all Women*, Esther Harding
*The Great Mother*, Eric Neumann
*Myths and Symbols in Indian Art and Civilization*, Zimmer
*Man and His Symbols*, Carl Jung
*Moon, Moon*, Anne Kent Rush

We usually do a Birth Ritual for a woman 2 or 3 weeks before her baby is due, in her home. Usually only women are present, and she invites whoever she'd like (friends, sisters, mother). The midwife "catching" her baby is usually the "mistress of ceremonies."

536

## OUR REASONS FOR DOING RITUALS:

To allow the pregnant woman to feel the power of the good will and love that the women close to her feel toward her and her baby. To feel the powerful sisterhood between women.

To give form to the spiritual bond between a pregnant woman and the midwives who will attend her birth. A way to deepen that bond by allowing her to come to know more fully, through ritual, her own and her midwives' feelings about the sanctity of birth. Laying groundwork for the birth to come.

To strengthen the bond between midwives by strengthening our faith in the primal power available to us through our intuition (the power of the Goddess). My experience is that when I need to be particularly perceptive or make decisions at a birth, I can more easily open, listen, and trust that I will receive the wisdom needed, when there has been a birth ritual. The birth experience has been consciously sanctified in some way for all of us.

## CREATING A RITUAL:

Very few of the things we do at rituals are practices that we took from ancient cultures. The personal meaning that the ritual has for you might be more powerful if you make up your own practices that stem from your own perception of the birth process. The rituals I do are usually focused on the Mother Goddess. For someone else that might not feel real. Our rituals keep growing with different people's ideas.

## THINGS WE DO:

*Singing* at different times throughout the ritual — usually we begin with singing. We sometimes pass the words of the songs around to those that don't know them and they learn them as we go along.

*Yarn circle:* We use yarn to weave ourselves together in a circle. It's nice to use yarn that was hand spun by a member of the group. Beginning and ending with the pregnant woman,

537

the yarn is woven through the circle—across one woman's belly, around the next woman's back. The yarn symbolizes an umbilical cord linking us all to each other and to the Goddess. We read the prayer beginning "As women have always woven" and sing songs as the yarn goes around. This idea is from the book *Moon, Moon Symbols.* The pregnant woman is surrounded by symbols of the stages of her pregnancy:

Flowers—conception—a promise of the fruit to come

A shell—pregnancy—a water home

Hollow gourd—

Our personal rigidity—our "edges" are cooked away in the birth process and we become pure channels—softened. Not only the mother, but everyone involved in the birth. The birth of the universe from the Formless One—so the dance of relationship/duality can take place.

Open seed pod and separate seed: after birth.

Don Juan speaks of the hole left in the luminosity of the parents' spirit after the birth of a child. (*The Second Ring of Power*—Castaneda.)

*The cutting of the yarn:* Scissors are passed around the circle. The person on your left (the side of intuition) cuts the yarn wrapped around you and ties it to your left wrist. This signifies taking the bond with the Goddess back into the world with you. The prayer beginning "We call on the Goddess" is read and songs are sung while the scissors are passed—the pregnant woman is cut last.

*Passing through the gates:* In many cultures rites of passage contain three stages:

Initiation (labor—surrender)

Transformation (the moment of birth)

Rebirth (into an altered existence—mother and child
separate)

Two women form an arch, the next woman ducks backward into their arch and their arms are brought down around her, which signifies initiation). She is hugged and kissed by both women forming the arch, they turn her around to face for-

538

ward—both of them whisper in one of her ears: "Through women you were born into this world," (transformation) "Through women you are born into this circle." Then they raise their arms to form the side of the arch she is facing and push her out through it with the other two arms (rebirth).

The next woman in line goes through this process and then these two women who have gone through the arch form a second arch next to the first two women and so on until the "initiation" arch is a long one to duck backward through (to the last couple each time). When everyone but the pregnant woman (who will be last) has gone through the two women forming the 1st arch both go through and then the pregnant woman goes through. This signifies her bond with the chain of ancestral women that she follows through the birth process. We sing while we do this and hum after awhile—songs we've used are "'Tis the gift to be simple" and "Turn, Turn, Turn." This idea comes from the book: *Moon, Moon.*

*Corn Meal Foot Rub:* Corn is a symbol of the nourishment of the Earth Mother. This is to help the pregnant woman in her ability to draw in the nourishment and strength she needs to mother through her stance on the earth—through her feet. Use blue corn meal if possible. Reflexology points can be used. It's sometimes nice to do a full body massage too.

*I Ching Hexagram:* The pregnant woman formulates a question and throws the coins and reads the answer if she chooses to. Always direct and fitting answers have been heard so far.

*Sharing of the Sacred Tea:* Herbs are thrown into boiled water and stirred; each herb is meant to bless the pregnant woman with a particular quality she'll need during labor. She can pick herbs she particularly likes. I've used: Eyebright—clarity; Squawvine—stength; Lady Slipper—endurance; Black Haw—peace of heart; Mother of the Meadow—honoring the goddess.

The pregnant woman's midwife takes the tea around the circle and pours a small amount in each person's left palm. Each person offers their left (intuition) palm up cradled in their right palm. The tea should be hot enough to hurt a little, but not burn. Each person touches the tea to their forehead, puts it to their mouth and tastes it, then puts the rest over the top of their head. This signifies sharing and dispersing of the pregnant woman's pain in labor by the chain of ancestral women. The pregnant woman is given the tea last.

*Circle of Love:* We join hands in a circle around the pregnant woman and sing "May the blessings of her love rest upon you." (This is a sufi song: "May the blessings of God rest upon you" which we changed into a Goddess song.) Each person in the circle, at the beginning of a new verse, goes into the center and places their hands on the pregnant woman where she would like to give her strength — bell, back, heart or wherever. There is usually crying and incredible love circulating.

After everyone has touched the pregnant woman and has returned to the circle we start moving around as a circle. First as the Full Moon — complete, shining forth, arms in a circle above the head — eyes shinging outward, large steps. Then Crescent Moon — left arm arched up, right arm arched down, eyes downcast and hidden, potentiality, enclosed within, small, light, graceful steps. Lastly as the Sun — arms straight out to the side, palms outward, eyes straight ahead, firm, strong steps, moving for nothing, adapting to nothing. Shining outward.

These walking meditations I learned from a Sufi woman.

*The "utensils"* used at rituals: Yarn, flower vase, gourd, shell, seed pod, vessel for corn meal, I Ching and coins, vessel for the tea, mat for the foot rub; all which become rather sacred and very special as they are used over and over. Most of the things I use were given to me by members of my family.

Open yourself when the spirit moves you, to what is meaningful for you and let it become a ritual. You needn't use any of the things we've done. You're welcome to use all of them. Sometimes an idea will come to you and later you'll find it is related to, or a repetition of, an ancient ritual. Talking about

540

all this really can't convey the feeling that ritual carries. You need to do and experience birth rituals to know how beautiful they can be.

Reprinted by permission of the author.

# A Hogan Song From Blessingway

*It is my hogan where, from the back corners beauty radiates,*
*it radiates from a woman.*
*It is my hogan where, from the rear center beauty radiates,*
*it radiates from a woman.*
*It is my hogan where, from the fireside beauty radiates,*
*it radiates from a woman.*
*It is my hogan where, from its side corners beauty radiates,*
*it radiates from a woman.*
*It is my hogan where, from the doorway on and on beauty*
*radiates, it radiates from a woman, it increases*
*its radius of beauty.*

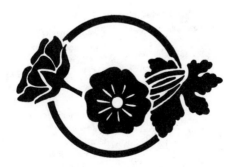

541

# Plant Index

542

# Plant Index Continued

Artemis Speaks *Plant Index Continued*

544

# Plant Index Continued

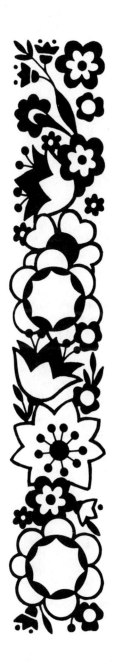

545

# General Index

546

# General Index Continued

# Artemis Speaks, *General Index Continued*

548

# General Index Continued

# Artemis Speaks, *General Index Continued*

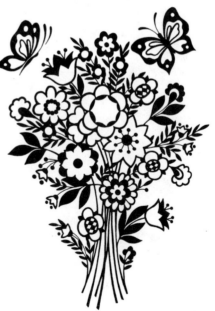